Fourth Edition

Medical Terminology
COMPLETE!

Bruce Wingerd

National University and San Diego State University,
San Diego, California

HEMATOLOGY

hemat/o

-logy

-ary

coron/o

NEURALGIA

CORONARY

neur/o

-algia

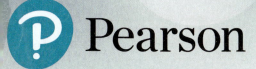

Pearson

330 Hudson Street, NY NY 10013

Vice President, Portfolio Management: Julie Levin Alexander
Director, Portfolio Management: Marlene McHugh Pratt
Executive Portfolio Manager: John Goucher
Content Producer: Melissa Bashe
Editorial Project Manager: Meghan DeMaio, SPi Global
Portfolio Management Assistant: Lisa Narine
Development Editor: Jennifer Maybin
Vice President, Content Production and Digital Studio: Paul DeLuca
Director, Digital Production: Amy Peltier
Digital Studio Producers, e-text: Ellen Viganola and Allison Longley
Digital Content Team Lead: Brian Prybella
Digital Content Project Lead: William Johnson
Field Marketing Manager: Brittany Hammond
Product Marketing Manager: Rachele Strober
Operations Specialist: MaryAnn Gloriande
Creative Digital Lead: Mary Siener
Text Designer: SPi Global
Cover Designer: SPi Global
Cover Art: FabrikaSimf/Shutterstock
Full-Service Project Management: Thomas Russell, SPi Global
Composition: SPi Global
Printer/Binder: LSC Communications, Inc.
Cover Printer: Phoenix Color/Hagerstown

DEDICATION

For Mala, who has shown so many thousands
of students how learning can be made
fun . . . including me.

Credits and acknowledgments for content borrowed from other sources and reproduced, with permission, in this textbook appear on the appropriate page within text.

Copyright © 2019, 2016, 2013, 2009 by Pearson Education, Inc. All rights reserved. Manufactured in the United States of America. This publication is protected by Copyright and permission should be obtained from the publisher prior to any prohibited reproduction, storage in a retrieval system, or transmission in any form or by any means, electronic, mechanical, photocopying, recording, or likewise. To obtain permission(s) to use material from this work, please submit a written request to Pearson Education, Inc., Permissions Department, 221 River Street, Hoboken, New Jersey 07030 or you may fax your request to 201-236-3290.

Notice: The author and the publisher of this book have taken care to make certain that the information given is correct and compatible with the standards generally accepted at the time of publication. Nevertheless, as new information becomes available, changes in treatment and in the use of equipment and procedures become necessary. The reader is advised to carefully consult the instruction and information material included in each piece of equipment or device before administration. Students are warned that the use of any techniques must be authorized by their medical advisor, where appropriate, in accordance with local laws and regulations. The publisher disclaims any liability, loss, injury, or damage incurred as a consequence, directly or indirectly, of the use and application of any of the contents of this book.

Many of the designations by manufacturers and seller to distinguish their products are claimed as trademarks. Where those designations appear in this book, and the publisher was aware of a trademark claim, the designations have been printed in initial caps or all caps.

Library of Congress Cataloging-in-Publication Data

Wingerd, Bruce D., author.
  Medical terminology complete! / Bruce Wingerd. — Fourth edition.
    p. ; cm.
  Includes index.
  ISBN 978-0-13-470122-6
  ISBN 0-13-470122-4
  I. Title.
  [DNLM: 1. Medicine—Programmed Instruction. 2. Terminology as
Topic—Programmed Instruction.   W 18.2]
  R123
  610.1'4—dc23
                                      2014042089
1 17

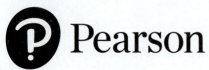

ISBN 10: 0-13-470122-4
ISBN 13: 978-0-13-470122-6

Welcome!

Welcome to *Medical Terminology Complete!* You have chosen an exciting time to begin a career as a healthcare professional. The healthcare industry is a dynamic field that is filled with opportunities for those who care about helping other people. Although many aspects of health care remain relatively constant, research breakthroughs occur each year to keep us moving forward in the war against human suffering. And you can be a part of this exciting process!

This book is designed to help you through the process of building a medical vocabulary. It teaches you the language by using a method known as *programmed learning*. With this approach, you read through the information at your own pace, one small box (or frame) at a time. Within most frames are blanks, which you fill in as you read. The answers to the blanks are provided in the left column, making it easy and quick to check your answer to make sure you are on the right track. To maximize your learning experience, it is best to cover the answers in the left column until you have filled in the blanks on your own. Challenge yourself! By filling in the blanks as you read, you become an active learner, which improves your chance of successfully mastering medical terminology. You'll have the opportunity to learn thousands of medical terms, and our simple goal is to provide you with the tools and confidence to help you master this brand new vocabulary.

You may be wondering about the title of this book: *Medical Terminology Complete!* Let us explain the two goals we had in mind as we developed this text.

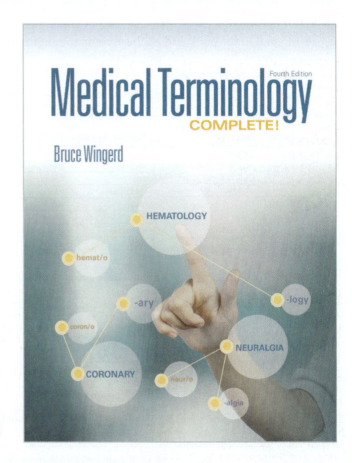

1. To place a **complete** resource at your fingertips. With its interactive format and its wealth of clear definitions, vivid images, practical examples, and challenging exercises, it's all that you need to become proficient in speaking and understanding the language of medicine.

2. To allow you to **complete** the exercises on every page. This book features a programmed method that prompts you, the reader, to fill in the content as you read. This approach keeps your pen or pencil on every page, so you stay engaged and retain more.

Now please turn the page to get a glimpse of what makes this book an ideal guide to your exploration of medical terminology.

Discover What Makes This Book Unique

This section provides you with a snapshot of what makes this book special. Consider this your user's manual to the book and all the accompanying resources that are available to you.

Diseases and Disorders of the Male Reproductive System

Here are the word parts that specifically apply to the diseases and disorders of the male reproductive system and are covered in the following section. Note that the word parts are color-coded to help you identify them: prefixes are yellow, combining forms are red, and suffixes are blue.

Prefix	Definition
an-	without, absence of
hyper-	excessive, abnormally high, above
para-	alongside, abnormal

Combining Form	Definition
andr/o	male
balan/o	glans penis
crypt/o	hidden
epididym/o	epididymis
hydr/o	water
orchi/o, orchid/o	testis
prostat/o	prostate gland
varic/o	dilated vein

Suffix	Definition
-cele	hernia, swelling, or protrusion
-ism	condition or disease
-itis	inflammation
-pathy	disease
-plasia	formation, growth

Color-Coded Word Parts

Prefixes, combining forms, and suffixes are each designated by a unique color—making it easier for you to visually recognize the distinctions between each word part, thereby aiding in your mastery of word building.

KEY TERMS A–Z

andropathy
an DROPP ah thee

anorchism
an OR kizm

an/orch/ism

balanitis
bal ah NYE tiss

benign prostatic hyperplasia
bee NINE * pross TAT ik * HIGH per PLAY zee ah

12.17 A combining form that means "male" and the suffix meaning "disease" may be combined to form a general term for a disease afflicting only males, _____. This constructed term includes three word parts, which can be represented as andr/o/pathy.

12.18 A word root that means "testis" is *orchi* or *orchid*. When the prefix meaning "without, absence of" is added along with the suffix *-ism*, the constructed term _____ is created. It means "condition of without testis" and refers to the absence of one or both testes. The constructed form of the term is written ____/_____/____. The term **anorchidism** may also be used with the same meaning.

12.19 Inflammation of the glans penis is a disorder called _____. It is a constructed term with two word parts, as you can see in balan/itis.

12.20 Among many men older than age 50, the prostate gland enlarges to constrict the urethra passing through it. Known as **benign prostatic hyperplasia**, symptoms include nocturia (nighttime urination) and a frequent need to void (■ Figure 12.4). It is not a form of cancer and does not spread to other tissues, but its symptoms are uncomfortable. _____ _____ _____ is also called **benign prostatic hypertrophy**; both are abbreviated **BPH**.

Key Terms A–Z

The most important terms are listed in alphabetical order, helping you to easily review those important terms before an exam.

Programmed Instruction

This format allows you to learn actively but at your own pace, filling in blanks as you read. Answers appear in the left column, making it easy and quick to check your answer to make sure you are on the right track. Programmed instruction works best when you cover the answers in the left column until you fill in the blanks. If you remember to do this, it will keep your studies challenging, and your learning experience will benefit.

Medically Accurate Illustrations

Concepts come to life with vibrant, clear, consistent, and scientifically precise images.

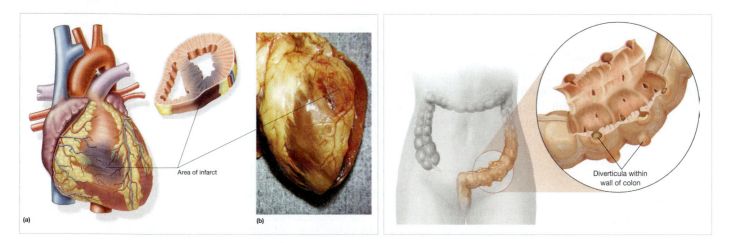

Image Labeling Frames

These frames provide you with opportunities to actively engage with the illustrations, helping to reinforce your knowledge of anatomy. They are included in the Chapter Review section at the ends of Chapters 5–15 and are new to this edition.

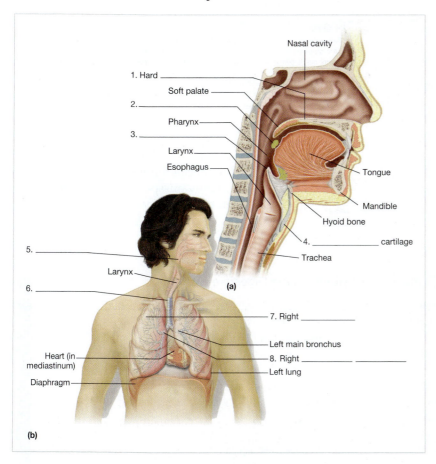

Word Building, Step by Step

At-a-glance tables provide a preview of the word parts and definitions you'll learn in each framed section that follows. Then, in the frame for each constructed term, word part reminders show how the individual word part meanings combine to form the constructed term. Word part breakdowns show, by using slash marks, how the constructed term is broken down. Word parts are colored here, too, for further word building reinforcement.

hypoparathyroidism

HIGH poh pair ah THIGH royd izm

hypo/para/thyroid/ism

15.25 The excessive production of PTH by the parathyroid glands is a disorder known as **hyperparathyroidism**. This lengthy term contains four word parts: hyper/para/thyroid/ism. Usually caused by a tumor, it results in excessive calcium levels in the blood, or hypercalcemia (Frame 15.23). In the opposite condition called _____, PTH levels are reduced and the condition of hypocalcemia (Frame 15.23) occurs. The constructed form of this term is ___/_____/_____/_____.

Did You Know?

These special frames reveal fascinating facts about the Latin or Greek origins of a medical term and provide interesting, relevant facts and figures.

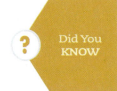

? Did You KNOW

IN SITU
The term *in situ* (pronounced in * SIGH tyoo) is a Latin phrase that literally means "in site." Its use in modern medicine refers to confinement to a site of origin. *Carcinoma in situ* describes a tumor that is confined to its organ of origin, rather than a metastatic tumor in a secondary site. For example, a tumor that originates and remains in the cervix is *in situ*, while a tumor that originates from the cervix but sheds cells to other organs such as the lungs or stomach is metastatic (or malignant).

WORDS TO Watch Out For

-pexy or *-plasty*?
The meanings of these two suffixes both relate to surgery—but they are very different forms of surgery. Remember that *-pexy* means "surgical *fixation, suspension*," and *-plasty* means "surgical *repair*." One way to remember the meaning of *-pexy* is that it uses an *x*, as does the word *fixation* in its definition. Similarly, a way to remember the meaning of *-plasty* is that it uses a *p*, as does the word *repair* in its definition.

Words to Watch Out For!

These special frames provide tips about commonly misspelled or error-prone terms and word parts.

Practice Exercises

These are exercises that follow each chapter subsection and provide opportunities to pause and review with practices such as *The Right Match, Linkup,* and *Break the Chain.*

PRACTICE: Signs and Symptoms of the Digestive System

The Right Match
Match the term on the left with the correct definition on the right.

_____ 1. dysphagia	a. backward flow of material in the GI tract
_____ 2. reflux	b. gas trapped in the GI tract
_____ 3. flatus	c. difficulty in swallowing
_____ 4. halitosis	d. infrequent or incomplete bowel movements
_____ 5. ascites	e. frequent discharge of watery fecal material
_____ 6. diarrhea	f. bad breath
_____ 7. nausea	g. from the French word for yellow
_____ 8. constipation	h. a symptomatic urge to vomit
_____ 9. jaundice	i. accumulation of fluid in the peritoneal cavity

Reinforcement Activities Conclude Each Chapter

CHAPTER REVIEW

Word Building

Construct medical terms from the following meanings. (Some are built from word parts, some are not.) The first question has been completed as an example.

1. inflammation of the larynx   _____*laryng*itis
2. absence of oxygen   _____oxia
3. inflammation of the bronchi   bronch_____
4. respiratory failure characterized by atelectasis   respiratory _____
5. physical exam that includes listening to body sounds   _____ (do this one on your own!)
6. deficient oxygen levels in the blood   hyp_____
7. difficulty breathing   _____pnea
8. excessive carbon dioxide levels in the blood   hyper_____
9. abnormal dilation of the bronchi   bronchi _____
10. lung inflammation due to dust inhalation   _____coniosis
11. cancer arising from cells within the bronchi   bronchogenic _____
12. an inherited disease of excessive mucus production   cystic _____
13. inflammation of the trachea   trache_____
14. the absence of respiratory ventilation   _____sphyxia
15. x-ray image of the bronchi   broncho_____
16. surgical puncture and aspiration of fluid from the pleural cavity   thora_____
17. measurement of oxygen levels in the blood   oxi_____

Word Building Exercises

These review opportunities provide practice in assembling word parts to form many of the medical terms you have just learned about in the chapter.

Define the Combining Form Exercises

This review gives you the opportunity to practice your new knowledge in the definitions of combining forms found in the chapter and provide an example of how a combining form may create a term (new to this edition).

Define the Combining Form

In the space provided, write the definition of the combining form, followed by one example of the combining form used to build a medical term in Chapter 10.

	Definition	Use in a Term
1. gastr/o	_____	_____
2. cholecyst/o	_____	_____
3. choledoch/o	_____	_____
4. enter/o	_____	_____
5. duoden/o	_____	_____
6. gingiv/o	_____	_____
7. col/o	_____	_____
8. pept/o	_____	_____

Complete the Labels

This review of basic anatomy asks you to complete the labeling of illustrations. The fully labeled illustrations are provided at the beginning of the chapter in the Anatomy and Physiology Terms section (new to this edition).

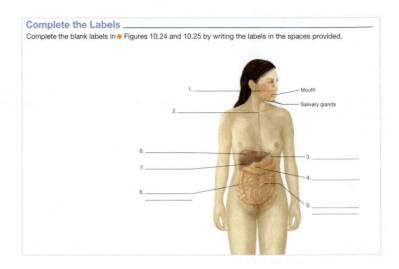

Complete the Labels

Complete the blank labels in ■ Figures 10.24 and 10.25 by writing the labels in the spaces provided.

Medical Report Exercises

These scenarios combine the use of medical case studies and comprehension questions to help you develop a firmer understanding of the terminology in a real-world clinical context.

MEDICAL REPORT EXERCISES

Anita Del Rio

Read the following medical report, then answer the questions that follow.

PGH

PEARSON GENERAL HOSPITAL

5500 University Avenue, Metropolis, New York
Phone: (211) 594-4000 • Fax (211) 594-4001

Medical Consultation: Pediatrics   **Date:** 09/07/2017

Patient: Anita Del Rio   **Patient ID:** 123456

Dob: 1/15/2004   **Age:** 13   **Sex:** Female   **Allergies:** NKDA

Provider: Jonathon McClary, MD

Subjective:

"I'm really tired most of the day, mostly between meals, and getting behind in school. I get real thirsty a lot, and it seems like I need to use the bathroom 20 times a day! Lately, I've also been getting headaches a lot and have trouble falling asleep at night."

13 y/o female complains of malaise, polydipsia, polyuria, cephalalgia, and insomnia. Although full of pep in the clinic during her visit, her mother supports her complaints and is very concerned with her lack of energy. No medical history available.

Objective:

Vital Signs: T: 98.6°F; **P:** 80; **R:** 22; **BP:** 120/75

Ht: 5'1"

Wt: 90 lb

General Appearance: Skin appears healthy, with no apparent masses or discolorations.

Heart: Rate at 80 bpm. Heart sounds with auscultation appear normal.

Lungs: Clear without signs of disease.

AbD: Bowel sounds normal all four quadrants.

HEENT: No abnormalities present.

Lab: Ketone bodies elevated, mild acidosis pH 7.3; FBS 220 confirmed with GTT

Assessment:

Diabetes mellitus type 1

Plan:

Treat as type 1 DM with regular insulin injection regimen and enroll with parent in diabetes management class.

Photo Source: Scott Griessel/Fotolia.

MyLab Medical Terminology™

What is MyLab Medical Terminology?

MyLab Medical Terminology is a comprehensive online program that gives you, the student, the opportunity to test your understanding of information, concepts, and medical language to see how well you know the material from the test results. MyLab Medical Terminology builds a self-paced, personalized study plan unique to your needs. Remediation in the form of etext pages, illustrations, exercises, audio segments, and video clips is provided for those areas in which you may need additional instruction, review or reinforcement. You can then work through the program until your study plan is complete and you have mastered the content. MyLab Medical Terminology is available as a standalone program or with an embedded etext.

MyLab Medical Terminology is organized to follow the chapters and learning outcomes in *Medical Terminology Complete!*, fourth edition. With MyLab Medical Terminology, you can track your own progress through your entire med term course.

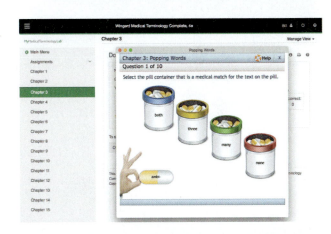

How do Students Benefit?

Here's how MyLab Medical Terminology helps you.

- Keep up with information presented in the text and lectures.
- Save time by focusing study and review on just the content you need.
- Increase understanding of difficult concepts with study material for different learning styles.
- Remediate in areas in which you need additional review.

Key Features of MyLab Medical Terminology

Pre-Tests and Post-Tests. Using questions aligned to the learning outcomes in *Medical Terminology Complete!*, multiple tests measure your understanding of topics.

Personalized Study Material. Based on the topic pre-test results, you receive a personalized study plan, highlighting areas where you may need improvement. It includes these study tools:

- Links to specific pages in the etext
- Images for review
- Interactive exercises
- Animations and video clips
- Audio glossary
- Access to full Personalized Study Material.

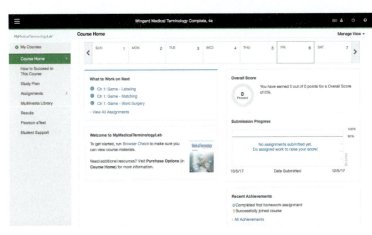

How do Instructors Benefit?

- Save time by providing students with a comprehensive, media-rich study program.
- Track student understanding of course content in the program guidebook.
- Monitor student activity with viewable student assignments.

Comprehensive Instructional Package

Perhaps the most gratifying part of an educator's work is the "aha" learning moment when the light bulb goes on and a student truly understands a concept—when a connection is made. Along these lines, Pearson is pleased to help instructors foster more of these educational connections by providing a complete battery of resources to support teaching and learning. Qualified adopters are eligible to receive a wealth of materials designed to help instructors prepare, present, and assess. For more information, please contact your Pearson sales representative or visit **www.pearsonhighered.com/educator**.

Preface

Medical Terminology Complete! presents the most current and accepted language of health care in a programmed learning approach. It has helped prepare thousands of students for careers in health professions by providing a self-guided tool for learning medical terminology. The book may be used as a text to support lectures and online courses or as an independent student workbook. The flexibility of its application is made possible by the book's text-like format combined with its self-guided learning program, self-assessment questions, and reinforcement exercises. To provide an optimum learning format, the text discussions are basic, clear, and concise. The programmed learning modules are simple and easy to follow, and the self-assessment questions and exercises provide reviews and clinical applications of the information at frequent intervals.

New to This Edition

Based on extensive feedback from students and instructors, we have revised *Medical Terminology Complete!* so that it provides an even more valuable teaching and learning experience than previous editions. Here are the enhancements we have made:

- All chapters have been carefully reviewed and edited to complete a shift from a biological perspective to a more clinical perspective, thereby providing improved clinical training for students poised to enter healthcare careers.

- All selected terms have been carefully screened for current accuracy, with outdated terms removed and new terms added to bring the text up-to-date.

- Many new photographs and several new illustrations have been added to help learners more easily visualize the concepts and meanings of selected terms.

- Additional Chapter Review exercises at the end of chapters 5-15 have been added to give students more practice with reviewing chapter terms, including **Define the Combining Form** and **Complete the Labels**.

- The online support has been improved to provide easier access and enhancements to interactive learning, making this edition a valuable learning tool for online courses in medical terminology.

The Programmed Approach

Each learning frame contains a clear and concise statement, usually describing a single medical term. This allows learners to focus on one term at a time. Each frame includes at least one blank space, which can be completed based on clues within the frame. The answer to the blank is provided in the left column. Students can either cover the answer column or leave it uncovered. Either way, the kinesthetic component of filling in the blank provides another level of learning that ensures retention.

Each body systems chapter presents the most important terms (or "Key Terms") in the answer column with color-coded word parts, where applicable, as well as a phonetic pronunciation. Prefixes appear in **yellow**; combining forms are **red**; and suffixes are **blue**.

An added benefit of this Key Terms answer column is that the terms are presented in alphabetical order, which provides a way for students to quickly review the priority terms. Other terms that are related to the Key Terms in the answer column, but not as vital for the student to understand, are presented in the main frame section in boldface type.

The self-study features enable students to learn with a minimum of instructor guidance. In addition to the programmed learning frames, other self-study features include blocks of review questions (**Practice**) that are placed at frequent intervals throughout each chapter. In these sections, students have the opportunity to test their understanding by answering questions in **The Right Match**, **Linkup**, and **Break the Chain** activities. Answers to these activities, along with those for the end-of-chapter review questions, appear in Appendix E located at www.pearsonhighered.com/healthprofessionsresources.

The book also includes boxes intended to promote additional interest in medical terminology. They include **Did You Know?** boxes, which reveal fascinating facts about the Latin or Greek origins of a medical term and provide interesting and relevant facts and figures that draw a connection between a particular term and its clinical point of interest, and **Words to Watch Out For!** boxes, which provide tips about commonly misspelled or error-prone terms and word parts.

Chapter Format

Each chapter begins with a brief list of **Learning Objectives**. In each chapter beginning with Chapter 5, a brief review of the structure and function of the particular body system discussed in the chapter follows the objectives. The section is titled **Anatomy and Physiology Terms**, and it begins with an at-a-glance table with the major combining forms and definitions for that body system. The Anatomy and Physiology section then presents a limited number of learning frames—enough to give students an opportunity to review essential anatomy and physiology, without overwhelming them or providing redundancy to students who have already taken an anatomy course as a prerequisite. The illustrations accompanying this section provide a visual review of anatomy.

The primary text of each chapter consists of a brief narrative introduction discussing the pathophysiology of the body system, followed by numerous programmed learning frames and **Practice** exercises that are divided into three sections:

- **Signs and Symptoms**
- **Diseases and Disorders**
- **Treatments, Procedures, and Devices**

An **Abbreviations** listing and a **Practice** exercise follow to conclude the teaching portion of the chapter.

Finally, a **Chapter Review** section provides several review exercises, including **Word Building** and **Medical Report Exercises** with two medical reports and case studies. New to this edition are additional chapter review exercises, including **Define the Combining Form** and **Complete the Labels**.

Organization of the Book

The organization of this text is unique in that it provides a slow, building approach to teaching medical terminology. Students can often be overwhelmed by this new language, so here's what we've done to address this and make the learning experience more comfortable for students:

- The text begins with three chapters devoted exclusively to word building and word parts. Chapter 1 provides an introduction to medical terminology and to the programmed learning approach. Basic definitions of terminology and word construction are first described here. Also, the importance of learning the most common Latin and Greek word parts is emphasized as a starting point. Chapter 2 provides an opportunity for students to learn the common suffixes that are in frequent use in building medical terms. Chapter 3 covers prefixes and their common uses in medical terms. We then present Chapter 4, which introduces anatomy and physiology word roots and combining forms, both of which create the foundation for the majority of medical terms. This chapter also introduces other foundational terms, such as anatomical and directional terms. This allows the student to take a slow, logical approach to learning word parts and word building.

- Then, the student can put that knowledge to work and learn about medical terms as they apply to each body system. The body system chapters progress from the least complex body system (integumentary) to the most complex body system (endocrine), with a sequence that parallels most courses in anatomy and physiology. This approach enhances learning by allowing students to build confidence as they work their way through the chapters.

Appendix A provides a complete glossary of all word parts that are presented in the text, along with their definitions. Appendix B lists abbreviations commonly used in the healthcare professions. Appendix C provides word parts for describing color, number, and plurals. In Appendix D (online), common terms used in pharmacology are included for your reference. Appendix E (online) provides the answers to the Practice exercises and to the end-of-chapter Chapter Review questions. All online materials can be found at *www.pearsonhighered.com/healthprofessionsresources*.

A glossary/index concludes the book, providing a quick and handy reference.

I invite and welcome your reactions, comments, and suggestions to be sent to me directly so that subsequent editions may reflect your educational needs even better.

Bruce Wingerd
National University and San Diego State University
San Diego, CA 92037
Bruce.Wingerd@natuniv.edu

About The Author

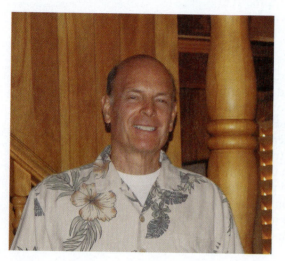

Bruce Wingerd is a member of the Biology Department at National University in San Diego, California. Previously, he has held teaching/administrative positions at Edison State College (now called Florida Southwestern State College), Broward College, and San Diego State University. Professor Wingerd's degrees are in the fields of zoology and physiology, and he has taught courses in medical terminology, human anatomy, advanced human anatomy, and anatomy and physiology for more than 30 years. He has written numerous textbooks, lab manuals, and multimedia learning resources in medical terminology, human anatomy, anatomy and physiology, histology, and comparative mammalian anatomy. Professor Wingerd's goal in teaching and writing is to provide students with learning tools that will help them reach their potential through education. He enjoys counseling students in the health sciences, developing novel approaches to teaching and learning, and leading faculty in the drive for excellence in education.

About the Illustrators

Marcelo Oliver is president and founder of Body Scientific International, LLC. He holds an MFA degree in Medical and Biological Illustration from the University of Michigan. For more than 15 years, his passion has been to condense complex anatomical information into visual education tools for students, patients, and medical professionals.

Body Scientific's lead artists in this publication were medical illustrators Carol Hrejsa, Liana Bauman, and Katie Burgess. They each hold Master of Science degrees in Biomedical Visualization from the University of Illinois at Chicago. Their contribution was the creation and editing of clear, effective, vibrant, and medically accurate artwork throughout.

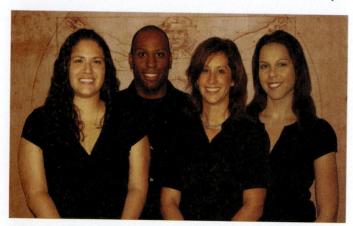

Acknowledgments

This book is the product of collective hard work from a talented team focused on creating a unique learning tool.

Our team received its original direction from then-Editor-in-Chief Mark Cohen, who provided the vision and energy to launch this project into its first edition and continue with improvements into the second edition. The third edition and now this new fourth edition were spearheaded and supported by our present Portfolio Manager, John Goucher, who shared in our collective vision for a unique learning tool. I am filled with gratitude for his support to produce a fourth edition. I also appreciate the efforts of Elena Mauceri of DynamicWordWorks, Inc. who brought an outstanding developmental editor to join our team for the third edition and now the fourth edition, Jennifer Maybin of Editor in the Woods, LLC. Jennifer made many helpful suggestions and contributions through her dedicated hard work on every line of the textbook, and her many contributions are highly appreciated.

Many other talented people worked hard to make this book a valuable teaching and learning resource. I extend to each of them my warmest gratitude:

Melissa Bashe, Content Producer, who coordinated the development of a world-class teaching and learning package.

Lisa Narine, Portfolio Management Assistant, who executed the complex process of managing our peer review program.

Marcelo Oliver and his team of medical illustrators at Body Scientific International, LLC, who created a dynamic, clear, and precise art program.

Meghan DeMaio, Editorial Project Manager for SPi Global, who directed the flow of textual and visual content throughout the production of the book and ancillary materials.

Patty Donovan and Thomas Russell, Production Editors for SPi Global, who oversaw the copyediting and page composition processes.

Our Development Team

The fresh, unique vision, format, and content contained within the pages of *Medical Terminology Complete!* comes as a result of an incredible collaboration of expert educators from around the United States. This book represents the collective insights, experience, and thousands of hours of work performed by members of this development team. Their influence will continue to have an impact for decades to come. Let us introduce the members of our team.

Fourth Edition Reviewers

Pamela Dobbins, MS
Shelton State Community College
Tuscaloosa, Alabama

Jodi Goodkin, PT, Med, CEAS
Broward College
Fort Meyers, Florida

Lisa Ritchie, EdD, RD, LD
Harding University
Searcy, Arkansas

Amy Samuel, CMA (AAMA), AHI (AMT)
University of Alaska, South East
Sitka, Alaska

Amy Snow, MS
Greenville Technical College
Greenville, South Carolina

Previous Edition Reviewers

Lynn Alexander, MEd, SBB (ASCP)
Winston-Salem State University
Winston-Salem, North Carolina

Martha Arnson, RN
Gwinnett Technical College
Lawrenceville, Georgia

Cindy Ault, MS, MT (ASCP)
Jamestown College
Jamestown, North Dakota

Mary Jo Belenski, EdD
Montclair State University
Montclair, New Jersey

Linda A. Bell, BS, MEd
Reading Area Community College
Reading, Pennsylvania

Bradley S. Bowden, PhD
Alfred University
Alfred, New York

Amy Bowersock, PhD
The University of Tampa
Tampa, Florida

Vera Brock, RNC, DSN
Georgia Highlands College
Rome, Georgia

Mary Elizabeth Browder, BA, AAS, CMA
Raymond Walters College/UC-Blue Ash
Cincinnati, Ohio

Joyce A. Bulgrin, MSA MT (ASCP)
University of Wisconsin–Stevens Point
Stevens Point, Wisconsin

Barbara Burri, MBA, BS, CVT, LVT
New Hampshire Community Technical College
Stratham, New Hampshire

Christina Campbell, PhD, RD
Montana State University
Bozeman, Montana

Sandra Carlson, RN, BSN, CNOR
Director, Surgical Technology
New Hampshire Community Technical College
Stratham, New Hampshire

Jean M. Chenu, MBA
Genesee Community College
Batavia, New York

Phyllis Clements, MA, OTR
Macomb Community College
Clinton Township, Michigan

Pam deCalesta, OD
Linn-Benton Community College
Albany, Oregon

Litta Dennis, BSN, MS
Illinois Central College
Peoria, Illinois

Rosemary DeSiervi, MEd
West Valley College
Saratoga, California

Sherry Gamble, RN, MSN
The University of Akron
Akron, Ohio

Steven B. Goldschmidt, DC, CCFC
North Hennepin Community College
Brooklyn Park, Minnesota
Inverhills Community College
Inver Grove Heights, Minnesota

Sandra Gustafson, MA Nursing, CNE
Hibbing Community College
Hibbing, Minnesota

Pamela Halter, MSN, RN
Kent State University at Tuscarawas
New Philadelphia, Ohio

Karen R. Hardney, MSEd
Chicago State University
Chicago, Illinois

Pamela Harmon, RT (R)
Triton College
River Grove, Illinois

Kathy Harward, RN, BSN
Florida Community College at Jacksonville
Jacksonville, Florida

Rachel M. P. Hopp, PhD
Houston Baptist University
Houston, Texas

Diana Houston, AAS
San Jacinto College North
Houston, Texas

James E. Hudacek, MSEd
Lorain County Community College
Elyria, Ohio

Louis M. Izzo, MS, CNMT
University of Vermont
Williston, Vermont

Marcie Jones, BS, CMA
Gwinnett Technical College
Lawrenceville, Georgia

Marie L. Kotter, PhD
Weber State University
Ogden, Utah

Susan P. Lathbury, MS
Broward College
Pembroke Pines, Florida

Paul Lucas, CMA, CPbt, PN, AS
Brown Mackie College
Fort Wayne, Indiana

Alice Macomber, RN, AS, RPT, RMA,
    CPI, AHI, LXMO
Keiser University
Port Saint Lucie, Florida

Mandy Mann, CMA
Big Bend Community College
Moses Lake, Washington

Laura Melendez, BS, RMA, BXMO
Southeastern College
Green Acres, Florida

Cheryl Meyer, RN, MSN
Delaware County Community
    College
Media, Pennsylvania

Deborah S. Molnar, PT, DPT, MSEd
SUNY Canton
Canton, New York

Sandra Mullins, EdD
Kentucky Community and Technical
    College System
Lexington, Kentucky

Sandra Mullins, EdD
Bluegrass Community and Technical
    College
Lexington, Kentucky

Lisa Nagle, BSed, CMA
Augusta Technical College
Augusta, Georgia

Anne Nez, RN, MSN
Central Wyoming College
Riverton, Wyoming

Arthur J. Ortiz, MA, LPN, LRCP
Southeast Community College
Lincoln, Nebraska

Elizabeth Pagenkopf, RN, BSN, MA
Harper College
Palatine, Illinois

Felicity F. Penner, BSc, MSPH
Southwestern Community College
Chula Vista, California

Daniel Podd, MPAS, RPAC
St. Johns University
Fresh Meadows, New York

Linda Reeves, MD
Virginia College Online
Hoover, Alabama

Carol Reid, MS, RN
Century College
White Bear Lake, Minnesota

Lisa Ritchie, EdD, MS.E, BS
Harding University
Searcy, Arkansas

Lawrence Rosenquist, MS, RN
Wilkes University
Wilkes-Barre, Pennsylvania

Donna M. Rowan, MAT, RMA
Harford Community College
Bel Air, Maryland

Mary T Senor, BS
Bergen Community College
Paramus, New Jersey

Paula Silver, BS, PharmD
ECPI University
Newport News, Virginia

Lorraine M. Smith, MBA
Fresno City College
Fresno, California

Steven C. Stoner, PharmD, BCPP
UMKC School of Pharmacy
Kansas City, Missouri

Roger Thompson, BS, RRT
Mountain Empire Community College
Big Stone Gap, Virginia

Garnet Tomich, BA
San Diego, California

Judy Traynor, MS, FNP, RN,
    CASAC
Jefferson Community College
Watertown, New York

Twila Wallace, MEd
Central Community College
Columbus, Nebraska

Margaret T. Warren, PhD, RN
Rockland Community College
Suffern, New York

Kathy Whitley, MSN, FNP
Patrick Henry Community College
Martinsville, Virginia

Lynn C. Wimett, RN, ANP, EdD
Regis University
Denver, Colorado

Kathy Zabel, BS, AAS
Southeast Community College
Lincoln, Nebraska

Previous Edition Ancillary Content Providers

Linda C. Campbell, CMT,
    FAAMT
The Andrews School
Oklahoma City, Oklahoma

Charlotte Creason, RHIA
Tyler Junior College
Tyler, Texas

Duane A. Dreyer, PhD
Miller-Motte College
Cary, North Carolina

Jennifer Esch, BS, PA-C
Bryant and Stratton College
Milwaukee, Wisconsin

Pamela A. Eugene, BAS, RT, (R)
Delgado Community College
New Orleans, Louisiana

Jodi Gootkin, PT, MEd
Edison State College
Fort Myers, Florida

Sherry Grover, PhD
Virginia College
Houston, Texas

Jean M. Krueger-Watson, PhD
Clark College
Vancouver, Washington

Trisha LaPointe, PharmD, BCPS
Massachusetts College of Pharmacy and
    Health Sciences
Boston, Massachusetts

Peggy Mayo, MEd MLT (ASCP)
Columbus State Community College
Columbus, Ohio

**Lynette S. McCullough, MCH,
    NREMT-P**
Southern Crescent Technical College
Griffin, Georgia

Donna Jeanne Pugh, BSN, RN
Florida Metropolitan University
Jacksonville, Florida

Linda Reeves, MD, FAAP
Virginia College Online
Birmingham, Alabama

Ann Wentworth, BAS, RT (R) (CT)
Jackson Community College
Jackson, Michigan

Kathy Zaiken, PharmD
Massachusetts College of Pharmacy and
    Health Sciences
Boston, Massachusetts

A Commitment To Accuracy

As a student embarking on a career in health care you probably already know how critically important it is to be precise in your work. Patients and coworkers will be counting on you to avoid errors on a daily basis. Likewise, we owe it to you—the reader—to ensure accuracy in this book. We have gone to great lengths to verify that the information provided in *Medical Terminology Complete!* is complete and correct. To this end, here are the steps we have taken:

1. **Editorial Review**—We have assembled a large team of developmental consultants (listed on the preceding pages) to critique every word and every image in this book. No fewer than 12 content experts have read each chapter for accuracy. In addition, some members of our developmental team were specifically assigned to focus on the precision of each illustration that appears in the book.
2. **Medical Illustrations**—A team of medically trained illustrators was hired to prepare each piece of art that graces the pages of this book. These illustrators have a higher level of scientific education than the artists for most textbooks, and they worked directly with the author and members of our development team to make sure that their work was clear, correct, and consistent with what is described in the text.
3. **Accurate Ancillaries**—The teaching and learning ancillaries are often as important to instruction as the textbook itself. Therefore, we took steps to ensure accuracy and consistency of these by reviewing every ancillary component. The author and editorial team studied every PowerPoint slide and online course frame to ensure the context was correct and relevant to each lesson.

Although our intent and actions have been directed at creating an error-free text, we have established a process for correcting any mistakes that may have slipped past our editors. Pearson takes this issue seriously and therefore welcomes any and all feedback that you can provide along the lines of helping us enhance the accuracy of this text. If you identify any errors that need to be corrected in a subsequent printing, please send them to:

> **Pearson Health Editorial**
> **Medical Terminology Corrections**
> **221 River Street**
> **Hoboken, NJ 07030**

Thank you for helping Pearson reach its goal of providing the most accurate medical terminology textbooks available.

Contents

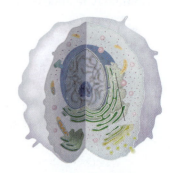

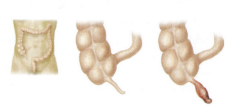

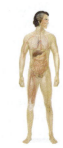

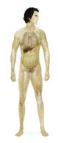
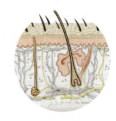
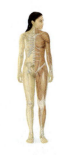
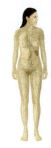

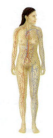
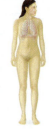
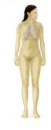
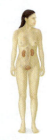

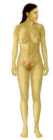
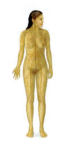

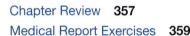

xxiii

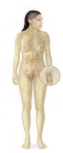

Chapter 15 ● The Endocrine System 503

*Appendix D and Appendix E can be found online at www.pearsonhighered.com/
healthprofessionsresources

Chapter 1

Introduction to Word Parts and Word Construction

Learning Objectives

After completing this chapter, you will be able to:

1.1 Use the technique of programmed learning and frames.

1.2 Apply the phonetic pronunciation guides that are used in frames.

1.3 Recognize that medical terminology has both constructed and nonconstructed terms.

1.4 Identify each of the three word parts (word roots, prefixes, and suffixes) used to construct medical terms.

1.5 Identify the function of a combining vowel that is added to a word root to form a combining form.

1.6 Recognize that many medical terms are constructed from word parts and can be deconstructed into their word parts.

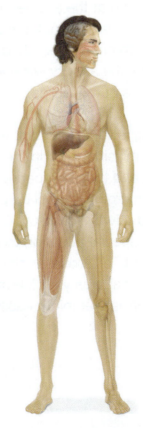

The Programmed Learning Approach

frame	**1.1** This textbook teaches you medical terminology by using the friendly technique of **programmed learning**. This technique has been used for many years to teach many subjects, such as math, world languages, and of course, medical terminology. It consists of blocks of information, known as frames, which contain one or more blanks. The blanks are provided for you to write in the missing word. In some cases, the missing word is easy to determine, and in other cases it becomes more of a challenge. In either case, the missing word is provided in the left margin of the _____, so you don't have to feel frustrated if you have trouble identifying or spelling the missing word correctly.
number	**1.2** As you can see, each frame consists of a block of information with the blank in the box on the right side of the page. Note the frame _____. This number enables you to locate and flip back to a previous frame with ease if needed.
blank	**1.3** The far left margin in each frame contains the missing word(s). As you proceed from frame to frame, you should write the missing word in the _____. To challenge yourself and make the best use of your time, try to work by first filling in the blank *without* looking at the answer. It works best to use a 3 × 5 card or something similar to block the answers in the margin; then after committing to an answer, check to see if your choice is correct. By doing so, the activity will engage your mind and help you to learn the meanings of the words.
spelling	**1.4** Spelling is very important when learning medical terminology. By writing the missing word in the blank without looking at it in the far left margin and then comparing your answer with the one provided in the far left margin, you will be practicing the _____ of the word. Always check your answer before moving to the next frame. Pay special attention to the "Did You Know?" and "Words to Watch Out For" boxes in this text. These alert you to helpful information that aids your learning and identifies tricky spelling issues or terms that might easily be confused.

phonetic foh-NET-ik	**1.5** In addition to spelling, correct pronunciation of medical terms is also important. To help you with pronunciation, the phonetic ("sounds like") form of the word is provided in parentheses whenever a new term is introduced; for example, _____ (_____) and pronunciation (proh NUN see AYE shun). You should say the new word aloud whenever possible, using the phonetic guide to assist you.
guides	**1.6** In the phonetic _____ that appear in this text, note that the syllables with the most spoken emphasis are shown in all capital letters. Here are some examples: ■ The term *cardiology* is pronounced (kar dee AHL oh jee). Note that the middle syllable *AHL* carries the most emphasis. ■ The term *gastrohepatic* is pronounced (GAS troh heh PAT ik). Note that the long *o* sound in the second syllable is demonstrated when spelled phonetically as *oh*, and the short *e* sound is demonstrated when spelled *eh*. ■ The term *osteopathic* is pronounced (oss tee oh PATH ik). Note that the long *e* sound in the second syllable is shown as *ee*.
pronunciation	You can also refer to the student website for audio samples of the pronunciation of each medical term presented in this text. Spend time listening to the _____ of each term presented in each chapter. Doing so will help you complete the pronunciation exercise in this chapter's "Talking Shop."

PRACTICE: The Programmed Learning Approach

The Right Match

Match the term on the left with the correct definition on the right.

_____ 1. pronunciations

_____ 2. spelling

_____ 3. blank

_____ 4. programmed learning

_____ 5. Words to Watch Out For boxes

a. alert you to terms that might easily be confused

b. learning technique that consists of blocks of information, known as frames, which contain one or more blanks for the student to fill in

c. by comparing your filled-in answer with the one provided in the far left margin, you will be practicing this

d. as you proceed from frame to frame, you should write the missing word into this

e. you can also refer to the student website for audio samples of these

Talking Shop

In the blank, write the letter of the pronunciation that matches the term. The first one is completed for you as an example. Visit the student website to hear the correct pronunciation of these terms.

Term

_f_ 1. cardiologist
____ 2. lymphoma
____ 3. pneumonia
____ 4. fracture
____ 5. meningitis
____ 6. meningocele
____ 7. epicardium
____ 8. nephrolithiasis
____ 9. psychologist
____ 10. hepatomegaly
____ 11. pediatrician
____ 12. bacteriuria

Pronunciation

a. pee dee ah TRISH an
b. men IN goh seel
c. limm FOH mah
d. ep ih KAR dee um
e. FRAK sher
f. kar dee AHL oh jist
g. NEFF roh lith EYE ah siss
h. HEPP ah toh MEG ah lee
i. bak teer ee YOO ree ah
j. noo MOH nee ah
k. sigh KAHL oh jist
l. MEN in JYE tis

Constructed and Nonconstructed Terms

language

medical terminology

1.7 Medical terminology is a language for medical health professionals. This _____ has rules of grammar, spelling, and pronunciation, just like any other language. Because medical terminology is the universal language of medicine, its terms must be understood by speakers of many languages in many parts of the world, especially in our age of globalization. For the purpose of learning the language of _____ _____, terms in this specialized language can be separated into two main categories: constructed terms and nonconstructed terms.

constructed terms

word

1.8 Many medical terms are **constructed terms**, which are made up of multiple word parts that are combined to form a new word. In most cases, the word parts are derived from Latin and Greek. The key to learning _____ _____ is to first learn the meaning of the various word parts. It may be helpful to think of constructed terms as if they were written in code. Once you have the key to a code, it becomes a fairly simple process to decode the messages or to use the code to form messages yourself. Similarly, once you learn the meanings of the individual _____ parts, you have the key to the medical terminology code. See ■ Figure 1.1.

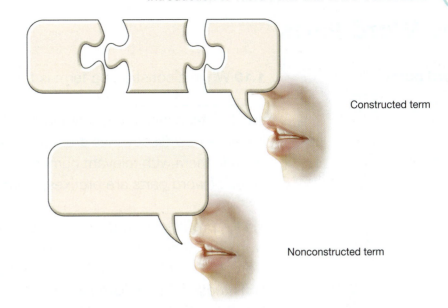

Constructed term

Nonconstructed term

■ **Figure 1.1**
Medical terms are either constructed words, which are composed of more than one word part, or nonconstructed words you must memorize, which include terms that are a single Latin or Greek word part, eponyms, acronyms, and so on.

eponym

nonconstructed terms

1.9 The second group of medical terms is **nonconstructed terms**, terms that are not formed from individual word parts. Nonconstructed terms include **eponyms**, which are terms derived from the names of people. For example, *eustachian tube* is an _____ because it is derived from the name of Bartolommeo Eustachio, who first discovered this small tube between the throat and the middle ear. Other forms of nonconstructed terms include **acronyms**, which are words derived from the first letters of words in a compound term, such as *LASIK* for **las**er-assisted **i**n situ **k**eratomileusis; and words derived from languages other than Greek or Latin, such as *jaundice*, which is derived from the French word for yellow, *jaune*. To learn _____ _____, you must commit them to memory.

PRACTICE: Constructed and Nonconstructed Terms

The Right Match

Match the term on the left with the correct definition on the right.

_____ 1. nonconstructed terms
_____ 2. constructed terms
_____ 3. medical terminology
_____ 4. eponym

a. term derived from a person's name
b. must be committed to memory
c. made up of word parts
d. the universal language of medicine

The Word Parts

word parts	**1.10** When a constructed term is formed, individual _____ _____ are assembled to create a term with a new meaning. This is very useful in medicine because new discoveries are made frequently, and the need to provide them with relevant names is important. The three primary types of word parts are prefixes, word roots, and suffixes.
prefix	**1.11** A **prefix** is a word part that is affixed to the beginning of a word. Its purpose is to expand or enhance the meaning of the word. Let's look at an example of a prefix in action, using the word *construction*. In our sample word, *con-* is the prefix. It means "with, together, jointly." Notice the hyphen following the prefix. You will know that a word part is a _____ by the hyphen that immediately follows it (e.g., *con-*).
word root	**1.12** A **word root** is a word part that provides the primary meaning of the term. The _____ _____ provides the basis for the term and is the part to which other word parts are attached. Nearly all terms have a word root, and some have more than one. In our sample word *construction*, *struct* is the word root. It means "make, build."
suffix	**1.13** A **suffix** is a word part that is affixed to the end of a word. The _____ often indicates the word's part of speech (noun, verb, adjective, adverb, etc.) or modifies the word's meaning. In our sample word *construction*, the suffix is *-ion*. It indicates that the word is a noun and it means "process." You will know that a word part is a suffix by the hyphen that immediately precedes it (for example, *-ion*).
three	**1.14** To summarize using our example, the word *construction* is composed of _____ word parts (■ Figure 1.2):

con- + struct + -ion

(prefix + word root + suffix)

We decipher the meaning of medical words by defining each of the word parts. First, we look at the meaning of the suffix, and then we look at the meaning of the prefix. Finally, we define the word root. Then we combine the meanings of all the word parts in the way that makes the most sense. Thus, con- + struct + -ion means "process of building together."

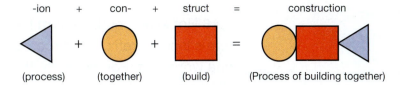

Figure 1.2
Most medical terms are formed by assembling word parts.

Did You KNOW

This text has a special color-coding system to help you recognize the individual word parts. Each time a word part is presented, it appears in a specific color:

- Prefixes are **yellow**
- Word roots and combining forms are **red**
- Suffixes are **blue**

word parts

1.15 The word *construction*, then, as we use it in medical terminology, refers to "building words out of word parts." This is what we do every time we write and speak. This is also what we do when we use medical terminology by speaking and writing medical terms. Understanding how to build words out of _____ _____ is essential to understanding the meaning of medical terms. Equally important is understanding how to deconstruct or break down a medical term into its component word parts. That is exactly what we did when we deciphered the meaning of our sample word *construction*. We broke the word down into its prefix, word root, and suffix parts and then combined the definitions of the word parts to derive the meaning of the term. Now let's break down a medical term into its word parts:

hypodermic
hypo- + derm + -ic
(prefix + word root + suffix)

hypo- is a prefix that means "deficient, abnormally low, below"
derm is a word root that means "skin"
-ic is a suffix that means "pertaining to"

Thus, the term *hypodermic* means "pertaining to below the skin." Notice that the meaning of the suffix comes first when describing the meaning of the term from its word parts.

word root

1.16 Not every medical term has all three word parts. Some medical terms lack a prefix, word root, or suffix, and some have more than one word root. For example, the term *gastroenteritis* (GAS troh en ter EYE tis) breaks down like so:

gastroenteritis

gastr + enter + -itis

(word root + word root + suffix)

gastr is a word root that means "stomach"
enter is a _____ _____ that means "small intestine"
-itis is a suffix that means "inflammation"

Thus, the term *gastroenteritis* means "inflammation of the stomach and small intestine." Notice the letter *o* between the two word roots. You will learn about the importance of its use very soon (Frame 1.18).

suffix

1.17 Some medical terms are made simply of a prefix and a suffix. The term *aphasia* is an example.

aphasia

a- + -phasia

(prefix + suffix)

a- is a prefix that means "without or absence of"
-phasia is a _____ that means "speaking"

Thus, the term *aphasia* means "absence of speaking."

combining vowel

1.18 A fourth word part is the **combining vowel**. It is used when a word root requires a connecting vowel in order to add a suffix that begins with a consonant, or to add another word root, when forming a term. The _____ _____ does not add to or alter the meaning of the word root; it simply assists us in pronouncing a term. In most cases, the combining vowel is the letter *o*, and in some cases it is the letter *i* or *e*.

combining form

1.19 Generally, it is best to learn a word root with its combining vowel. This word root plus combining vowel form is called a **combining form**. Whenever possible, the combining forms are presented in this text to ease your building and deconstructing of medical terms, some of which are shown in ■ Figure 1.3. The method for writing a _____ _____ is to use a slash between the word root and the combining vowel, such as

cardi/o
(word root/combining vowel)

The combining vowel in *cardi/o* is *o*.

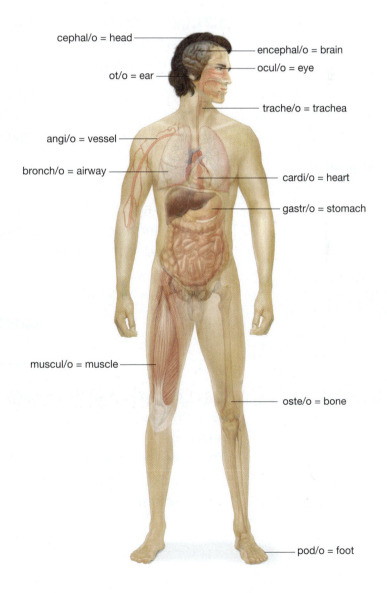

cephal/o = head

encephal/o = brain

ocul/o = eye

ot/o = ear

trache/o = trachea

angi/o = vessel

bronch/o = airway

cardi/o = heart

gastr/o = stomach

muscul/o = muscle

oste/o = bone

pod/o = foot

■ **Figure 1.3**
The human body, with many of the common combining forms.

o

1.20 You learned from Frame 1.18 that the most common combining vowel is the letter _____. As practice, let's take a look at a medical term you may be familiar with:

cardiology

This term is made up of three word parts: a word root, a combining vowel, and a suffix. The combining form is *cardi/o* and the suffix is *-logy*. *Cardi/o* means "heart" and *-logy* means "study or science of." Thus, when we define the word parts of the term *cardiology* and then combine their definitions in a logical way, we know it means "the study or science of the heart." It may help to write the constructed form of the term, which is written with slashes separating each word part:

cardi/o/logy

1.21 Let's practice deconstructing medical terms and using word parts to decipher their meaning. Here are some more medical terms that you may already know.

dermatologist
dermat/o + -logist
(combining form + suffix)

combining form

dermat/o is a _____ _____ that means "skin"
-logist is a suffix that means "one who studies."
Thus, the term *dermatologist* means "one who studies the skin." The constructed form is written dermat/o/logist.

1.22 Another example is:

tonsillectomy
tonsill + -ectomy
(word root + suffix)

tonsill is a word root that means "almond or tonsil"

suffix

-ectomy is a _____ that means "surgical excision, removal"
Thus, the term *tonsillectomy* means "surgical removal of tonsil (shaped like an almond)." The constructed form is written tonsill/ectomy.

1.23 Another example is:

microscopic

micro- + scop + -ic

(prefix + word root + suffix)

micro- is a prefix that means "small"
scop is a word root that means "viewing instrument"
-ic is a suffix that means "pertaining to"

Thus, the term *microscopic* means "pertaining to the viewing instrument for investigating small things," or "visible only by means of a microscope." The constructed form is written _____/_____/_____.

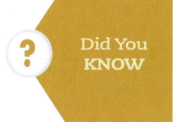

micro/scop/ic

? Did You KNOW

THE ORIGINS OF MEDICAL TERMS

Just as Greek and Latin have played a critical role in the formation and meaning of words in many languages such as English, French, Italian, Spanish, Portuguese, and others, these two ancient languages have contributed to the development of the language of medicine and many related disciplines. The ancient Greek, Hippocrates, is considered the father of modern medicine because he was among the first to explore the identification and treatment of disease (■ Figure 1.4). Hippocrates and other early Greek scholars explored and observed the human body and its functions, and they wrote about their discoveries using everyday words from their native language. Later, the Romans advanced medicine with their own experiments and observations. They added Latin terms to the growing body of medical language.

For example, the fallopian tube that connects the ovary with the uterus is known as a *salpinx* (plural, *salpinges*). This is an ancient Greek word meaning "trumpet." The organ in the female body was named for its trumpetlike shape. From this descriptive Greek word, we can build many medical terms such as *salpingitis* ("inflammation of the fallopian tube"), *salpingoplasty* ("surgical repair of the fallopian tube"), *salpingo-oophorectomy* ("surgical

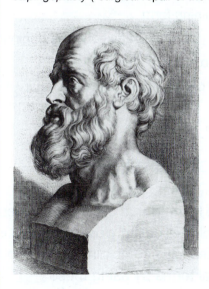

■ **Figure 1.4**
The Greek father of medicine, Hippocrates, who originated many medical terms.
Source: Courtesy of the National Library of Medicine.

continued

removal of the ovary and fallopian tube"), and many others. See Table 1.1 ■ for examples of word roots that originate from Greek and Latin.

Sometimes the origins of medical terms relate to history, poetry, mythology, geography, physical objects, and ideas. For example, the medical term *psychology* has its origins in the meaning of the Greek word *psyche* ("mind, soul"). Further investigation leads to the Greek myth of a princess named Psyche who falls in love with the god of love, Eros. Knowing the myth of Psyche and Eros may help you remember the meaning of the term *psyche* when you encounter it.

We briefly explore the origins of medical terms in other "Did You Know?" features throughout the text. Look for these boxes to expand your understanding of medical terminology and provide a useful way to remember meanings.

Table 1.1 ■ Word Roots from Greek and Latin

Root	Origin	Definition	Medical Term Example
lith	*lithos*, Greek	stone	*cholelithiasis* condition of having gallstones
maxim	*maximus*, Latin	biggest, highest	*gluteus maximus* the biggest (outermost) gluteus muscle in the buttocks
derm	*derma*, Greek	skin	*dermatitis* inflammation of the skin
path	*pathos*, Greek	disease	*pathogen* disease-causing agent

PRACTICE: The Word Parts

The Right Match

Match the term on the left with the correct definition on the right.

_____ 1. prefix

_____ 2. word root

_____ 3. *-ectomy*

_____ 4. *o*

_____ 5. *cardi/o*

_____ 6. constructed term

a. the most common combining vowel

b. a combining form

c. a word part that is affixed to the beginning of a word

d. a term built from word parts

e. a word part that provides the primary meaning of the term

f. a suffix

Forming Words From Word Parts

word parts

1.24 You have learned that constructed medical terms are created from building blocks called word parts and include word roots, prefixes, suffixes, and combining forms. You will now learn how to form medical terms by using these _____ _____.

combining vowel

1.25 One rule to remember when forming words from word parts is the proper use of the combining vowel. The combining vowel is not always used at the end of a word root to create a combining form. As a general rule, the _____ _____ is used to connect a word root with a suffix that begins with a consonant.

cardi/o/logy

1.26 For example, let's use the word root for heart, *cardi*. As you know, *cardiology* means "study or science of the heart." The constructed form of this term is written _____/_____/_____. Notice that it contains the combining vowel *o* and the suffix begins with a consonant (an *l*). Another term that includes the word root for heart is *carditis*, which means "inflammation of the heart." The constructed form of this term is written card/itis. Notice that the suffix begins with a vowel (*i*) and there is no combining vowel. If you wanted to change the suffix to *-pathy*, which means "disease," to form the term that means "disease of the heart," how would you write the new term? Because the suffix *-pathy* begins with a consonant (*p*), you would include the combining vowel (*o*) to form a new term, which is

cardiopathy

_____. The constructed form of this term is written cardi/o/pathy.

combining vowel
consonant

1.27 There are exceptions to this rule, so it is not absolute. You will learn these exceptions as you learn the material in this book. For now, just keep in mind that you need to include the _____ _____ when the suffix begins with a _____.

word roots

1.28 A second rule to remember when forming new constructed terms involves combining two word roots. Constructed medical terms use combining vowels to unite two _____ _____. For example, when describing an injury that involves both the muscular and skeletal systems, the two word roots (*muscul* and *skelet*) are united by placing the combining vowel between them. To make the term complete, the suffix *-al* is added to form the term *musculoskeletal*. Literally, the term means "pertaining to muscles and the skeleton," and its constructed form is written

muscul/o/skelet/al

_____/_____/_____/_____.

cardiopulmonary

1.29 Another example of this use of combining vowels occurs when forming the term describing a condition of the heart and lungs. As you know, the word root for heart is *cardi*. The word root for lung is *pulmon*. The suffix *-ary* ("pertaining to") is added to form the term *pulmonary*. A combining vowel is added to unite the two word roots, creating the new term _____, which can be written as cardi/o/pulmon/ary.

epi/cardi/um

1.30 A third rule to remember when forming constructed words from word parts applies when prefixes are added to other word parts. Generally, a prefix requires no change when another word part unites with it to form a new term. For example, *epi-* is a prefix that means "upon, over, above, on top." When this prefix is combined with the word root *cardi*, which means "heart," and the suffix *-um*, which means "pertaining to," it forms the new term *epicardium* that means "pertaining to on top of the heart." The constructed form of this new term is written _____/_____/____. Notice that the prefix *epi-* did not change.

1.31 Finally, because most medical terms are composed of Latin or Greek word parts, changing a singular medical term into a plural form is handled differently than in most English-language words where an *s* is simply added to the end. Here are some helpful points:

vertebrae

- If the term ends in *a*, the plural is usually formed by adding an *e*. For example, the plural form of the term *vertebra* is _____.

diagnoses

- If the term ends in *is*, the plural form is usually formed by changing the *is* to *es*. For example, the plural form of *diagnosis* is _____.

- If the term ends in *itis*, the plural form is *itides*. For example, the plural form of *gastritis* is *gastritides*.

myocardia

- If the term ends in *on* or *um*, the plural form drops the *on* or *um* and adds *a*. For example, the plural form of *ganglion* is *ganglia* and *myocardium* is _____.

fibromata

- If the term ends in *ma*, the plural form is changed to *mata*. For example, the plural form of *fibroma* is _____.

episiotomies

- If the term ends in *y*, the plural form drops the *y* and adds the ending *ies*. For example, the plural form of *episiotomy* is _____.

fungi

- If the term ends in *us*, the plural form drops the *us* and adds the ending *i*. For example, the plural form of *fungus* is _____.

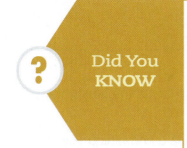

RULES TO REMEMBER

- A prefix comes before the word root or combining form.

- A suffix is a word ending and comes after the word root(s) or combining form(s).

- The word root or combining form provides the primary meaning of the term.

- The combining vowel for most word roots is *o*. The vowels *i* and *e* are also used as combining vowels for some word roots. If the combining form is to be joined with another word root or combining form that begins with a consonant, retain the combining vowel. When adding a suffix starting with a vowel to a combining form, drop the combining vowel.

- Prefixes do not require combining vowels to join with other word parts. Rarely, a prefix will drop its ending vowel to combine with another word part.

- Medical terms are deciphered by breaking them into word parts, and then defining first the suffix, then the prefix, then the word root(s) or combining forms.

The following list of word parts includes prefixes, word roots/combining vowels (combining forms), and suffixes. These are provided for you to practice constructing and deconstructing medical terms in the exercises that follow. You will be asked to learn these terms and their definitions later in this text. For now, concentrate on practicing the principles of constructed medical terms that you learned in the previous frames.

Prefix	Definition
anti-	against, opposite of
brady-	slow
endo-	within
epi-	upon, over, above, on top
neo-	new
pre-	to come before

Word Root/ Combining Vowel	Definition
append/o, appendic/o	appendix
bi/o	life
cardi/o	heart
cerebr/o	brain, cerebrum
derm/o, dermat/o	skin
electr/o	electricity
encephal/o	brain
gastr/o	stomach
hem/o	blood
hepat/o	liver
hyster/o	uterus
laryng/o	voice box, larynx
leuk/o	white
mamm/o, mast/o	breast
ment/o	mind
nat/o	birth
neur/o	nerve
path/o	disease
proct/o	rectum or anus
psych/o	mind
rhin/o	nose
tonsill/o	almond, tonsil
vas/o	vessel

Suffix	Definition
-al	pertaining to
-ectomy	surgical excision, removal
-emia	condition of blood
-gram	a record or image
-ia	condition of
-iatry	treatment, specialty
-ic	pertaining to
-itis	inflammation
-logist	one who studies
-logy	study or science of
-pathy	disease
-philia	loving, affinity for
-plasty	surgical repair
-scope	instrument used for viewing
-tic	pertaining to

PRACTICE: Forming Words from Word Parts

The Right Match

Match the term on the left with the correct definition on the right.

_____ 1. combining vowel

_____ 2. *-al*

_____ 3. prefix

_____ 4. consonant

a. adding this word part to a word root requires no combining vowel

b. a suffix

c. if a suffix begins with this type of letter, use a combining vowel

d. used to connect a word root with another word root or a suffix

Break the Chain

Analyze these medical terms:

    a) Separate each term into its word parts and label each word part using **p** = prefix, **r** = root, **cv** = combining vowel, and **s** = suffix.

    b) For the Bonus Question, write the requested word part or definition in the blank that follows.

The first set has been completed for you as an example.

1. a) cardiology   ***cardi/o/logy***
                                r cv s

    b) *Bonus Question:* What is the definition of the suffix? ***study or science of***

2. a) appendicitis   _____/_____
                                  /

    b) *Bonus Question:* What is the definition of the suffix? _____

3. a) hepatitis   _____/_____
                                  /

    b) *Bonus Question:* What is the definition of the word root? _____

4. a) neonatology   _____/_____/_____/_____
                                  /   /   /

    b) *Bonus Question:* Does this term contain a word root? _____

5. a) mammoplasty   _____/_____/_____
                                  /   /

    b) *Bonus Question:* What is the definition of the suffix? _____

6. a) electrocardiogram   _____/_____/_____/_____/_____
                                  /   /   /   /

    b) *Bonus Question:* How many word roots/combining forms does this term have? _____

7. a) prenatal   _____/_____/_____
                                  /   /

    b) *Bonus Question:* What is the definition of the prefix? _____

Fill It In

Complete the following sentences with the correct plural endings. The first one is completed for you as an example.

1. The plural form of appendicitis is appendic*itides*.
2. In one day, the surgeon performed several mammoplast_____.
3. The pericardium of the heart includes two layers, the parietal and visceral pericardi_____.
4. The patient was diagnosed with multiple sarcoma tumors, or sarco_____.
5. The diseased heart was found to have many cardiopath_____.

Linkup

Link the word parts in the list to create the terms that match the definitions. You may use word parts more than once. Remember to add combining vowels when needed—and that some terms do not use any combining vowel. The first one is completed for you as an example.

Prefixes	Word Roots/Combining Vowel	Suffixes
endo-	encephal/o	-ectomy
neo-	hyster/o	-gram
	mamm/o	-itis
	mast/o	-logist
	nat/o	-logy
	neur/o	-pathy
	path/o	-plasty
	rhin/o	-scope

Definition	Term
1. inflammation of the brain	encephalitis
2. study or science of newborns	_____
3. disease of the nerves	_____
4. surgical removal of a breast	_____
5. surgical repair of the nose	_____
6. instrument for viewing within	_____
7. x-ray image of a breast	_____
8. one who studies disease	_____
9. surgical removal of the uterus	_____

CHAPTER REVIEW

Word Building

Construct medical terms from the following meanings. (All are built from word parts. Refer to the word parts table on page 15 for word part meanings.) The first question has been completed for you as an example.

1. disease within the nose   endorhino***pathy***_____
2. surgical removal of the tonsils   tonsill_____
3. surgical repair of a fallopian tube   salpingo_____
4. inflammation of the skin   _____itis
5. study or science of the nose   _____logy
6. pertaining to the mind   _____al
7. disease of the nerves   _____pathy
8. inherited defect in blood coagulation   _____philia
9. inflammation of the larynx   laryng_____
10. study or science of the skin   dermato_____
11. instrument used for viewing the larynx   _____scope
12. study or science of life   _____logy

Define the Combining Form

1. cardi/o _____
2. hem/o _____
3. neur/o _____
4. gastr/o _____
5. path/o _____

6. cerebr/o _____
7. hepat/o _____
8. psych/o _____
9. dermat/o _____
10. rhin/o _____

MyLab Medical Terminology™

MyLab Medical Terminology is a premium online homework management system that includes a host of features to help you study. Registered users will find:

- A multitude of quizzes and activities built within the MyLab platform
- Powerful tools that track and analyze your results—allowing you to create a personalized learning experience
- Videos, flashcards, and audio pronunciations to help enrich your progress
- Streaming lesson presentations and self-paced learning modules
- A space where you and your instructors can view and manage your assignments

Chapter 2

Understanding Suffixes

 Learning Objectives

After completing this chapter, you will be able to:

2.1 Define and spell the suffixes often used in medical terminology.

2.2 Identify suffixes in medical terms.

2.3 Use suffixes to build medical terms that pertain to medical specialties, symptoms, and diseases.

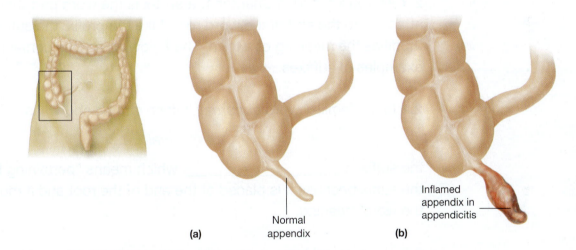

(a)   Normal appendix

Inflamed appendix in appendicitis

(b)

Getting Started with Suffixes

Review the following list of common suffixes and their definitions. This will help you to recognize suffixes and their meanings.

Suffixes	Definition
-al	*pertaining to*
-ic	*pertaining to*
-itis	*inflammation*
-logy	*study or science of*
-meter	*measure, measuring instrument*
-ous	*pertaining to*
-pathy	*disease*
-scope	*instrument used for viewing*
-scopy	*process of viewing*

2.1 As you learned in Chapter 1, a **suffix** is the word part that is attached to the end of the word root. Like the prefix, the suffix modifies the meaning of a term. The following frames contain examples of suffixes.

-al

2.2 In the familiar word *abnormal*, which can be shown as:

ab/norm/al

the suffix is _____, which means "pertaining to." It is the suffix because it is placed at the end of the root and it modifies the word meaning.

-itis

2.3 The medical term *endocarditis* can be shown as

endo/card/itis

It means "inflammation within the heart." The suffix is _____, which means "inflammation." It is a suffix because it is placed at the end of the root and it modifies the word meaning.

-pathy

2.4 The medical term *arthropathy* can be shown as:

arthr/o/pathy

It means "disease of the joint." The suffix is _____, which means "disease."

-itis	**2.5** The medical term *gastritis* can be shown as: *gastr*/*itis* It means "inflammation of the stomach." The suffix is _____, and the word root *gastr* means "stomach."

Suffix Introduction

Complete the following frames to expand the suffixes you know.

pertaining to **pertaining to** **pertaining to**	**2.6** The suffixes *-ic*, *-ous*, and *-al* all share the same meaning, which is "pertaining to." This can be seen in the terms: *cardiac*, which means "_____ _____ the heart"; *fibrous*, which means "_____ _____ fiber"; and *dermal*, which means "_____ _____ the skin."
inflammation	**2.7** Because the suffix *-itis* means "inflammation," the term *esophagitis* means "_____ of the esophagus."
study or science of	**2.8** Because the suffix *-logy* means the "study or science of," the term *cardiology* means "the _____ _____ _____ _____ the heart."
measures	**2.9** Because the suffix *-meter* means "measure or measuring instrument," a thermometer is an instrument that _____ temperature.
disease	**2.10** Because the suffix *-pathy* means "disease," the term *cardiopathy* means any "_____ of the heart."
viewing	**2.11** The suffix *-scope* indicates an instrument that is used for viewing. A laparoscope is an instrument used for _____ the abdomen.

| process | **2.12** Because the suffix *-scopy* means "process of viewing," the term *laparoscopy* indicates a _____ in which an instrument (in this case, a laparoscope) is used to view the abdomen. (See ■ Figure 2.1.) |

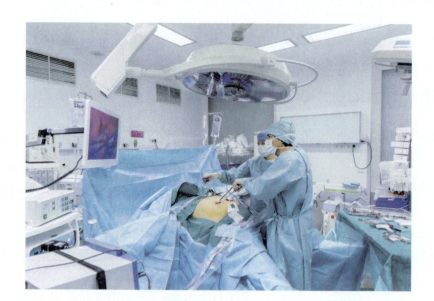

■ **Figure 2.1**
Laparoscopy is a surgical procedure of the abdominal cavity using a laparoscope, which is a tubular instrument inserted into the cavity. It includes a small camera for viewing the procedure on a monitor and surgical tools for working on internal organs.
Source: S4svisuals/Shutterstock.

PRACTICE: Suffix Introduction

The Right Match

Match the suffix on the left with the correct definition on the right.

_____ 1. -meter   a. disease

_____ 2. -al   b. pertaining to

_____ 3. -scopy   c. inflammation

_____ 4. -itis   d. pertaining to

_____ 5. -logy   e. process of viewing

_____ 6. -ous   f. study or science of

_____ 7. -pathy   g. measure, measuring instrument

_____ 8. -scope   h. pertaining to

_____ 9. -ic   i. instrument used for viewing

Suffix Linkup

Link the suffixes in the list to create the terms that match the definitions. The first one is completed for you as an example.

Suffix	Definition		Suffix	Definition
-scopy	*process of viewing*		-logy	*study or science of*
-meter	*measure, measuring instrument*		-itis	*inflammation*

Definition   **Term**

1. study or science of the heart   cardio**logy** _____

2. an instrument that measures temperature   thermo _____

3. a procedure in which an instrument (in this case, a laparoscope)   laparo _____
   is used to view the abdomen

4. inflammation of the stomach   gastr _____

Suffixes That Indicate an Action or State

Complete the following frames to learn about suffixes that indicate an action or state.

running	**2.13** In the term *syndrome*, the suffix *-drome*, which means "run or running," and the prefix *syn-*, which means "together," combine to literally mean "_____ together." The medical term is formally defined as a group of symptoms that together are characteristic or indicative of a specific disorder, condition, or disease.
-emesis	**2.14** In the term *hematemesis*, the word root *hemat*, which means "blood," is modified by the suffix _____, which means "vomiting." The term *hematemesis* means "vomiting of blood."
softening	**2.15** The suffix *-malacia* means "softening" as in the term *cardiomalacia*, which is the _____ or degeneration of heart tissue, usually from insufficient blood supply or tissue degeneration.
view	**2.16** In the term *biopsy*, the suffix *-opsy* means "view of"; the term is defined as the removal and examination (or _____) of living tissue.
oxygen	**2.17** In the term *hypoxia*, the suffix *-oxia* means "condition of oxygen." Because the prefix *hypo-* means "deficient, below," the constructed term indicates that the level of _____ in the tissues is below normal.
loving or affinity for	**2.18** The suffixes *-phil* and *-philia* mean "loving or affinity for," as in the term *hemophilia*, which literally means "_____ _____ _____ _____ blood." The medical meaning of the term is an inherited condition of uncontrolled blood loss.

eating or swallowing	**2.19** The suffix *-phagia* means "eating or swallowing." In the term *dysphagia*, the prefix *dys-*, meaning "bad, abnormal, painful, or difficult," adds to the meaning of the term; together these word parts combine literally to mean "painful or difficult eating or swallowing." Similarly, the medical use of the term is a difficulty in _____ _____ _____.
speaking	**2.20** The suffix *-phasia* means "speaking." In the term *aphasia*, the prefix *a-*, which means "without or absence of," adds to the meaning of the term; together these word parts combine to literally mean "without or absence of _____." The term is defined as an absence or impairment of speech.

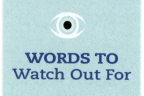

WORDS TO Watch Out For

-phagia or *-phasia*?

Don't confuse the suffix *-phagia* with the suffix *-phasia*. Although they are spelled almost the same, their meanings are very different: *-phagia* means "eating or swallowing"; *-phasia* means "speaking." To help you remember, try associating the *g* in *-phagia* with the *g* in *gastr/o* (the combining form for "stomach") and the *s* in *-phasia* with the *s* in speaking.

growth	**2.21** The suffix *-physis* means "growth." In the term *hypophysis*, it combines with the prefix *hypo-*, which means "deficient, below," to literally mean "_____ below." The hypophysis is the pituitary gland, which is located below the brain.
paralysis	**2.22** In the term *quadriplegia*, the suffix *-plegia* means "paralysis." When it is combined with the prefix *quadri-*, which means "four," the whole term means "_____ of four limbs."
tumor	**2.23** In the term *osteoma*, the suffix *-oma* means "tumor"; when combined with the word root *oste*, the combined word parts mean "_____ of bone."
standing still	**2.24** The suffix *-stasis* means "standing still." In the term *homeostasis*, the combining form *home/o* is included to build the term and means "sameness, unchanging." The literal meaning of the word parts, "sameness, _____ _____," gives an idea of continual balance; the term is defined as the process of maintaining internal stability despite changes in the environment.

PRACTICE: Suffixes That Indicate an Action or State

The Right Match

Match the suffix on the left with the correct definition on the right.

_____ 1. -plegia
_____ 2. -oma
_____ 3. -emesis
_____ 4. -phasia
_____ 5. -oxia
_____ 6. -physis
_____ 7. -malacia
_____ 8. -philia

a. tumor
b. speaking
c. growth
d. condition of oxygen
e. paralysis
f. softening
g. loving or affinity for
h. vomiting

Suffix Linkup

Link the suffixes in the list to create the terms that match the definitions.

Suffix	Definition
-drome	run, running
-opsy	view of
-phagia	eating or swallowing

Suffix	Definition
-philia	loving or affinity for
-stasis	standing still

Definition

1. a group of symptoms that together are characteristic or indicative of a specific disorder, condition, or disease
2. the removal and examination (or view) of tissue
3. a condition of uncontrolled blood loss
4. a difficulty in swallowing
5. the tendency of an organism or system to maintain internal stability

Term

syn_____

bi_____

hemo_____

dys_____

homeo_____

Suffixes That Indicate a Condition or Disease

Complete the following frames to learn about suffixes that indicate a condition or disease.

pain	**2.25** In the term *arthralgia*, the suffix *-algia*, which means "condition of pain," combines with the root *arthr* to mean "_____ in a joint."
weakness	**2.26** The suffix *-asthenia*, which means "weakness," makes the term *myasthenia* mean the "_____ of muscle."

closure or absence	**2.27** The suffix *-atresia* means "a closure or the absence of a normal body opening," so the term *hysteratresia* is the _____ _____ _____ of the uterine cavity.
hernia	**2.28** Because the suffix *-cele* means "hernia, swelling, or protrusion," when it is added to the combining form *mening/o*, meaning "membrane," it builds the word *meningocele*, which is a _____ of the meninges of the brain or spinal cord, resulting in tissue that protrudes through an abnormal opening in the skull or vertebral column. (See ■ Figure 2.2.)

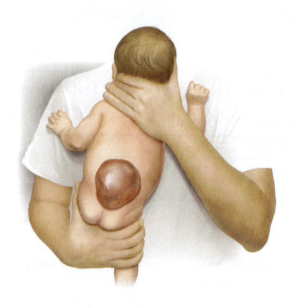

■ **Figure 2.2**
Illustration of a child born with spina bifida, with a large meningocele.

pain	**2.29** Because the suffix *-dynia* means "pain," the term *tenodynia* means "_____ in a tendon."
condition	**2.30** The suffix *-ia* means "condition of," so when it is added to the term that means "no appetite," we build the term *anorexia*, which literally means "a _____ in which there is no appetite."
condition	**2.31** The suffix *-osis* also means "condition of." In the term *adenosis*, the word root for gland is included to form the meaning "_____ of a gland."
condition	**2.32** Another suffix with the meaning "condition or disease" is *-ism*. Thus, because the combining form *albin/o* means "white," the term *albinism* means "a _____ of white," or the lack of skin pigment.

inflammation	**2.33** The suffix -*itis* means "inflammation." Adding this ending to the word root that means "stomach" forms the term *gastritis*, which means "_____ of the stomach."
tumor	**2.34** The suffix -*oma* means "tumor." Adding this suffix to the word root for fat, which is *lip*, forms the term *lipoma*, meaning "_____ of fat tissue."
disease	**2.35** The suffix -*pathy* is very common and means "disease," as in the terms *neuropathy*, *gastropathy*, and *adenopathy*. In the latter, it makes the term mean "_____ of a gland."
deficiency	**2.36** Because -*penia* means "deficiency or abnormal reduction in number" and the combining form *leuk/o* means "white," the term *leukopenia* means "a _____ of white blood cells."
fear	**2.37** The suffix -*phobia* is well known and means "fear." Because the combining form for "water" is *hydr/o*, the constructed term *hydrophobia* means "_____ of water."
growth	**2.38** Because -*plasia* means "formation, growth," *neoplasia* means "new formation or _____," and refers to a tumor.
abnormal discharge	**2.39** Because -*rrhagia* means "abnormal discharge," the term *rhinorrhagia* means "_____ _____ of the nose or nosebleed."
discharge	**2.40** The suffix -*rrhea* means "discharge." Because the combining form *rhin/o* means "nose," the term *rhinorrhea* refers to a nasal _____ (or runny nose).
rupture	**2.41** Because -*rrhexis* means "rupture," an *amniorrhexis* is a _____ of the membrane known as the *amnion*, which encloses a fetus.
hardening	**2.42** The suffix -*sclerosis* means "condition of hardening." In the term *arteriosclerosis*, the artery walls are _____ and losing their elasticity.
sudden, involuntary muscle contraction	**2.43** The word *spasm* and the suffix -*spasm* both indicate a sudden, involuntary muscle contraction. Thus, the term *bronchospasm* indicates a _____ _____ _____ _____ of the wall of the bronchi.

PRACTICE: Suffixes That Indicate a Condition or Disease

Suffix Linkup

Link the suffixes in the list to create the terms that match the definitions.

Suffix	Definition
-asthenia	weakness
-cele	hernia, swelling, protrusion
-dynia	condition of pain
-ia	condition of
-itis	inflammation
-oma	tumor

Suffix	Definition
-penia	abnormal reduction in number, deficiency
-plasia	formation, growth
-rrhagia	abnormal discharge
-rrhea	discharge
-rrhexis	rupture

Definition

1. a nosebleed
2. pain in a tendon
3. rupture of the amnion
4. a tumor of fat tissue
5. a deficiency of white blood cells
6. a condition in which a person has no appetite
7. growth or formation of a tumor
8. debility and weakness of muscle
9. a discharge from the nose
10. hernia or swelling of the meninges of the brain or spinal cord that protrudes through a hole in the skull or vertebral column
11. inflammation of the stomach

Term

rhino_____
teno_____
amnio_____
lip_____
leuko_____
anorex_____
neo_____
my_____
rhino_____
meningo_____

gastr_____

The Right Match

Match the suffix on the left with the correct definition on the right.

_____	1. -spasm	a.	rupture
_____	2. -algia	b.	disease
_____	3. -rrhexis	c.	sudden involuntary muscle contraction
_____	4. -ism	d.	formation, or growth
_____	5. -oma	e.	condition of pain
_____	6. -sclerosis	f.	fear
_____	7. -pathy	g.	condition of hardening
_____	8. -dynia	h.	condition or disease
_____	9. -plasia	i.	abnormal discharge
_____	10. -rrhagia	j.	tumor
_____	11. -phobia	k.	condition of pain

Suffixes That Indicate Location, Number, or a Quality

Complete the following frames to learn about suffixes that indicate location, number, or a quality.

toward	**2.44** Because the suffix *-ad* means "toward," the term *cephalad* means "_____ the head."
blood	**2.45** The suffixes *-emia* and *-hemia* mean "condition of blood." The prefix *poly-* means "excessive, over, many," and the root *cyt* means "cell." These word parts combine in the term *polycythemia*, which is a condition in which there is an overproduction of red _____ cells.
vertebrae	**2.46** A word ending in *a* is a singular form, which is made plural by adding an *e* to the end, *-ae*. For example, a *vertebra* is a bone of the spine, or vertebral column. The vertebral column includes 24 _____ in an adult.
pertaining to	**2.47** There are numerous suffixes that mean "pertaining to." They include: ■ *-ac* ■ *-al* ■ *-ar* ■ *-ary* ■ *-ic* ■ *-ous* Here are some examples of terms using these suffixes: ■ *cardiac*, which means "pertaining to the heart" ■ *cervical*, which means "pertaining to the cervix or neck" ■ *ocular*, which means "pertaining to the eyes" ■ *pulmonary*, which means "_____ _____ the lungs" ■ *cephalic*, which means "pertaining to the head" ■ *nervous*, which means "pertaining to the nerves"

PRACTICE: Suffixes That Indicate Location, Number, or a Quality

The Right Match

Match the suffix on the left with the correct definition on the right.

_____ 1. -ad   a. singular

_____ 2. -emia   b. plural

_____ 3. -a   c. pertaining to

_____ 4. -ac   d. toward

_____ 5. -ae   e. condition of blood

Suffix Linkup

Link the suffixes in the list to create the terms that match the definitions. You may use them more than once.

Suffix	Definition
-a	singular
-ac	pertaining to
-ad	toward
-al	pertaining to
-ar	pertaining to
-ary	pertaining to
-hemia	condition of blood
-ic	pertaining to
-ous	pertaining to

Definition	Term
1. pertaining to the heart	cardi_____
2. pertaining to the cervix or neck	cervic_____
3. pertaining to the eyes	ocul_____
4. pertaining to the lungs	pulmon_____
5. pertaining to bacteria	bacteri_____
6. pertaining to the head	cephal_____
7. pertaining to the nerves	nerv_____
8. toward the head	cephal_____
9. a condition in which there is an overproduction of red blood cells	polycyt_____

Suffixes That Indicate a Medical Specialty

Complete the following frames to learn about suffixes that indicate a medical specialty.

treatment	**2.48** Because the suffix *-iatry* means "treatment or specialty" and *pod* is a word root that means "feet," the term *podiatry* refers to the field of health care involving the diagnosis and _____ of diseases of the feet.
studies	**2.49** The suffix *-logist* means "one who studies" and the combining form *audi/o* means "hearing," so the term *audiologist* describes a specialist who _____ and treats hearing disorders.
study	**2.50** Similarly, the suffix *-logy* means "study or science of"; hence, the term *pathology* is the _____ of diseases and the structural and functional changes they cause. A *pathologist* is a physician who often manages a lab where specimen samples are analyzed for diagnostic purposes.
practice	**2.51** The suffix *-practic* comes from the Greek word *praktikos*, which means "a practice." Hence, the term *chiropractic* is the healthcare _____ involving the diagnosis and treatment of musculoskeletal disorders by manipulation of the spinal column and other body structures.

PRACTICE: Suffixes That Indicate a Medical Specialty

The Right Match

Match the suffix on the left with the correct definition on the right.

_____ 1. -iatry	a. practice
_____ 2. -logist	b. study or science of
_____ 3. -logy	c. treatment, specialty
_____ 4. -practic	d. one who studies

Suffix Linkup

Link the suffixes in the list to create the terms that match the definitions.

Suffix	Definition
-iatry	*treatment, specialty*
-logist	*one who studies*
-logy	*study or science of*
-practic	*practice*

Definition

1. a specialist who studies and treats hearing disorders
2. the study of diseases and the structural and functional changes caused by them
3. the healthcare profession involving the practice of diagnosing and treating musculoskeletal disorders by manipulation of the spinal column and other body structures
4. the healthcare field involving the diagnosis and treatment of diseases of the feet

Term

audio_____

patho_____

chiro_____

pod_____

Suffixes That Indicate a Procedure or Treatment

Complete the following frames to learn about suffixes that indicate a procedure or treatment.

puncture	**2.52** The suffix *-centesis* means "surgical puncture." When it is included with *thorac/o*, the combining form for "chest, thorax," we form the term *thoracocentesis*, which is often shortened to *thoracentesis*. It is a medical procedure in which a surgical _____ is made into the chest cavity, usually to remove unwanted excess fluid.
broken apart	**2.53** The suffixes *-clasia*, *-clasis*, and *-clast* all mean to "break apart." So the term *osteoclasis* describes a surgical procedure in which a bone is artificially fractured (or _____ _____) to correct deformity.
fusion	**2.54** An *arthrodesis* is a procedure that involves the surgical fixation or fusion of two or more joints using either bone grafts or metal rods. The suffix *-desis* means "surgical fixation or _____."
excision	**2.55** The suffix *-ectomy* means "surgical _____," or "removal." For example, a chondrectomy is the excision of cartilage, and a thyroidectomy is the excision of the thyroid gland in the neck. (See ■ Figure 2.3.)

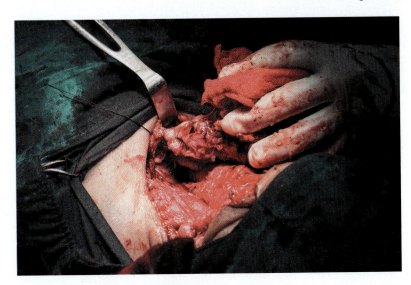

■ **Figure 2.3**
Thyroidectomy. In this minor surgery, the anterior neck is opened to remove a diseased thyroid gland. The gland is the large structure that has been pulled to the side prior to its removal.
Source: Chanawit Sitthisombat/123RF.com.

recording

2.56 The suffixes *-gram*, *-graph*, and *-graphy* are closely related: *-gram* means "a record or image," *-graph* means "an instrument for recording," and *-graphy* is a "recording process." When the combining forms for electrical and heart, *electr/o* and *cardi/o*, are combined and these suffixes are included, the resulting terms are:

■ *electrocardiogram*, a record of the electrical events of the heart

■ *electrocardiograph*, an instrument for _____ the electrical events of the heart

■ *electrocardiography*, the process of recording an electrocardiogram

measuring

2.57 Because the suffix *-meter* means "measure, measuring instrument," a *thermometer* is an instrument used for _____ temperature.

measurement

2.58 Similarly, the suffix *-metry* means "measurement, process of measuring." Hence, *oximetry* is the _____ or process of measuring oxygen levels in the bloodstream.

fixation

2.59 The suffix *-pexy* means "surgical fixation, suspension," and the combining form of the word "breast" is *mast/o*. Together they form the term *mastopexy*, which means "a surgical _____ or lifting of the breasts."

protective

2.60 The suffix *-phylaxis* means "protection" as in the term *prophylaxis*, which means "_____ treatment to prevent disease."

surgical repair	**2.61** The suffix *-plasty* means "surgical repair," so the term *gastroplasty* means "a _____ _____ of the stomach." (See ■ Figure 2.4.)

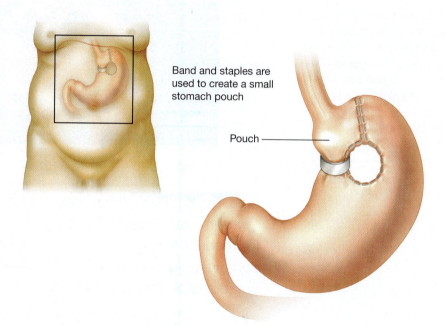

Band and staples are used to create a small stomach pouch

Pouch ————

■ **Figure 2.4**
Gastroplasty. Illustration of a surgical repair of the stomach as a treatment for obesity, in which a band and staples are inserted to create a small pouch that serves to reduce stomach volume.

suturing	**2.62** Because *-rrhaphy* means "suturing," the term *herniorrhaphy* means "the _____ of a hernia (an abnormal protrusion)."
instrument **viewing**	**2.63** The suffixes *-scope* and *-scopy* are very similar: *-scope* means "a viewing instrument" and *-scopy* means "the process of viewing." So the term *gastroscope* means "an _____ for examining and treating the stomach," whereas a *gastroscopy* indicates the _____, or examination, process itself.
surgical	**2.64** The suffix *-stomy* means "surgical creation of an opening," so the term *gastrostomy* means "the _____ creation of an opening into the stomach."
cutting instrument	**2.65** The suffixes *-tome* and *-tomy* are closely related. The suffix *-tome* refers to a cutting instrument and *-tomy* refers to an incision. So the *craniotome* is the _____ _____ used during a *craniotomy*, which is performed to access the brain.

surgical crushing	**2.66** The suffix *-tripsy* means "surgical crushing," as in the term *lithotripsy*, which means "_____ _____ of unwanted stones" that may form in the kidneys or gallbladder.
process	**2.67** The suffix *-ion* means "process," as in the term *ovulation*, which is the _____ of ovulating, or releasing an oocyte (egg cell) from an ovary.

PRACTICE: Suffixes That Indicate a Procedure or Treatment

The Right Match

Match the suffix on the left with the correct definition on the right.

_____ 1. -centesis

_____ 2. -graphy

_____ 3. -clast

_____ 4. -tomy

_____ 5. -metry

_____ 6. -desis

_____ 7. -stomy

_____ 8. -scopy

_____ 9. -pexy

_____ 10. -rrhaphy

_____ 11. -ectomy

_____ 12. -plasty

a. measurement, process of measuring

b. surgical creation of an opening

c. fusion

d. process of viewing

f. suturing

e. recording process

g. break apart

h. process of cutting into

i. surgical puncture

j. excision or surgical removal

k. surgical repair

l. surgical fixation, suspension

Suffix Linkup

Link the suffixes in the list to create the terms that match the definitions.

Suffix	Definition
-centesis	surgical puncture
-clasis	break apart
-desis	surgical fixation, fusion
-gram	a record or image
-graphy	recording process
-ion	process
-meter	measure, measuring instrument
-pexy	surgical fixation, suspension
-phylaxis	protection
-plasty	surgical repair
-scope	instrument used for viewing
-tome	cutting instrument
-tomy	incision, to cut
-tripsy	surgical crushing

Definition

Term

1. a medical procedure in which a surgical puncture is made into the chest cavity to remove fluid   thoraco_____

2. a surgical procedure in which a joint is artificially fractured (or broken apart) to correct deformity   osteo_____

3. to surgically crush or pulverize kidney stones or gallstones   litho_____

4. the cutting instrument used during a craniotomy   cranio_____

5. a procedure that involves the surgical fixation or fusion of two or more joints using either bone grafts or metal rods   arthro_____

6. the image or recording of the electrical activity of the heart   electrocardio_____

7. the process of recording an electrocardiogram   electrocardio_____

8. an instrument used for measuring oxygen levels in the blood   oxi_____

9. the process of ovulating   ovulat_____

10. a surgical fixation or lifting of the breasts   masto_____

11. protective treatment against disease   pro_____

12. surgical repair of the stomach   gastro_____

13. an instrument for examining and treating the stomach   gastro_____

14. a procedure of cutting into the cranium with a craniotome   cranio_____

CHAPTER REVIEW

Word Building

Construct medical terms from the following meanings. The first question has been completed for you as an example.

1. disease of the joint   arthro**pathy**_____

2. pertaining to the nerves   nerv_____

3. group of symptoms that together are characteristic or indicative of a   syn_____
   specific disorder, condition, or disease

4. surgical procedure in which a bone is artificially fractured (or broken   osteo_____
   apart) to correct deformity

5. benign tumor made of fat tissue   lip_____

6. condition of uncontrolled blood loss   hemo_____

7. specialist who studies and treats hearing disorders   audio_____

8. study of diseases and the structural and functional changes they cause   patho_____

9. vomiting of blood   hemat_____

10. painful or difficult eating or swallowing   dys_____

11. protective treatment against disease   pro_____

12. surgical puncture into the chest cavity to remove fluid   thoraco_____

13. healthcare field involving the diagnosis and treatment of diseases   pod_____
    of the feet

14. softening or degeneration of heart tissue   cardio_____

15. to surgically crush unwanted stones that may form in the kidneys or   litho_____
    gallbladder

16. pain in a tendon   teno_____

17. surgical repair of the stomach   gastro_____

18. condition in which a person has no appetite   anorex_____

19. hernia of the meninges of the brain or spinal cord that protrudes through   meningo_____
    a hole in the skull or vertebral column

20. level of oxygen in the tissues is below normal   hyp_____

21. instrument for examining and treating the stomach   gastro_____

22. pertaining to the cervix or neck   cervic_____

23. healthcare practice (diagnosis and treatment) of musculoskeletal   chiro_____
    disorders by manipulation of the spinal column and other body structures

24. procedure that involves the surgical fixation or fusion of two or more joints   arthro_____
    using either bone grafts or metal rods

25. removal and examination (or view) of tissue   bi_____

26. debility and weakness of muscle   my_____

27. instrument that measures oxygen levels in blood   oxi_____

28. inflammation of the esophagus   esophag_____

29. process of using an instrument to view the abdomen   laparo_____

30. without or absence of speaking   a_____

Practice with Suffixes

Circle the suffixes in the following terms, then define the suffix in the space provided.

1. endoscopy _____
2. oximeter _____
3. cardiac _____
4. microbiology _____
5. endocrinopathy _____
6. gastritis _____
7. lymphoma _____
8. hemophilia _____
9. paraplegia _____
10. rhinorrhagia _____
11. cervical _____
12. gastroplasty _____
13. colonostomy _____
14. pathologist _____

MyLab Medical Terminology™

MyLab Medical Terminology is a premium online homework management system that includes a host of features to help you study. Registered users will find:

- A multitude of quizzes and activities built within the MyLab platform
- Powerful tools that track and analyze your results—allowing you to create a personalized learning experience
- Videos and audio pronunciations to help enrich your progress
- Streaming lesson presentations (Guided Lectures) and self-paced learning modules
- A space where you and your instructors can view and manage your assignments

Chapter 3

Understanding Prefixes

 Learning Objectives

After completing this chapter, you will be able to:

3.1 Define and spell the prefixes commonly used in medical terminology.

3.2 Identify prefixes in medical terms.

3.3 Use prefixes to build medical terms.

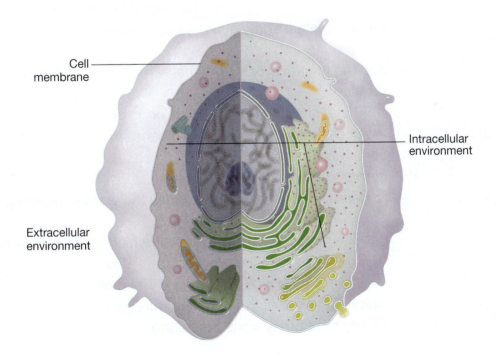

Cell membrane

Intracellular environment

Extracellular environment

Getting started with Prefixes

Review the following list of some common prefixes and their definitions. This will help you become more familiar with prefixes.

Prefixes	Definition
a-	without, absence of
ab-	away from
bi-	two
endo-	within
hyper-	excessive, abnormally high, above
hypo-	deficient, abnormally low, below
intra-	within
post-	to follow after
pre-	to come before
sub-	under, beneath, below

fix	**3.1** A **prefix** is the word part that is placed before the root to modify its meaning. The word *prefix* literally means "to _____ at the beginning of a word." The following frames contain some examples of prefixes.
away from **prefix**	**3.2** The familiar word *abnormal*, which can be shown with its word parts as: <div align="center">*ab/norm/al*</div>includes the prefix *ab-*, which means "away from." Therefore, *abnormal* means "_____ _____ normal." The word part *ab-* is the _____ because it is placed before the root to modify the word's meaning.
intra-	**3.3** The medical term *intravenous*, which can be shown as: <div align="center">*intra/ven/ous*</div>means "pertaining to within a vein." The prefix is _____, which means "within." It is the prefix because it is placed before the root to modify the word's meaning.
hyper-	**3.4** The word *hypertension* can be shown as: <div align="center">*hyper/tens/ion*</div>The prefix is _____, which means "excessive, abnormally high, or above." Because *tens/o* is the combining form that means "pressure," *hypertension* means "high pressure," usually referring to the condition of abnormally high blood pressure.

Prefix Introduction

Complete the following frames to expand the prefixes you know.

convulsions	**3.5** The prefix *anti-* means "against or opposite of" as in the term *anticonvulsive*, which is a type of drug used to stop _____.
a-	**3.6** The one-letter prefix that means "without or absence of" is _____. An example of its use is found in the term *aphasia*, which means "absence of speech."
together	**3.7** The prefix *con-* means "with, together, or jointly." For example, when twins are *conjoined*, the *con-* prefix indicates that the twins are joined _____.
conception	**3.8** *Contra-* means "counter or against" as in the term *contraception*, which literally means "against _____, or birth."

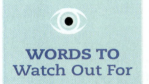

WORDS TO Watch Out For

contra- or **con-**?

Don't confuse the prefix *contra-* with the prefix *con-*. Their meanings are very different. *Contra-* means "counter or against"; the prefix *con-* means "with, together, or jointly."

changed	**3.9** *Meta-* means "after or change" as in the term *metabolism*, which is the process by which foods are _____ into energy for use by the body and energy is used to change molecules into new substances.

PRACTICE: Prefix Introduction

The Right Match

Match the prefix on the left with the correct definition on the right.

_____	1. meta-	a.	against or opposite of
_____	2. a-	b.	after or change
_____	3. contra-	c.	without or absence of
_____	4. con-	d.	counter or against
_____	5. anti-	e.	with, together, or jointly

Prefix Linkup

Link the prefixes in the list to create the terms that match the definitions. The first one is completed for you as an example.

Prefix	Definition
a-	*without or absence of*
con-	*with, together, or jointly*
contra-	*counter or against*
meta-	*after or change*

Definition

Term

1. prevention of conception
   _____ *contra*ception
2. the process by which foods are changed into energy for use by the body and the use of energy to change molecules into new substances
   _____bolism
3. when twins are joined together
   _____joined
4. the absence of speech
   _____phasia

Prefixes That Indicate Number or Quantity

Complete the following frames to learn about prefixes that indicate number or quantity.

both	**3.10** The prefix *ambi-* means "both"; the term *ambidextrous* is the ability to use _____ hands equally.
bifocal	**3.11** The prefix *bi-* means "two." For example, _____ means "pertaining to two focal points," as in eyeglasses that correct for both near vision and far vision.
two	**3.12** The Latin word *cuspis* means "a point." In heart anatomy, a *cusp* is a pointed flap that forms a heart valve, so the term *bicuspid* refers to a heart valve with "_____ cusps."
both	**3.13** The prefix *bi-* is also in the term *bilateral*. It means "pertaining to two sides," and its use in medicine refers to _____ sides of the body.
double	**3.14** The prefix *di-* means "double." Because *-plegia* means "paralysis," *diplegia* is a _____ paralysis, or the loss of muscle function of the two arms or the two legs.
double	**3.15** The prefix *dipl-* also means "double." In the term *diplopia*, the prefix *dipl-* indicates that a person with the condition perceives a single object as two images; it is also called _____ vision because *-opia* is a suffix that means "condition of vision."

half	**3.16** Because the prefix *hemi-* means "half," *hemiplegia* is a paralysis of half the body; in other words, on _____ or one side of the body.
one	**3.17** The prefix *mono-* means "one." *Monoplegia* means "paralysis of _____ limb or muscle/muscle group."
many	**3.18** The prefix *multi-* means "many, more than once, or numerous." A *multipolar* neuron is a nerve cell that includes _____ branches, called *dendrites*, at one end of the cell. (See ■ Figure 3.1.)

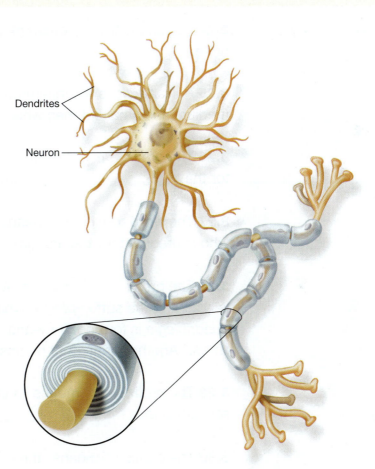

Dendrites

Neuron

■ **Figure 3.1**
Illustration of a multipolar neuron, with many branching dendrites at one end of the cell.

many	**3.19** When a woman's chart indicates *multipara*, it means that she has given birth _____ times.
never	**3.20** The terms *nullipara* and *nulligravida* share the prefix *nulli-*, which means "none." *Nullipara* means "the condition of never having given birth, or no births"; *nulligravida* means "_____ having been pregnant or no pregnancies."

all	**3.21** Because the prefix *pan-* means "all," the term *pandemic* refers to a disease occurring over a wide geographic area. Also, *pansinusitis* is inflammation of _____ paranasal sinuses on one or both sides of the nose.
poly-	**3.22** The term *polyphagia* includes the prefix _____. The prefix means "excessive, over, or many." Because the suffix *-phagia* means "eating," *polyphagia* means "excessive eating."
excessive	**3.23** *Polydipsia* is the condition of _____ thirst.
excessive	**3.24** *Polyuria* is the condition of _____ production of urine.
many	**3.25** *Polyarteritis* is the inflammation of _____ medium and small arteries where they branch.
first	**3.26** The prefix *primi-* means "first." A woman who has given birth for the _____ time is a *primipara*.
primi-	**3.27** The word root *gravid* means "pregnant." Therefore, a woman who is pregnant for the first time is a _____ *gravida*.
four	**3.28** The prefix *quadri-* means "four." Therefore, when this prefix is added to the suffix *-plegia*, which means "paralysis," the term *quadriplegia* is formed. It means "paralysis of _____ limbs." Another prefix that means "four" is *tetra-*.
partially	**3.29** The prefix *semi-* means "half or partial." The term *semiconscious* means "_____ conscious."
three	**3.30** The prefix *tri-* means "three," as in *tricycle*. The term *tripara* means "a woman who has given birth _____ times."
three	**3.31** The *tricuspid* valve is a valve of the heart containing _____ cusps, or pointed flaps. The *tricuspid* valve controls blood flow between the right atrium and the right ventricle of the heart.
one	**3.32** The prefix *uni-* means "one," similar to *mono-*. Therefore, a *unipara* woman has given birth to _____ child.

PRACTICE: Prefixes That Indicate Number or Quantity

The Right Match

Match the prefix on the left with the correct definition on the right.

_____	1. di-	a.	excessive, over, or many
_____	2. ambi-	b.	half
_____	3. quadri-	c.	first
_____	4. hemi-	d.	half or partial
_____	5. bi-	e.	two
_____	6. primi-	f.	double
_____	7. tri-	g.	both
_____	8. pan-	h.	four
_____	9. semi-	i.	one
_____	10. uni-	j.	one
_____	11. multi-	k.	never or none
_____	12. poly-	l.	all
_____	13. mono-	m.	many, more than once, or numerous
_____	14. nulli-	n.	three

Prefix Linkup

Link the prefixes in the list to create the terms that match the definitions.

Prefix	Definition
ambi-	both
mono-	one
nulli-	none
poly-	excessive, over, or many
quadri-	four
tetra-	four
tri-	three

Definition	Term
1. paralysis of one limb or muscle/muscle group	_____plegia
2. never having been pregnant or no pregnancies	_____gravida
3. the ability to use both hands equally	_____dextrous
4. excessive eating	_____phagia
5. the valve that consists of three cusps that control blood flow between the right atrium and the right ventricle	_____cuspid
6. a condition of paralysis of all limbs	_____plegia

Prefixes That Indicate Location or Timing

Complete the following frames to learn about prefixes that indicate location or timing.

away	**3.33** The prefix *ab-* means "away from," so the term *abduction* means "movement _____ from the midline of the body."
toward	**3.34** The prefix *ad-* means "toward," so the term *adduction* means "movement _____ the midline of the body."
anatomy	**3.35** The prefix *ana-* means "up, toward"; the word root *tom* means "to cut"; and the suffix *-y* means "process of." So, the literal meaning of the term _____ means "process of cutting up." The term *anatomy* was first used when the study of the human body was limited to the dissection of cadavers (lifeless bodies). We now use the term to mean "structure."
before	**3.36** The terms *prenatal* and *antenatal* share the root *nat*, which means "birth." Both terms mean "before birth," so both prefixes, *pre-* and *ante-*, have the same meaning, which is "_____" or "to come before."
through	**3.37** The term *dialysis* literally means "to loosen through" because the prefix *dia-* means "_____," and the suffix *-lysis* means "to loosen or dissolve." The term *dialysis* refers to the procedure that filters blood as it moves through a machine, a procedure that temporarily replaces the normal function of the kidneys.
apart **away**	**3.38** The prefix *dis-* means "apart or away." In the term *dislocation*, the prefix indicates that the dislocated part is _____ or _____ from its normal position in the body.
outside	**3.39** *Ec-* and *ecto-* mean "outside or out." An *ectopic pregnancy* is one in which the fertilized egg implants somewhere _____ the uterus.
within	**3.40** The prefix *endo-* means "within." Thus, the term *endogastric* means "_____ the stomach." (See ■ Figure 3.2.)

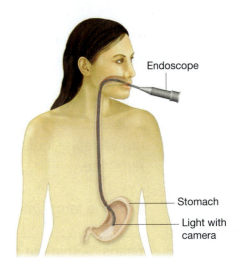

Endoscope

Stomach

Light with camera

■ **Figure 3.2**
Endogastric procedure using an endoscope to observe the internal stomach lining.

upon, over, above, on top of	**3.41** The prefixes *ep-* and *epi-* mean "upon, over, above, or on top." The *epidermis* is the outermost layer of skin because it is _____, _____, _____, or _____ _____ _____. the dermis layer.
inward	**3.42** The condition in which an eye is turned inward is called *esotropia*. To form this term, we add the prefix *eso-*, which means _____, and the suffix *-tropia*, which means "condition of turning."
away from	**3.43** The prefixes *ex-* and *exo-* mean "outside or away from," so in the condition *exotropia*, the eye is turned _____ _____ its normal position.
extra- **outside**	**3.44** The common prefix shared by the terms *extracellular*, *extracorporeal*, and *extrauterine* is _____, which means "outside." Therefore, *extracellular* means "outside the cell" (see ■ Figure 3.3), *extracorporeal* means "outside the body," and *extrauterine* means "_____ the uterus."

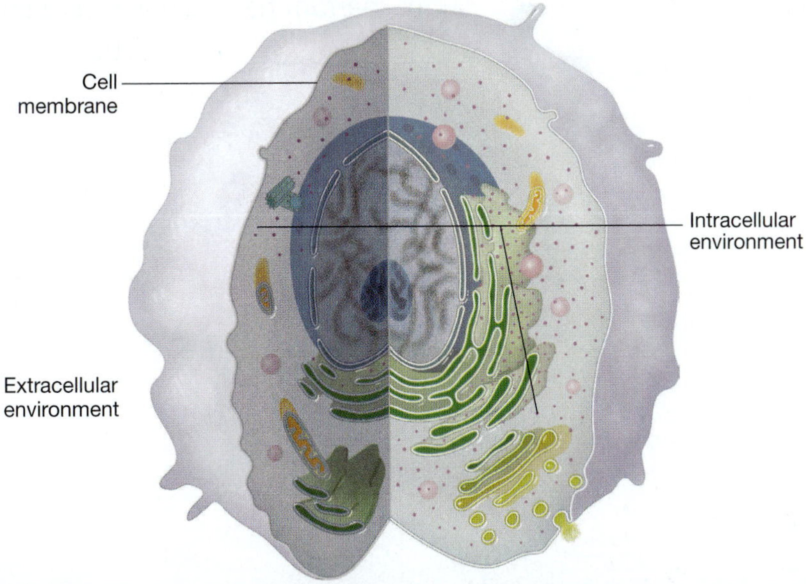

Cell membrane

Intracellular environment

Extracellular environment

■ **Figure 3.3**
A typical human cell. The environment within the cell is known as the intracellular environment and the one outside the cell is the extracellular environment.

below	**3.45** *Infer-* has the meaning "below," as in the term *inferior*. The term *inferior* indicates a position _____ another point of reference.
between	**3.46** Because the prefix *inter-* means "between," the term *intervertebral* indicates a position _____ the vertebrae.
intra- **within**	**3.47** The terms *intracellular* and *intrauterine* share the prefix _____, which means "within." Therefore, *intracellular* means "within the cell" (see Figure 3.3) and *intrauterine* means "_____ the uterus."
within	**3.48** Because *intra-* means "within," the term *intradermal* means "_____ the skin."
abnormal	**3.49** The prefix *para-* means "alongside or abnormal." Its use in the term *paracusis* indicates _____ hearing or a disorder in hearing.
around	**3.50** The prefix *peri-* means "around." In the term *pericardium*, this prefix indicates the membrane that covers the area _____ the heart.
after	**3.51** The prefix *post-* means "to follow after." If we add this prefix to a suffix that means birth, *-partum*, the term *postpartum* is formed, which means "to follow _____ birth."
after	**3.52** Notice that the terms *postnatal* and *postpartum* share the prefix *post-*, which means "to follow after." Because the term *natal* and suffix *-partum* have similar meanings, both terms mean "to follow _____ birth."

hypo-

subcutaneous

3.53 The prefixes *sub-* and *hypo-* both mean "below." To build a term that means "below the skin," add the prefix _____ to the Latin term for skin, *dermis*. The resulting term is *hypodermis*. An alternate term for the area below the skin attaches the prefix *sub-* to another word for skin, *cutaneous*. The resulting term is _____. (See ■ Figure 3.4.)

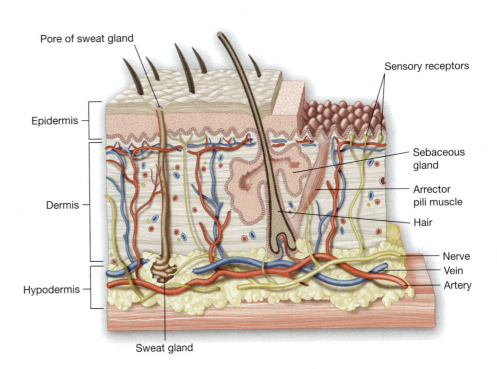

Pore of sweat gland

Sensory receptors

Epidermis

Sebaceous gland

Arrector pili muscle

Hair

Dermis

Nerve

Vein

Artery

Hypodermis

Sweat gland

■ **Figure 3.4**
Skin layers. The epidermis is on top of the dermis, and the hypodermis (or subcutaneous layer) is below the dermis.

above

3.54 The prefixes *super-* and *supra-* share the meaning "above"; the term *superior* indicates a position _____ another point of reference, and the term *supraorbital* is the area above an eye orbit.

together

3.55 The prefixes *sym-* and *syn-* also share a meaning, which is "together or joined." For example, a *symptom* is an experience that is added together with others to form an estimate of a disease, and *syndrome* is a group of symptoms or signs that occur _____.

PRACTICE: Prefixes That Indicate Location or Timing

The Right Match

Match the prefix on the left with the correct definition on the right.

_____ 1. ab-	_____ 12. dis-
_____ 2. dia-	_____ 13. peri-
_____ 3. ad-	_____ 14. ex-, exo-
_____ 4. endo-	_____ 15. inter-
_____ 5. ante-	_____ 16. eso-
_____ 6. extra-	_____ 17. sub-
_____ 7. ep-, epi-	_____ 18. post-
_____ 8. ana-	_____ 19. pre-
_____ 9. infer-	_____ 20. super-, supra-
_____ 10. ec-, ecto-	_____ 21. sym-, syn-
_____ 11. para-	

a. to come before
b. up or toward
c. apart or away
d. outside
e. away from
f. outside or away from
g. toward
h. within
i. inward
j. through
k. upon, over, above, or on top

l. to follow after
m. between
n. alongside or abnormal
o. below
p. around
q. outside or out
r. before
s. together or joined
t. under, beneath, below
u. above

Prefix Linkup

Link the prefixes in the list to create the terms that match the definitions.

Prefix	Definition
ab-	away from
ana-	up, toward
ante-	before
dia-	through
ecto-	outside, out
exo-	outside, away from

Prefix	Definition
infer-	below
para-	alongside, abnormal
pre-	to come before
sub-	under, beneath, below
syn-	together, joined

Definition	Term
1. process of cutting up; current meaning is "structure"	_____tomy
2. away from the midline of the body	_____duction
3. a pregnancy in which the fertilized egg implants somewhere outside the uterus	_____pic
4. a procedure that filters blood	_____lysis
5. a condition in which the eye turns away from its normal position	_____tropia
6. a position below another point of reference	_____ior
7. a disorder in hearing	_____cusis
8. below the skin	_____cutaneous
9. a group of symptoms or signs that occur together	_____drome
10. before birth	_____natal

Prefixes That Indicate a Specific Quality about a Term

Complete the following frames to learn about prefixes that indicate a specific quality about a term.

without	**3.56** Because the prefix *a-* means "without or absence of," the term *aseptic* means "sterile," or "pertaining to _____ pathogenic organisms."
a-	**3.57** Similarly, *asymptomatic* means "pertaining to not having symptoms" because the prefix _____ means "without."
without	**3.58** The prefix *an-* also means "without or absence of." Thus, the term *anoxia* means "_____ oxygen."
slow	**3.59** Because the prefix *brady-* means "slow" and *cardi/o* is the combining form for "heart," the term *bradycardia* means "abnormally _____ heart rate."
slow	**3.60** The term *bradykinesia* combines the prefix *brady-*, which means "slow," and the combining form *kinesi/o*, which means "motion," to create the meaning "condition of _____ motion."
around	**3.61** The term *circumference* contains the prefix *circum-*, which means "around." The term *circumcision* literally translates as a "process of cutting _____." *Circumcision* is a surgery that cuts around the base of the foreskin to remove it from the penis.
dys-	**3.62** The term *dyslexia* has the prefix _____, which means "bad, abnormal, painful, or difficult." It is a learning disability involving impaired reading, spelling, and writing ability.
good	**3.63** The prefix *eu-* means "normal or good." It is a prefix in the term *eupnea*, where it alters the meaning of the root word that means "breath," *pnea*, to create the meaning "normal or good breathing." It is also a prefix in the term *euthyroid*, where it alters the meaning of the word *thyroid*, an endocrine gland in the neck, to literally mean "normal or _____ thyroid," or in clinical language, a normally functioning thyroid gland.
different	**3.64** The prefixes *heter-* and *hetero-* both mean "different." Therefore, a *heterosexual* person prefers to have sex with someone of a gender _____ from themselves.

hyper-	**3.65** The terms *hyperacidity*, *hyperemesis*, *hyperkinesia*, and *hyperthermia* share the common prefix _____, which means "excessive, abnormally high, or above."
excessive	**3.66** *Hyperthyroidism* is a condition of _____ levels of thyroid hormones in the body.
low	**3.67** The prefix *hypo-* means "deficient, abnormally low, or below." *Hypothyroidism* is a condition of abnormally _____ levels of thyroid hormones in the body, causing reduced energy and weight gain.
hyper-	**3.68** Notice that the prefix *hypo-* has a meaning opposite to that of the prefix _____.
abnormally	**3.69** In the term *hypocalcemia*, *hypo-* indicates that the level of calcium in the blood is _____ low.
low	**3.70** The term *hypothermia* means a "state of abnormally _____ body temperature."
large	**3.71** The prefix *macro-* means "large." The combining form *cyt/o* means "cell," and the suffix *-osis* means "condition of." When these word parts are combined, the term *macrocytosis* is created, which refers to a condition of blood cells that are abnormally _____.
bad	**3.72** The prefix *mal-* means "bad," so the term *malabsorption* literally means "_____ absorption."
large	**3.73** The prefix *mega-* is familiar to many people and is in common use today. It shares the meaning "large or great" with the prefix *megalo-*. So, the term *megalocyte* literally means "_____ cell."
small	**3.74** The prefix *micro-* means "small." When we add the suffix *-scopy*, which means "process of viewing," we form the term *microscopy*, which refers to the procedure of observing objects too _____ to be seen with the unaided human eye.

neo-	**3.75** The term *neonate* refers to a newborn, specifically a baby within the first 28 days of life. The prefix _____ means "new," and the combining form *nat/o* means "birth."
false	**3.76** The prefix *pseudo-* means "false," as in the term *pseudocyesis*, which means "_____ pregnancy."
rapid	**3.77** The prefix *tachy-* means "rapid, fast." When we add the combining form *cardi/o*, which means "heart" with the suffix *-a* to form the singular, the term *tachycardia* is formed. It means "a _____ heart rate."
through **across** **crossing** **across**	**3.78** The prefix *trans-* means "through, across, or beyond," as in *transvaginal*, which means "_____ or _____ the vagina." *Transexual* means to "go through the process of _____ over to another gender," and *transverse* means to "lie _____ or in a crosswise direction."
beyond normal	**3.79** The prefix *ultra-* means "beyond normal," as in *ultrasound*, which is a noninvasive diagnostic procedure that provides images of internal structures by bouncing inaudible, or _____ _____, sound waves through the body (■ Figure 3.5).

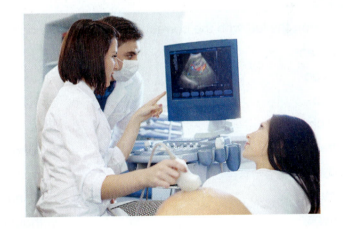

■ **Figure 3.5**
Ultrasound imaging. In this noninvasive procedure, inaudible sound waves are bounced through the body, detected by a sensor, and interpreted by a computer to reveal internal structures, such as a fetus within the uterus.
Source: Olesia Bilkei/Shutterstock.

PRACTICE: Prefixes That Indicate a Specific Quality about a Term

Prefix Linkup

Link the prefixes in the list to create the terms that match the definitions.

Prefix	Definition
a-	without or absence of
brady-	slow
circum-	around
dys-	bad, abnormal, painful, or difficult
hyper-	excessive, abnormally high, above
mal-	bad

Prefix	Definition
megalo-	large, great
neo-	new
pseudo-	false
trans-	through, across, or beyond
ultra-	beyond normal

Definition

1. false pregnancy
2. sterile, having no pathogenic organisms
3. a newborn; specifically, a baby within the first 28 days of life
4. abnormally slow heart rate
5. a surgery to remove the foreskin from the penis
6. a person who goes through the process of crossing over to another gender
7. a learning disability involving impaired reading, spelling, and writing ability
8. a condition of excess levels of thyroid hormones in the body
9. bad absorption
10. an abnormally large cell
11. a diagnostic procedure using sound waves

Term

_____cyesis
_____septic
_____nate
_____cardia
_____cision
_____sexual
_____lexia
_____thyroidism
_____absorption
_____cyte
_____sound

The Right Match

Match the prefix on the left with the correct definition on the right.

_____ 1. a-, an-

_____ 2. hypo-

_____ 3. neo-

_____ 4. tachy-

_____ 5. trans-

_____ 6. dys-

_____ 7. macro-

_____ 8. hyper-

_____ 9. circum-

_____ 10. brady-

_____ 11. micro-

_____ 12. eu-

_____ 13. mal-

_____ 14. pseudo-

_____ 15. heter-, hetero-

_____ 16. mega-, megalo-

a. bad

b. slow

c. small

d. false

e. around

f. normal or good

g. deficient, abnormally low, below

h. without or absence of

i. different

j. rapid, fast

k. bad, abnormal, painful, or difficult

l. large or great

m. large

n. through, across, or beyond

o. new

p. excessive, abnormally high, above

CHAPTER REVIEW

Word Building

Construct medical terms from the following meanings. The first question has been completed for you as an example.

1. excessive or abnormally high sensitivity to painful stimuli   _____ ***hyper***algesia

2. a substance that stops convulsions   _____convulsive

3. process by which foods are changed into energy for use by the body and energy is used to change molecules   _____bolism

4. condition of seeing a single object as two images   _____opia

5. paralysis of half the body   _____plegia

6. has given birth more than once   _____para

7. has never given birth   _____para

8. a disease that is widespread globally   _____demic

9. paralysis of corresponding parts on both sides of the body   _____plegia

10. inflammation of many medium and small arteries   _____arteritis

11. having given birth for the first time   _____para

12. movement toward the midline of the body   _____duction

13. procedure that filters blood   _____lysis

14. body part that is apart or away from its normal position   _____located

15. pregnancy in which the fertilized egg implants somewhere outside the uterus   _____pic

16. within the layers of the skin   _____dermal

17. membrane that covers around the heart   _____cardium

18. a group of symptoms or signs occurring together   _____drome

19. pertaining to not having symptoms   _____symptomatic

20. a state of sterility, having no pathogens   _____sepsis

21. slow movement   _____kinesia

22. removal of the foreskin from the penis   _____cision

23. "normal" or "good" breathing   _____pnea

24. abnormally low level of calcium in the blood   _____calcemia

25. false pregnancy   _____cyesis

26. rapid heart rate   _____cardia

27. twins that are joined together   _____joined

28. literally, "against conception"   _____ception

29. ability to use both hands equally   _____dextrous

30. pertaining to two focal points   _____focal

31. paralysis of one limb or muscle/muscle group   _____plegia

32. paralysis of four limbs   _____plegia

33. partially conscious   _____conscious

34. a woman who has given birth three times   _____para

35. a woman who has given birth to one child   _____para

36. away from the midline of the body   _____duction

Practice with Prefixes

Circle the prefixes in the following terms, then define the prefix in the space provided.

Definition

1. intracellular   _____

2. antispasmodic   _____

3. hypertonic   _____

4. bifocal   _____

5. hemiplegia   _____

6. pansinusitis   _____

7. polyuria   _____

8. tricuspid   _____

9. dislocation   _____

10. epidermis   _____

11. intrauterine   _____

12. hypokinesia   _____

13. neonate   _____

14. tachycardia   _____

MyLab Medical Terminology™

MyLab Medical Terminology is a premium online homework management system that includes a host of features to help you study. Registered users will find:

- A multitude of quizzes and activities built within the MyLab platform
- Powerful tools that track and analyze your results—allowing you to create a personalized learning experience
- Videos, flashcards, and audio pronunciations to help enrich your progress
- Streaming lesson presentations and self-paced learning modules
- A space where you and your instructors can view and manage your assignments

Chapter 4

The Human Body in Health and Disease

 Learning Objectives

After completing this chapter, you will be able to:

4.1 Define and spell the word parts used to create terms for the human body.

4.2 Identify the building blocks, organ systems, and cavities of the body.

4.3 Identify the anatomical planes, regions, and directional terms used to describe areas of the body.

4.4 Break down and define the important terms associated with the anatomy and physiology of the human body.

4.5 Define the introductory terms associated with medical terminology.

4.6 Identify the five major diagnostic imaging procedures.

4.7 Understand and interpret a Medical Report.

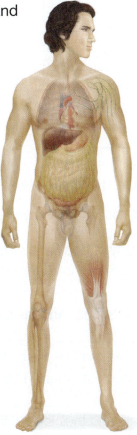

disease

4.1 A study of medical terminology includes learning about the human body in a healthy state to better understand the mechanisms of _____ and its terminology. In this chapter, you learn some basics about body organization and some general principles of function, which are necessary for understanding many of the medical terms that you encounter later in the book.

Organization of the Body

As the next step in learning the terminology of the human body, in this section you explore how the body is organized and many of the terms that are used to describe its organization. The combining forms that are presented in this chapter are listed here for you to preview.

Combining Form	Definition	Combining Form	Definition
abdomin/o	abdomen	infer/o	below
anter/o	front	inguin/o	groin
brachi/o	arm	later/o	side
cardi/o	heart	lumb/o	loin, lower back
caud/o	tail	medi/o	middle
cephal/o	head	organ/o	tool
cervic/o	neck	pelv/o	bowl, basin
chondr/i	gristle, cartilage	physi/o	nature
cran/o, crani/o	skull	pleur/o	pleura, rib
cyt/o	cell	poster/o	back
dist/o	distant	proxim/o	near
dors/o	back	super/o	above
femor/o	thigh, femur	thorac/o	chest, thorax
gastr/o	stomach	tom/o	to cut
glute/o	buttock	umbilic/o	navel, umbilicus
hom/o, home/o	same	ventr/o	belly
ili/o	flank, hip, groin		

Anatomy and Physiology Introduction

Complete the following frames to learn the basics of anatomy and physiology.

anatomy
  ann AH toe mee

structure

4.2 The study of body structure is called **anatomy**. The term is constructed from three word parts, as shown when it is written as ana/tom/y. The prefix *ana-* means "up, toward," the word root *tom* means "to cut," and the suffix *-y* means "process of." Thus, _____ literally means "the process of cutting up." The word was first used by the ancient Greeks, who used cadaver dissection to explore body structure. Today, we use the term to describe the study of body _____, which includes the identification of body components and their locations relative to one another.

physiology fiz ee AHL oh jee **functions**	**4.3** The combining form *physi/o* means "nature," and the suffix *-logy* means "study or science of." Combining these word parts forms the term _____, which literally means "study of nature." Thus, physiology refers to the study of the nature of living things. It is concerned with body _____ and seeks answers to the question, "How does it work?"
physiology **homeostasis** HOE mee oh STAY siss	**4.4** The functions of the body perform work to keep the body alive and as healthy as possible. Many body functions respond to a change, like a cold breeze or exposure to a virus, by making internal adjustments in the body. The goal of these functions is to keep the internal body in a constant, stable state despite changes in the world around us. The process of maintaining internal stability is a central concept of human _____ and is called **homeostasis**. This word is composed of three word parts, as shown when it is written as home/o/stasis. The combining form *home/o* means "sameness, unchanging" and *-stasis* is a suffix that means "standing still." Thus, _____ means "maintaining internal stability."
cell **tissues** **organs** **systems**	**4.5** The structure of the body may be described in terms of building blocks, in which small, simple blocks combine to form larger, more complex blocks until the ultimate structure, the whole body, is assembled. Notice in ■ Figure 4.1 that the simplest building block of the body is known as the **atom**. The atom is the simplest organized substance known, although it too is composed of smaller particles. Atoms may bind together to form **molecules**, which in turn combine to form large, nonliving structures such as parts of cells called **organelles**. These structures are assembled to form the next level of complexity, the living **cell**. The _____ is the most basic form of life in the body. Cells may be arranged into similar groups to form the next level, the **tissues**. There are four main categories of _____: epithelial tissue, connective tissue, muscle tissue, and nervous tissue. Two or more different tissues combine to form an **organ**, which maintains a certain shape and performs a general function. For example, the stomach, the brain, and the pancreas are _____. Organs are associated with other organs with a common goal of performing a general function, such as digestion, transportation of oxygen, or maintenance of the water balance in the body. A group of organs sharing a general function is called a **system**. There are 11 _____ of the body, which are summarized and illustrated in Table 4.1 ■.

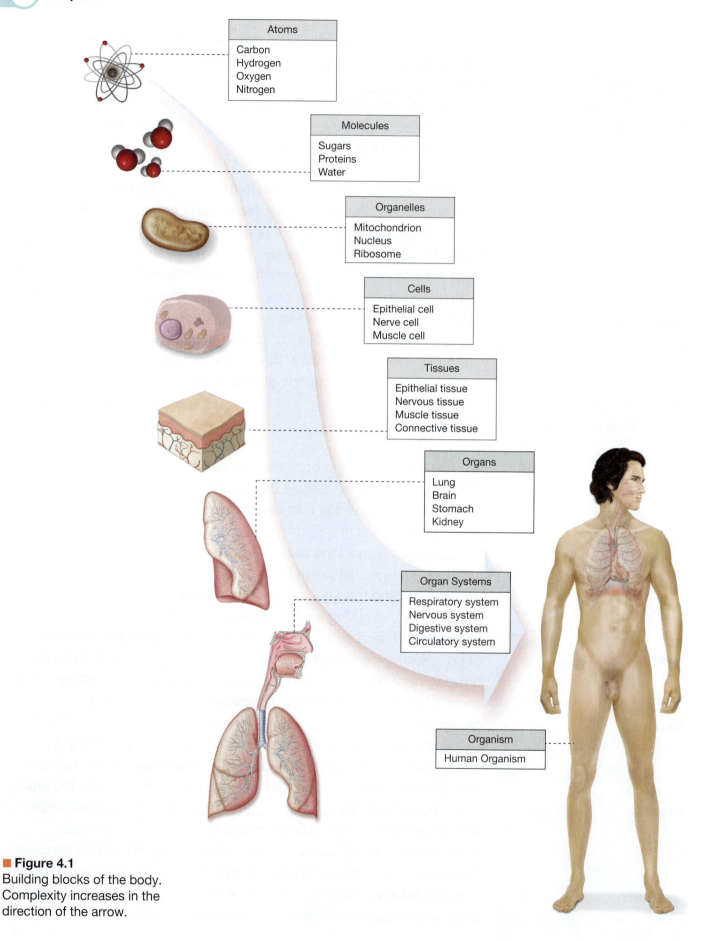

Figure 4.1
Building blocks of the body.
Complexity increases in the
direction of the arrow.

Table 4.1 ■ Systems of the Body

Cardiovascular System	Function	Lymphatic System	Function
Major arteries (in red), Heart, Major veins (in blue)	Transports substances to and from body cells.	Tonsils, Thymus, Lymphatic vessels, Spleen, Lymph nodes	Removes unwanted substances and recycle fluid to the bloodstream.
Respiratory System	**Function**	**Digestive System**	**Function**
Pharynx, Nose, Larynx, Trachea, Bronchi, Right lung, Left lung	Exchanges gases between the external environment and blood.	Pharynx, Mouth, Salivary glands, Esophagus, Liver, Gallbladder, Colon, Stomach, Pancreas, Small intestine	Prepares foods for absorption into the bloodstream and eliminate solid wastes.
Urinary System	**Function**	**Female Reproduction**	**Function**
Kidneys (2), Ureters (2), Urinary bladder, Urethra	Removes nitrogenous waste and excess water and salt from the bloodstream.	Mammary glands, Fallopian tube, Uterus, Ovary, Vagina	Produces female gametes for fertilization and provide support for prenatal development.

(continued)

Table 4.1 ■ Systems of the Body *(continued)*

Male Reproduction	Function	Nervous System	Function
Vas deferens Testis Prostate Urethra Penis	Produces male gametes for fertilization and a means to inseminate a female.	Brain Spinal cord Nerves	Controls homeostasis by sensing changes in the environment, processing information, and initiating body responses.

Endocrine System	Function	Musculoskeletal System	Function
Pituitary gland Thyroid gland Thymus Adrenal glands Pancreas Ovary (female) Testis (male)	Controls homeostasis by releasing hormones into the bloodstream, which alter body functions.	Bone Muscle Joint Tendon	Muscles produce movement of body parts; bones and joints support and protect soft body parts, store minerals, and form blood cells.
		Integumentary System	**Function**
		Hair Skin Nails	Protects the body from fluid loss, injury, and infection.

anatomical

4.6 Directional terms are words used to describe the relative location of the body or its parts. Because the body can move into many positions, such as sitting, standing, lying on one side, or lying on the back, we need a point of reference before we can describe the locations of body parts. The body position that is commonly used as a reference is known as the **anatomical position**. It is an erect posture with the face forward, arms at the sides, palms of the hands facing forward, and legs apart with the feet pointing forward (■ Figure 4.2). Directional terms are always based on the _____ position, regardless of the actual body position of the individual. Because healthcare professionals often assist a patient lying in bed, two optional terms of position are in common clinical use. If the patient is lying on the back with the face upward, the position is called **supine**, and if the patient is lying on the belly side, the position is called **prone**.

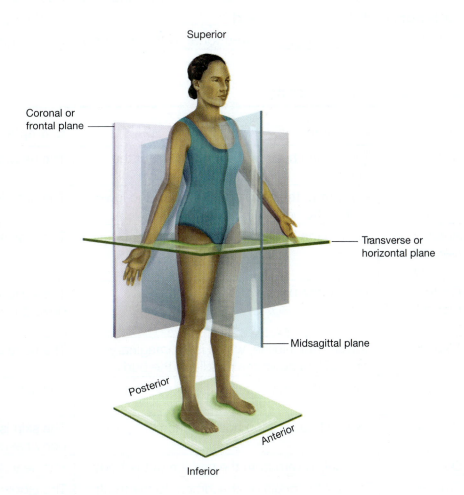

■ **Figure 4.2**
Body planes, shown with the figure in the anatomical position.

pertaining to

superior

dorsal

anterior

4.7 The most commonly used directional terms are constructed from word parts, and each includes one word root and one suffix. The suffixes are either *-ior* or *-al*, both with the same meaning of "_____ _____." The word roots include *super*, which means "above"; *infer*, which means "below"; *anter*, which means "front"; *poster*, which means "back"; *medi*, which means "middle"; *later*, which means "side"; *proxim*, which means "near"; *dist*, which means "distant"; *ventr*, which means "belly"; *dors*, which means "back"; and *caud*, which means "tail." Thus, the term _____ means "pertaining to above" and refers to a body part located above, or toward the head end, relative to another body part. For example, you would say that the nose is superior to the chest. Also, the term *dorsal* means "pertaining to the back." For example, you would say that the shoulder blades are _____ to the chest. Because posterior also means "pertaining to the back," *dorsal* and *posterior* are interchangeable terms. This is also true of *ventral* and _____. Table 4.2 ■ provides a summary of the directional terms and additional examples of how they are used.

Table 4.2 ■ Directional Terms

Term	Definition	Example
Superior super/ior	Toward the head end or upper part of the body	The head is *superior* to the neck.
Inferior infer/ior	Away from the head end or toward the lower part of the body	The neck is *inferior* to the head.
Anterior (ventral) anter/ior	Toward the front or belly side	The eyes are on the *anterior* side of the head.
Posterior (dorsal) poster/ior	Toward the back	The vertebral column (or backbone) extends down the *posterior (dorsal)* side.
Medial medi/al	Toward the midline, which is an imaginary vertical line down the middle of the body	The nose is *medial* to the ears.
Lateral later/al	Toward the side	The ears are *lateral* to the nose.
Superficial super/ficial	External, toward the body surface	The skin is *superficial* to the muscles and body cavities.
Deep	Internal, inward from the surface of the body	The heart lies *deep* to the rib cage.
Proximal proxim/al	Toward the origin of attachment to the trunk	The elbow is *proximal* to the wrist.
Distal dist/al	Away from the origin of attachment to the trunk	The knee is *distal* to the hip and thigh.

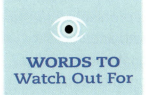

When to Drop the Combining Vowel

Remember the rule from Chapter 1: When a combining form is joined with a word part that begins with a vowel, the combining vowel is dropped, as is the case in the directional terms that appear in Table 4.2.

anatomical planes

sagittal

regions

4.8 A **plane** is an imaginary flat field that is used as a point of reference for viewing three-dimensional objects. Anatomical planes divide the body into imaginary sections that are useful in describing the location of body parts relative to one another. Three major _____ _____ are in common use.

A **frontal** or **coronal plane** is a vertical plane passing through the body from side to side, dividing the body into anterior and posterior portions. A **sagittal** (SAJ ih tal) **plane** is a vertical plane dividing the body into right and left portions. A _____ plane dividing the body down the center into equal portions is called *midsagittal*, and one dividing the body into unequal portions is known as *parasagittal*. Finally, a **transverse plane** is a horizontal plane dividing the body into superior and inferior portions. The three major anatomical planes are shown in Figure 4.2.

4.9 The **regions** of the body are areas that have been named to give healthcare workers the ability to communicate possible problems that may be revealed during a physical examination. The most commonly used names of _____ are constructed from one word root and one suffix, similar to directional terms (see Frame 4.7). For example, the **thoracic** region is the area of the chest. The term is constructed from the word root *thorac*, which means "chest, thorax," and the suffix *-ic*, which means "pertaining to." Also, the **abdominal** region is the area of the abdomen; the word root *abdomin* means "abdomen," and the suffix *-al* means "pertaining to." The regions are further described in Table 4.3 ■.

Table 4.3 ■ Regions of the Body

Major Body Regions	Subdivisions
Head	Face, cranium
Neck	Anterior neck, posterior neck
Upper appendages	Shoulder, axilla (armpit), brachium (upper arm), elbow, antebrachium (forearm), carpus (wrist), manus (hand), digits (fingers)
Trunk	Thorax, abdomen, pelvis, back
Lower appendages	Gluteus (buttock), femorus (thigh), knee, crus (leg), tarsus (ankle), pes (foot), digits (toes)

abdominal
ab DOMM ih nahl

hypogastric
HIGH poh GASS trik

4.10 To aid healthcare professionals in pinpointing problems associated with the large region of the abdomen with accuracy, the _____ region is further divided into nine smaller regions. The name of each abdominal region is a constructed term descriptive of its location. The regions are illustrated in ■ Figure 4.3a and include the **epigastric** (epi/gastr/ic, which means "on top of the stomach"), _____ (hypo/gastr/ic, which means "below the stomach"), **umbilical** (umbilic/al, which means "pertaining to the navel)", right and left **hypochondriac** (hypo/chondr/i/ac, which means "below the cartilage" of the ribs), right and left **iliac** (ili/ac, which means "pertaining to the hip or groin"), and right and left **lumbar** (lumb/ar, which means "pertaining to the loin"). A second set of abdominal divisions is also shown in ■ Figure 4.3b, in which the abdomen is divided into four quadrants. The quadrants are the **right upper quadrant (RUQ)**, **left upper quadrant (LUQ)**, **right lower quadrant (RLQ)**, and **left lower quadrant (LLQ)**. Referring to these quadrants by name is common in clinical practice.

■ **Figure 4.3**
The abdomen and abdominal regions. (a) The nine abdominal regions are mapped according to imaginary lines, as shown. (b) The abdomen may also be divided into four quadrants. The organs are superimposed in the figure.

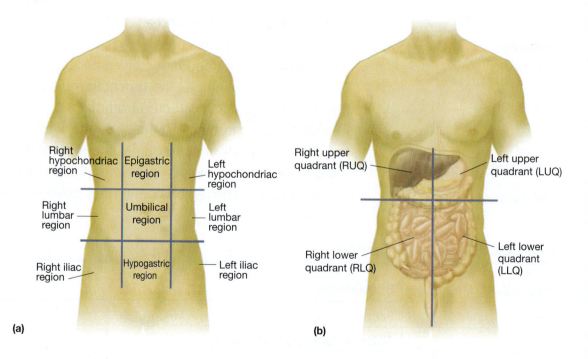

(a)

Right hypochondriac region
Epigastric region
Left hypochondriac region
Right lumbar region
Umbilical region
Left lumbar region
Right iliac region
Hypogastric region
Left iliac region

(b)

Right upper quadrant (RUQ)
Left upper quadrant (LUQ)
Right lower quadrant (RLQ)
Left lower quadrant (LLQ)

appendages
ap PEN dah jiz

cavities

4.11 When looking at the body as a whole, you will notice that its basic design consists of a central **trunk**, or torso, with attached **appendages**, or limbs. The _____ are the head, arms, and legs. The trunk and head are not solid structures like the arms and legs, but include spaces that are partially filled with organs, connecting structures, and fluids. The spaces are called **cavities**, and their internal contents are known as **viscera**. The cavities are surrounded by a moist membrane that helps control the spread of infections and keeps the internal organs moist and lubricated. Thus, the _____ are membrane-lined spaces filled with viscera.

dorsal cavity

4.12 There are two main cavities, the **dorsal cavity** and the **ventral cavity**. Each of these contains smaller cavities, which are illustrated in ■ Figure 4.4. As you can see from the figure, the _____ _____ (colored red) includes the **cranial cavity**, which houses the brain, and the **spinal** (vertebral) **cavity**, which contains the spinal cord.

ventral cavity

inferior

abdominopelvic cavity

4.13 The _____ _____ in the anterior part of the body (colored purple in Figure 4.4) is much larger than the dorsal cavity. A muscular partition called the **diaphragm** (DYE ah fram) divides the ventral cavity into an upper and lower cavity. The cavity that is superior to the diaphragm is the **thoracic cavity**, and the cavity _____ to the diaphragm is the **abdominopelvic cavity**. You learned in Frame 4.9 that the term *thoracic* is composed of two word parts and is written thorac/ic. The term *abdominopelvic* contains four word parts and is written abdomin/o/pelv/ic. As the names suggest, the thoracic cavity lies within the chest, and the _____ _____ lies within the abdominal and pelvic areas.

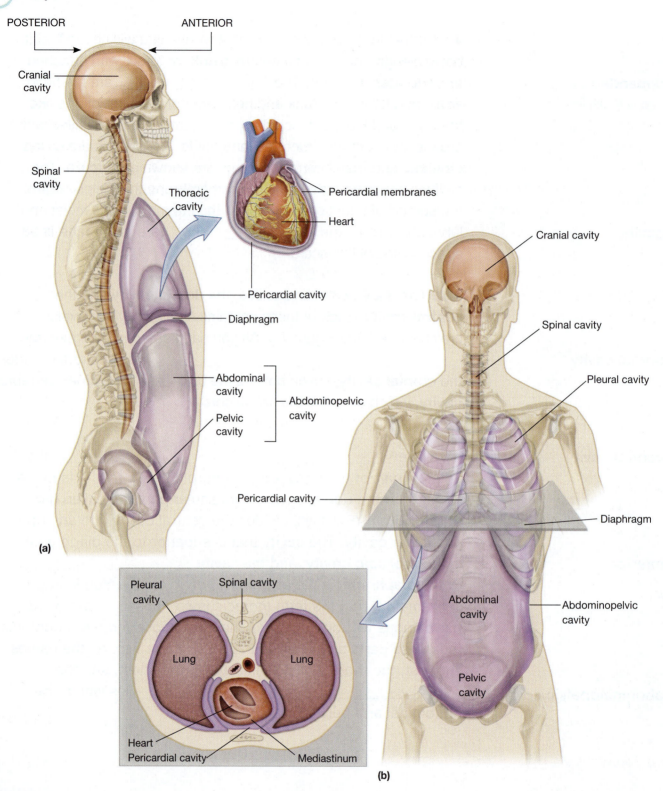

POSTERIOR   ANTERIOR

Cranial cavity

Spinal cavity

Thoracic cavity

Pericardial membranes

Heart

Pericardial cavity

Diaphragm

Abdominal cavity

Abdominopelvic cavity

Pelvic cavity

(a)

Cranial cavity

Spinal cavity

Pleural cavity

Pericardial cavity

Diaphragm

Abdominal cavity

Abdominopelvic cavity

Pelvic cavity

(b)

Pleural cavity

Spinal cavity

Lung

Lung

Heart

Pericardial cavity

Mediastinum

■ **Figure 4.4**

Body cavities. The dorsal cavities are shown in red, and the ventral cavities are in purple. (a) Lateral view of a sagittal section through the body. The insert shows the heart surrounded by the pericardial membranes. (b) Anterior view of a frontal section through the body. The insert is a transverse section through the thoracic cavity.

pericardial cavity	**4.14** The thoracic cavity contains several smaller cavities. The **pericardial cavity** lies along the midline of the thoracic cavity. The term *pericardial* consists of three word parts, peri/cardi/al, and literally means "pertaining to around the heart." Thus, the _____ _____ surrounds the heart. The other cavities within the thoracic cavity are the two **pleural cavities**. The term *pleural* is written pleur/al and contains two word parts, *pleur*, which means "pleura, rib," and -*al*, which means "pertaining to."
mediastinum mee dee ah STY num	**4.15** In addition to the pericardial cavity and the two pleural cavities, the thoracic cavity includes the area between the two lungs. Because it lies along the midline and is deep to the breastbone or sternum, it is called the **mediastinum**. The _____ contains the heart, the large blood vessels located above the heart, and a gland called the thymus gland.
abdominal **pelvic**	**4.16** As you have learned, the abdominopelvic cavity is the large cavity of the abdominal and pelvic regions. It contains an upper and lower area, which are not divided by a partition. The upper area is the **abdominal cavity**, which contains the liver, stomach, pancreas, spleen, and most of the small and large intestines. Recall that _____ literally means "pertaining to the abdomen." At the level of the iliac crest (the tips of the hip bones), the **pelvic cavity** begins and continues to the base of the abdominopelvic cavity. The pelvic cavity contains the urinary bladder, internal reproductive organs, and parts of the small and large intestines. The word _____ may be separated into its two word parts, pelv/ic, and literally means "pertaining to a bowl or basin," which accurately describes this bowl-shaped cavity.

PRACTICE: Anatomy and Physiology Introduction

The Right Match

Match the combining form on the left with the correct definition on the right.

_____ 1. abdomin/o

_____ 2. anter/o

_____ 3. brachi/o

_____ 4. caud/o

_____ 5. cephal/o

_____ 6. cervic/o

_____ 7. cran/o, crani/o

a. skull

b. neck

c. tail

d. back

e. distant

f. front

g. abdomen

_____ 8. cyt/o   h. arm

_____ 9. dist/o   i. cell

_____ 10. dors/o   j. head

_____ 11. femor/o   k. below

_____ 12. gastr/o   l. groin

_____ 13. glute/o   m. loin, lower back

_____ 14. hom/o, home/o   n. tool

_____ 15. ili/o   o. stomach

_____ 16. infer/o   p. middle

_____ 17. inguin/o   q. flank, hip, groin

_____ 18. lumb/o   r. buttock

_____ 19. medi/o   s. thigh

_____ 20. organ/o   t. same

Correct the Spelling

This exercise tests your ability to spell terms correctly. The list on the left column includes terms that are misspelled. In the right column, write in the correct spelling of the term.

1. abdominole   _____

2. thorasik   _____

3. parakardeal   _____

4. fizeology   _____

5. sagitall   _____

6. superfishal   _____

7. homiostaysis   _____

8. diafram   _____

Word Root Linkup

Link the word roots in the list to create the terms that match the definitions.

Word Root	Definition
abdomin	*abdomen*
cardi	*heart*
chondr	*gristle, cartilage*
pelv	*bowl, basin*
physi	*nature*

Definition

1. refers to the study of the nature of living things

2. the area of the abdomen

3. below the cartilage

4. pertaining to around the heart

5. literally means "pertaining to a bowl or basin," which accurately describes this bowl-shaped cavity

Term

_____/o/logy

_____/al

hypo/_____/i/ac

peri/_____/al

_____/ic

Medical Terms Introduction

As the next step in learning the terminology of the human body, in this section you explore introductory medical terms and diagnostic procedures. Here are two combining forms that you will see in this section.

Combining Form	Definition
chron/o	time
path/o	disease

Complete the following frames to learn some introductory medical terms and diagnostic procedures.

homeostasis **disease** dih ZEEZ	**4.17** The body's goal is to keep itself alive and healthy. Each system performs functions that endeavor to keep the body in a constant, stable state by adjusting to changes. As you learned in Frame 4.4, this is the process of maintaining homeostasis. When body functions fail to maintain _____, a condition of instability results that is called **disease**. In general, the term _____ refers to a state of the body in which homeostasis has faltered for any reason.
pathology path AHL oh jee	**4.18** The study of disease is a field of medicine called **pathology**. This term is derived from the Greek word for suffering or disease, *pathos*, creating the combining form *path/o*. The term is completed by adding the suffix *-logy*, which means "study or science of." A **pathologist** is a physician who specializes in _____, or the study of disease. In most cases, a pathologist does not treat individual patients, but manages a clinical lab that evaluates data about patients to assist other healthcare professionals.
diagnosis DYE ag NO sis	**4.19** When examining a patient who is complaining of an illness, the healthcare professional must first identify the illness before it can be treated. Identification of the illness is called a **diagnosis**. This is a constructed word containing the word parts *dia-*, which means "through," and *-gnosis*, which means "knowledge." The _____ must be established before a treatment program can be created.
symptoms SIMP tumz	**4.20** To make a diagnosis, a healthcare professional listens to the patient to learn about clues that might suggest the nature of the illness. Experiences of the patient resulting from a disease are called **symptoms**. They are usually sensations—such as pain, heat, cold, or pressure—but can also be the loss of sensations, such as numbness or loss of appetite. Other _____ include dizziness, loss of balance, and mental confusion.

sign

4.21 Before a diagnosis can be made, a healthcare professional often examines the patient for physical signs of disease. A **sign** is a finding that can be discovered by an objective examination, such as a physical exam or lab exam. For example, a thermometer inserted into the mouth or ear canal will indicate the presence of an elevated body temperature, or **fever**, which is a common _____ of an infectious disease.

acute
ah KYOOT

4.22 As part of a diagnosis, a disease is commonly classified by its expected duration: a brief or a long duration. The term **acute** describes a disease of short duration. For example, a head cold is usually an _____ disease because of its short duration. The medical term for a head cold is **acute coryza** (kor EYE zah). Although an acute disease is relatively brief, many such diseases can have severe effects that can become life-threatening, so keep in mind that the term does not imply a mild disease.

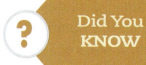

Did You KNOW

ACUTE

The term *acute* is derived from the Latin word *acutus*, which means "sharp." It describes how a symptom or sign that is of short duration strikes quickly, such as would result from a stinging stab from a sharp instrument.

chronic
KRON ik

4.23 A term frequently used to describe diseases that are of long duration is **chronic**. The term is derived from the Greek word for time, *kronos*; these _____ diseases usually develop slowly and last for many years. An example of a chronic disease is the skin condition **psoriasis** (soh RYE ah siss), which lasts a lifetime.

infection
in FEKK shun

etiology
ee tee AHL oh jee

4.24 Diseases may also be classified on the basis of their cause or origin. One of the most common forms of disease is **infection**, a disease caused by microorganisms such as bacteria, viruses, fungal parasites, or protozoans. The presence of _____ results in the development of **infectious disease**. The cause of a disease is called its **etiology**, which literally means "the study or science of cause." For example, the _____ of the infectious disease malaria is a microscopic protozoan called *Plasmodium*, which is passed to us by the bite of an infected *Anopheles* mosquito.

trauma
TRAW mah

4.25 Disease may also be caused by physical injury or **trauma**. For example, a fractured bone is a common _____ arising from an automobile collision. It is a disease because it upsets homeostasis—in this case, homeostasis of the bone and surrounding tissues. Disease resulting from trauma is called **traumatic disease**.

prognosis
prog NOH sis

4.26 Once a reliable diagnosis is made, the healthcare professional may predict the probable course of the disease and its probable outcome. This prediction is called a **prognosis**. _____ is a constructed word containing the word parts *pro-*, which means "before," and *-gnosis*, "knowledge."

diagnostic imaging

4.27 As you may suspect, making an accurate diagnosis is an essential part of medicine. As a result of improving technologies, making a diagnosis has become a more efficient and reliable practice than in the past. The most important improvements have been in the way instruments are able to observe the internal structure and functions of the body without the need for open surgical procedures. These noninvasive procedures are called **diagnostic imaging**. The five major types of _____ _____ are endoscopy, CT scan, PET scan, MRI, and ultrasound.

endoscopy
end AH skoh pee

4.28 The use of a long, flexible tube that can be inserted into a patient is called **endoscopy**. This constructed term includes two word parts: *endo-*, which means "within," and *-scopy*, which means "process of viewing." During the _____, a healthcare professional may observe the internal cavities and organs of the patient with the attachment of a camera at the far end of the tube (■ Figure 4.5). The tube may also contain surgical attachments, enabling a surgeon to manipulate internal body parts while viewing a monitor.

■ **Figure 4.5**
Endoscopy. This is a minimally invasive surgical procedure because it reduces patient recovery time and the risk of infection by avoiding the opening of body cavities. Instead, a fiberoptic tube with a camera is inserted into a body opening, such as the mouth (shown here), allowing the surgeon to observe internal organs and cavities on a monitor.
Source: Beloborod/Shutterstock.

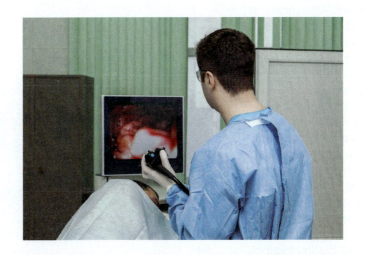

CT scan

4.29 A **CT (CAT) scan** is a diagnostic procedure that combines multiple x-rays and computer enhancement to produce three-dimensional images of internal body structures (■ Figure 4.6). The term _____ _____ is an acronym for **computed tomography scanning**. As a result of the computer enhancement, cross-sectional images or "slices" of body regions are produced. CT scans are useful, speedy, and relatively low cost when cross-sectional images of organs in the chest or abdomen, muscles, and joints are needed, as in the evaluation of trauma.

■ **Figure 4.6**
CT scan. The patient is undergoing the scan in the procedure room while the radiologic technician is monitoring the instrument behind the glass wall. The CT scan image is visible on the monitor.
Source: Linda Bartlett/National Cancer Institute.

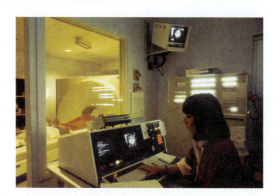

PET scan

4.30 A **PET scan** is a procedure that detects the journey of a radioactive-labeled substance, such as glucose (sugar), through the body. The PET scan instrument contains scanners that respond to radiolabeled glucose and computers that create an image to track the pathway of the glucose as it is metabolized by body cells. As a result, the _____ _____ reveals areas of the body that have an unusually high metabolic rate, such as tumors (■ Figure 4.7). The term *PET* is an acronym for **positron emission tomography**.

■ **Figure 4.7**
PET scan. (a) Photograph of a PET scan instrument. After receiving a radiolabeled mixture (usually in the form of an ingested drink), the patient lies on the table while the table moves into the doughnut-shaped scanner. *Source: Ververidis Vasilis/Shutterstock.* (b) The scanner detects the radiolabeled mixture while it is metabolized by the patient, and interprets the data to form an image like the one shown. Areas of metabolically active cells may glow yellow (shown here) or use other colors to highlight their presence.
Source: Monet_3k/Shutterstock.

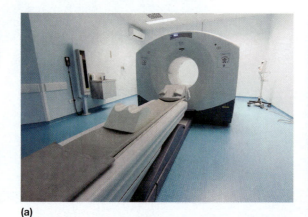

(a)

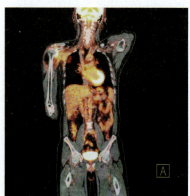

(b)

MRI

4.31 Among all the diagnostic imaging techniques available, the **MRI** has generated the most excitement in the medical community because it offers the clearest, most complete images of internal anatomy. The term *MRI* is an acronym for **magnetic resonance imaging**. The instrument includes magnets that respond to hydrogen atoms in the body by sending signals to a computer, which analyzes the information to produce three-dimensional images (■ Figure 4.8). Unlike CT and PET scans, MRI does not use radioisotopes and is thereby safer to use. The _____ can be used to diagnose many forms of cancer, joint disease, and trauma.

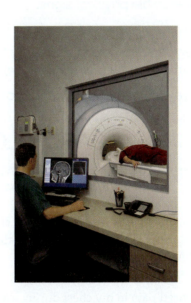

■ **Figure 4.8**
MRI. The patient enters the MRI instrument through the "doughnut" opening, while a technician monitors progress in an adjacent room. An MRI of the head is visible on the monitor.
Source: James Steidl/ Shutterstock.

ultrasound imaging

4.32 Ultrasound imaging, or **sonography**, involves the pulsation of harmless sound waves through a body region. As the waves travel through tissues of varying density, they produce echoes that can be detected by a probe and interpreted by a computer (■ Figure 4.9). Because of its harmless nature, _____ _____ has proven useful in prenatal care by providing an early glimpse of the developing fetus (a child before birth) in the uterus.

■ **Figure 4.9**
Ultrasound imaging. The use of sound waves produces a computer-enhanced image of the pregnancy status on the monitor, giving the parents an exciting early view of their child and healthcare professionals a valuable tool for mapping the progress of the pregnancy.
Source: Monkey Business Images/Shutterstock.

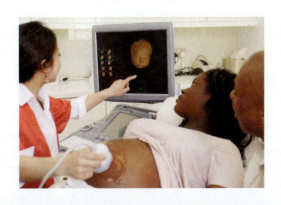

UNDERSTANDING MEDICAL REPORTS

As you approach the ends of Chapters 5–15, you will come upon a section titled **Medical Report Exercises**. In each of these chapters, the exercises present a clinical issue that is very similar to the type of patient concerns you will encounter while working in medical health care. Each exercise begins with information about the patient, which is obtained by way of an interview that includes a physical exam of the patient. The patient information is recorded and becomes a part of the patient's **medical record**, or **chart**, and is available for the health professionals assigned to the patient's care. To help prepare you for a career in health care, the format of the medical record is presented using the popularized SOAP standard, which is an acronym for **S**ubjective, **O**bjective, **A**ssessment, and **P**lan. Here's what each of these terms means:

Subjective: What the patient has experienced regarding his or her present illness, usually recorded in his or her actual words as symptoms. This may also be called History of the Present Illness (abbreviated *Hx* or *HPI*).

Objective: The unbiased facts of the illness, usually based on the results of the physical exam (abbreviated *PE*) and recorded as measurable physical signs.

Assessment: The diagnosis (abbreviated *Dx*) made by the medical team of the patient's illness.

Plan: The medical strategies employed in improving the patient's health, such as any lab or imaging procedures, surgery, or medications (abbreviated *Rx*).

Here is what the SOAP version of a medical record often looks like.

CARDIOLOGY SERVICES

5500 University Avenue, Metropolis, New York
Phone: (211) 594-4000 • Fax (211) 594-4001

Date: 07/15/2017
Patient: Williams, James   **Patient ID:** 123456
Dob: 3/20/1978   **Age:** 39   **Sex: Male**   **Allergies:** NKDA (no known drug allergy)
Provider: Robert A. Young, MD

S   **Subjective:**

"Lately I have noticed pain in my chest during exercise, and I feel out of breath more quickly than usual. I am extremely worried."

39 y/o male describes chest pain and shortness of breath during workouts. Noted patient clenching his jaw and fist while describing his chest pain and shortness of breath. Patient denied radiating pain, nausea, or vomiting. The chest pain "disappeared" within a few seconds after exercising. He indicated he has no family or personal history of heart disease.

O   **Objective:**

Vital Signs: T (body temperature): 98.2°F; **P** (pulse rate): 60; **R** (breathing rate): 20; **BP** (blood pressure): 160/90
Ht: 5'10"
Wt: 210 lb
General Appearance: Slightly overweight. Noted no obvious signs of physical distress such as edema, pallor, or diaphoresis. Overall health appears WNL (within normal limits).
Heart: Rate at 60 beats per minute, with no extra sounds, regular rhythm, no murmurs.
Lungs: Lungs clear, no rales or wheezes.
Abd: Bowel sounds normal all four quadrants; no tenderness or masses.
MS: Joints and muscles symmetric; no swelling, masses, or deformity.

A   **Assessment:**

Chest pain (angina pectoris).

P   **Plan:**

Evaluate heart function and cause of chest pain with stress ECG. Rx to include beta-blocker and, to reduce BP (blood pressure), ACE inhibitor. Consult for possible angioplasty.

CHAPTER REVIEW

Word Building

Construct medical terms from the following meanings. (Some are built from word parts; some are not.) The first question has been completed for you as an example.

1. identification of an illness   dia/**gnosis**_____

2. maintaining internal stability   home/o/_____

3. common synonym of CAT scan   _____ scan

4. of long duration   _____/ic

5. the study of disease   _____/o/logy

6. a disease of short duration   _____ (do this one on your own!)

7. divides the body into superior and inferior portions   _____ plane

8. body cavity inferior to the diaphragm   _____/_____/_____/ic cavity

9. procedure using a long flexible tube   _____/scopy

10. term for a finding following an objective examination   _____

11. formed from similarly grouped cells   _____

12. area of the chest   _____/ic region

13. MRI   magnetic _____ imaging

14. on top of the stomach   _____/_____/ic

15. pertaining to the lung   _____/al

16. divides the body vertically into right and left portions   _____ plane

17. pertaining to the navel   _____/al

18. science or study of the cause of disease   _____/o/logy

19. study of body structure   _____/tom/y

20. study of nature   _____/o/logy

Define the Combining Form

	Definition	Use in a Term
1. abdomin/o	_____	_____
2. crani/o	_____	_____
3. infer/o	_____	_____
4. poster/o	_____	_____
5. proxim/o	_____	_____
6. super/o	_____	_____
7. thorac/o	_____	_____
8. tom/o	_____	_____
9. pleur/o	_____	_____
10. pelv/o	_____	_____

MyLab Medical Terminology™

MyLab Medical Terminology is a premium online homework management system that includes a host of features to help you study. Registered users will find:

- A multitude of quizzes and activities built within the MyLab platform
- Powerful tools that track and analyze your results—allowing you to create a personalized learning experience
- Videos and audio pronunciations to help enrich your progress
- Streaming lesson presentations (Guided Lectures) and self-paced learning modules
- A space where you and your instructors can view and manage your assignments

Chapter 5

The Integumentary System

Learning Objectives

After completing this chapter, you will be able to:

5.1 Define the word parts used to create medical terms of the integumentary system.

5.2 Break down and define common medical terms used for symptoms, diseases, disorders, procedures, treatments, and devices associated with the integumentary system.

5.3 Build medical terms from the word parts associated with the integumentary system.

5.4 Pronounce and spell common medical terms associated with the integumentary system.

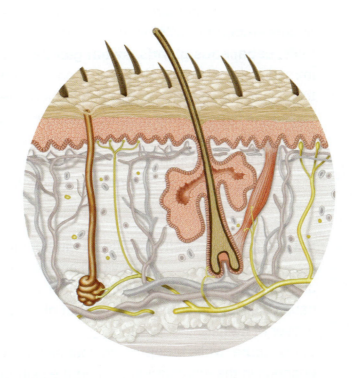

Anatomy and Physiology Terms

Review the combining forms that specifically apply to the anatomy and physiology of the integumentary system. Note that the combining forms are colored red to help you identify them when you see them again later in the chapter.

Combining Form	Definition
aden/o	gland
aut/o	self
cutane/o	skin
cyan/o	blue
derm/o, dermat/o	skin

Combining Form	Definition
follicul/o	little follicle
kerat/o	hard
onych/o	nail
seb/o	sebum, oil

integumentary
IN teg yoo MEN tar ee

epidermis

subcutaneous
sub kyoo TANE ee us

5.1 The _____ system forms the entire surface area of the body. It is dominated by the largest organ of the body, the **skin**. The skin is composed of two distinct layers: an inner, deep layer composed of connective tissue known as the **dermis** and an outer layer of epithelium called the **epidermis**. The term *dermis* means "skin," and the term _____ means "on top of skin." The integumentary system also includes smaller accessory organs embedded within the skin, such as **hair** and **hair follicles**, **nails**, **sebaceous glands**, **sweat glands**, and **sensory receptors**. Immediately below the skin is an area of connective tissue that binds the skin to the muscles and is rich in blood vessels and nerves. Called the **hypodermis** or **subcutaneous layer**, it is a region of the body that commonly receives injections. The term *hypodermis* means "below the skin." Because *cutane/o* also means "skin," _____ also means "below the skin."

protection

regulate

sensation

5.2 The primary function of the integumentary system is protection. _____ is provided against outside temperature changes, dehydration, and infectious microorganisms that may cause disease. In addition, the sweat glands, blood vessels, and a layer of fat help the skin to _____ internal body temperature, while receptors in your skin provide the ability to detect changes in the environment, giving the skin the added function of _____.

5.3 Review the anatomy of the integumentary system by studying the illustration of the skin in ■ Figure 5.1 and the illustration of nails in ■ Figure 5.2.

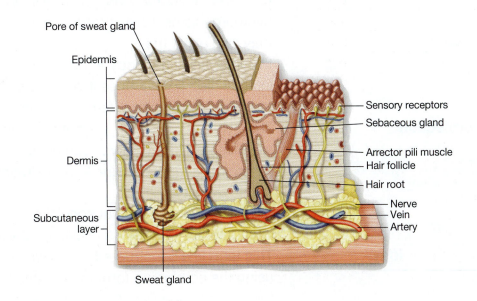

■ **Figure 5.1**
Anatomy of the skin. Illustration of a section of skin showing key structures.

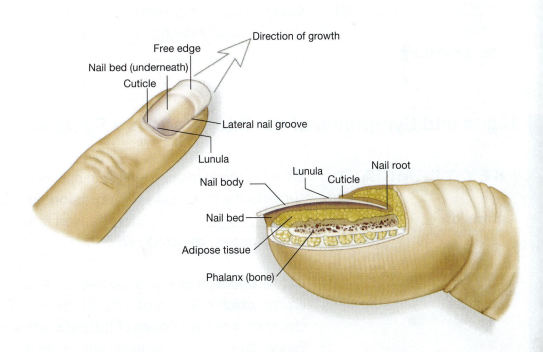

■ **Figure 5.2**
Nail structure, top view and side view.

Medical Terms of the Integumentary System

organ

skin

protection

5.4 The integumentary system can experience many types of challenges to its homeostasis. As the outermost organ of the body, the skin is more exposed to the extremes of the external environment than any other _____, subjecting it to temperature fluctuations, physical injury, and invasion by unwanted microorganisms. Many types of inherited and acquired diseases may also afflict the _____. In many cases, it is the first part of the body to display signs and symptoms of an internal disorder because it is the body part with which we are most familiar—we often see, feel, and touch our skin throughout the day. The _____ that it provides to your overall health is significant: A loss of skin, such as occurs in a severe burn, can lead to severe consequences due to dehydration and infection, even death.

dermat/o/logy

5.5 The medical field that specializes in the health and disease of the integumentary system is known as **dermatology** (derm ah TAHL oh jee). This term is a constructed word, written _____/_____/_____, using the combining form that means "skin," *dermat/o*, to carry the primary meaning. A physician specializing in dermatology is commonly known as a **dermatologist** (derm ah TAHL oh jist).

integumentary

5.6 In the following sections, we review the prefixes, combining forms, and suffixes that combine to build the medical terms of the _____ system.

Signs and Symptoms of the Integumentary System

KEY TERMS A–Z

abrasion
  ah BRAY zhun

5.7 A common injury to the skin caused by scraping produces a superficial wound called an **abrasion**. Practice spelling this term: _____. It is derived from the Latin word *abrasus*, which means "to scrape off."

abscess
  AB sess

5.8 An **abscess** is a localized elevation of the skin containing a cavity, which is a sign of a local infection. The _____ cavity contains a mixture of bacteria, white blood cells, damaged tissue, and fluids collectively known as **pus** and is surrounded by inflamed tissue. Several medical terms may be used to describe the production of pus. They are **suppuration** (suhp ah RAY shun), **purulence** (PEWR yoo lens), and **pyogenesis** (PIE oh JENN eh SISS).

? **Did You KNOW**

ABSCESS
Many medical terms of the integumentary system are derived directly from Latin or Greek words with descriptive meanings. For example, the word *abscess* is derived from the original Latin word *abscessus*, which means "a going-away" (which is what you hope to happen soon to the abscess if one appears on your skin, since they can be very painful).

cellulite SELL yoo light	**5.9 Cellulite** is a local uneven surface of the skin and is a sign of subcutaneous fat deposition. _____ is relatively common in women on the thighs and buttocks.
cicatrix SIK ah trix	**5.10** An injury to the skin resulting in a break through the epidermis and into the dermis or deeper layers of skin requires the process of healing. During this process, epidermal cells migrate to the wound and produce new cells while cells within the dermis produce additional protein fibers. If the wound is too large for the epidermal cells to close the breakage, additional protein fibers (collagen) will be produced to seal the wound. In this case, the wound becomes closed by the formation of **scar tissue**. A clinical term for scar is **cicatrix**. _____ is a Latin word that means "scar." The plural form is **cicatrices** (sik ah TRYE sees).
comedo KOM ee doh	**5.11** The clinical term for **pimple** is **comedo**. It is a local elevation of the skin arising from a minor infection of sebaceous (oil) glands. Bacteria feed on the oil, attracting the movement of white blood cells and their products and resulting in the localized inflammation. In Latin, the word _____ means "glutton," referring to the fact that the lesion is caused by the action of "gluttonous" bacteria. The plural form is **comedones** (KOM ee DOH neez).
contusion kon TOO zhun	**5.12** Commonly known as a **bruise**, a **contusion** (kon TOO zhun) is a discoloration and swelling of the skin resulting from tissue damage to the blood vessels of the dermis or deeper tissues. Thus, a _____ is a common sign following a physical trauma, such as an automobile accident or a blow to the face.
cyanosis sigh ah NO siss	**5.13** The combining form for the color blue is *cyan/o*. Adding the ending *-osis*, which means "condition of," produces the term _____. It is a blue tinge of color to an area of the skin and is a sign of a cardiovascular or respiratory disturbance. **Cyanosis** is usually apparent most clearly in the lips and fingertips. A patient exhibiting this sign is called **cyanotic**.

cyst sist	**5.14** Derived from the Greek word *kystis* that means "bladder," a **cyst** is a closed sac or pouch on the surface of the skin that is filled with liquid or semisolid material. Notice that the *c* in the term _____ sounds like an *s*.
edema eh DEE mah	**5.15** An injury often leads to inflammation, which includes swelling. Swelling occurs when fluid accumulates in a confined space, such as beneath the skin. The clinical term for fluid accumulation is **edema**. It is derived from the Greek word *oidema*, which means "swelling." Caused by the leakage of fluid across capillary walls, _____ is a common sign of injury and infection.
erythema ehr ih THEE mah	**5.16** The Greek word that means "blush" is *erythema*. We use the same word for any redness of the skin. It is a common sign of injury or infection. The correct spelling is the same as the original Greek word; it is spelled _____.
fissure FISH er	**5.17** The clinical term for a narrow break or slit in the skin is **fissure**. It is derived from the Latin word for a split or crack, *fissura*, and is illustrated in ■ Figure 5.3 with other signs of skin disease. Write the correct spelling of this term: _____.

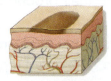

A macule is a discolored spot on the skin; freckle

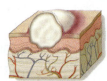

A pustule is a small, elevated, circumscribed lesion of the skin that is filled with pus; whitehead

 allergy

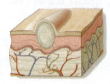

A wheal is a localized, evanescent elevation of the skin that is often accompanied by itching; urticaria

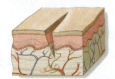

An erosion or ulcer is an eating or gnawing away of tissue; decubitus ulcer

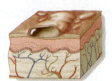

A papule is a solid, circumscribed, elevated area on the skin; pimple

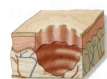

A fissure is a crack-like sore or slit that extends through the epidermis into the dermis; athlete's foot

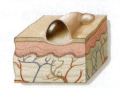

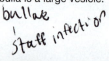

A vesicle is a small fluid-filled sac; blister. A bulla is a large vesicle.

bullae
Staff infection

■ **Figure 5.3**

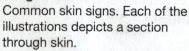

Common skin signs. Each of the illustrations depicts a section through skin.

furuncle
FOO rung kl

5.18 If an abscess is associated with a hair follicle, the local swelling on the skin is called a **furuncle**. Commonly known as a **boil**, it is derived from the Latin word for boil, *furunculus*. A photograph of a _____ is provided in ■ Figure 5.4.

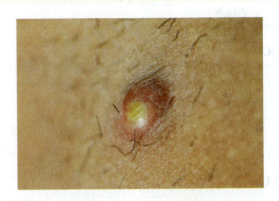

■ **Figure 5.4**
Furuncle.
Source: FCG/Shutterstock.

induration
in doo RAY shun

5.19 A local hard area on the skin, or perhaps elsewhere in the body, is known as an **induration**. This word is derived from the Latin word *induratio*, which means "the process of becoming firm or hard." An _____ is usually a sign of an excessive deposit of collagen or calcium.

jaundice
JAWN diss

[handwritten: Yellow skin from waste protien billirubin]

5.20 The French word for yellow is *jaune*. It is the origin of the clinical term for an abnormal yellow coloration of the skin and eyes, **jaundice**. In most cases, _____ is a sign of liver or gallbladder disease. The yellowing results from an abnormal release of bile pigments by the liver.

keloid
KEE loyd

[handwritten: overgrown scar]

5.21 You have learned that a cicatrix (scar) may be formed when skin undergoes repair from an injury (see Frame 5.10). An overgrowth of scar tissue that forms an elevated lesion on the skin is known as a **keloid**. This large scar, or _____, is often discolored, which sets it apart from adjacent, normal skin (■ Figure 5.5). The term is derived from a Greek word for "spot," *kelis*.

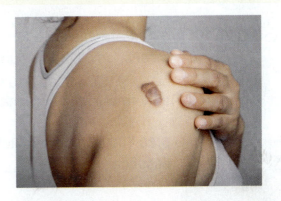

■ **Figure 5.5**
Keloids. A single keloid is visible on the shoulder of this patient as an elevated, pigmented lesion.
Source: WEERACHAT/Shutterstock.

laceration *Cut* LASS err AY shun	**5.22** A **laceration** is the common result of an injury caused by a tear or perhaps a cut by a sharp object with an irregular surface. A _____ penetrating the dermis and extending for more than one inch often requires stitching with sutures to close the wound.
macule *Small flat skin legion* MAK yool	**5.23** A discolored flat spot on the skin surface, such as a **freckle**, is clinically called a **macule**, which means "little spot" in Latin. A _____ is a sign of sun damage to the skin, and the tendency to develop them is genetically determined. A macule is illustrated in Figure 5.3.
nevus *mole* NEE vus	**5.24** Similar to a macule but darker in color, a **nevus** is a pigmented spot that is commonly called a **mole** (■ Figure 5.6). It is actually a sign of a benign tumor, and if its edges become irregular or the color changes, the _____ should be examined as a suspected malignancy known as a **melanoma** (see Frame 5.51).

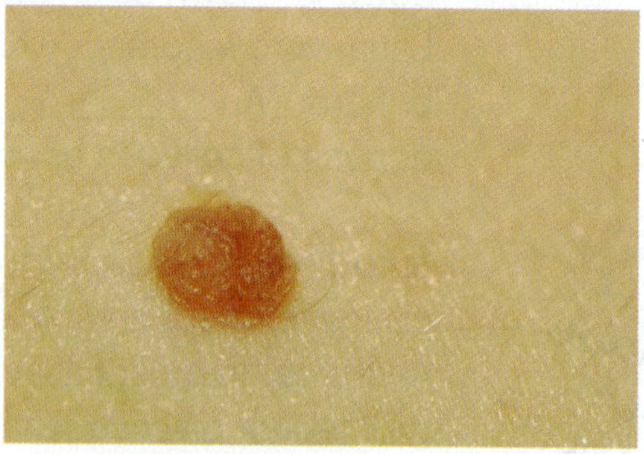

■ Figure 5.6
Nevus.
Source: D. Kucharski, K. Kucharska/Shutterstock.

pallor *pale skin* PAL or	**5.25 Pallor** is an abnormally pale color of the skin. Derived from the Latin word *pallor* that means "paleness," _____ is a sign of an internal condition causing a decreased flow of blood to the skin.
papule *Small, solid raised legion* PAP yool	**5.26** A **papule** is a general term describing any small, solid elevation on the skin (see Figure 5.3). An example of a _____ is a comedo, or pimple. The term is derived from the Latin word *papula*, which means a "small pimple."
petechiae *tiny red dot (from blood infection meningitis)* peh TEE kee eye	**5.27 Petechiae** is a term derived from a Latin word that means "small red or purple dots." The presence of dot-sized _____ on the surface of the skin is a sign of the abnormal rupture of small blood vessels in the dermis.
pruritus *itching* proo RYE tuss	**5.28** The symptom of itchy skin is known as **pruritus**. As you might suspect, _____ means "an itching" in Latin.

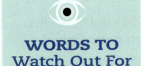

WORDS TO
Watch Out For

Pruritus

You might think at first glance that *pruritus* ("an itching") is a constructed term that uses the suffix *-itis*, meaning "inflammation." This isn't the case, however. Make a note of the spelling of this non-constructed Latin term. The correct spelling of prurit**us** has a *u* near the end.

---

purple/red skin

purpura
PER pew rah

5.29 The Greeks used the word *porphyra* to name a shellfish that releases a purple dye. In time, it was changed to name the color purple. Dermatologists use a form of the word, **purpura**, for a symptom of purple-red skin discoloration. _____ is usually the result of a hemorrhage (one or more broken blood vessels) that spread blood through the skin.

---

pustule
PUS tyool

5.30 You learned from Frame 5.8 that pus is a fluid containing bacteria, white blood cells, and their products. A general term for an elevated area of the skin filled with pus is **pustule**. An example of a _____ is a whitehead with pus. A pustule is illustrated in Figure 5.3.

---

erodes skin

ulcer
ULL ser

5.31 An **ulcer** is an erosion through the skin or mucous membrane (see Figure 5.4). The term is derived from the Latin word that means "a sore," *ulcus*. A common form of ulcer arises from lack of movement when lying supine for an extended period of time. It is called a **decubitus** (dee KYOO bih tus) _____. Because a decubitus ulcer may arise in patients confined to bedrest for long periods of time, the erosion is commonly called a **bed sore**.

---

allergic rash of wheals that come and go

urticaria
er tih KARE ree ah

5.32 A common allergic skin reaction to medications, foods, infection, or injury produces small fluid-filled skin elevations, known as **urticaria** (■ Figure 5.7). Derived from the Latin word *urtica*, this sign is commonly known as **hives**. _____ is usually accompanied by itching, or pruritus (see Frame 5.28).

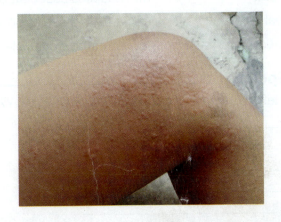

■ **Figure 5.7**
Urticaria, or hives, is an allergic reaction resulting in small skin vesicles (Frame 5.34).
Source: Ipen/Shutterstock.

wart **verruca** ver ROO kah	**5.33** A **wart** is a sign of infection by a papilloma virus. The wart, or **verruca** from its original Latin, is an effort by the skin to rid itself of the virus and is observed as a skin elevation with a thickened epidermis. A _____ can be treated with antiviral medication.
(chicken pox) **vesicle** VESS ih kl	**5.34** A **vesicle** is a small elevation of the epidermis that is filled with fluid containing little or no pus (see Figure 5.3). A blister is an example of a _____ that results from injury to the skin.
wheal WEEL *allergy reaction*	**5.35** A temporary, itchy elevation of the skin, often with a white center and red perimeter, is called a **wheal**. A _____ is a symptom of an allergic reaction of the skin and is illustrated in Figure 5.3.

PRACTICE: Signs and Symptoms of the Integumentary System

The Right Match

Match the term on the left with the correct definition on the right.

_____	1. cellulite	a.	localized skin swelling that is a sign of infection
_____	2. abscess	b.	abnormal yellow coloration of the skin
_____	3. cicatrix	c.	a local uneven surface of the skin caused by fat deposition
_____	4. abrasion	d.	an erosion through the skin or mucous membrane
_____	5. jaundice	e.	itchy skin
_____	6. nevus	f.	clinical term for scar
_____	7. pruritus	g.	a pigmented spot on the skin; a mole
_____	8. ulcer	h.	scraping injury to the skin
_____	9. cyst	i.	a wart
_____	10. erythema	j.	elevated area of the skin filled with pus
_____	11. furuncle	k.	temporary, itchy elevation of the skin
_____	12. pustule	l.	redness of the skin
_____	13. verruca	m.	abscess associated with a hair follicle; a boil
_____	14. wheal	n.	a closed sac or pouch filled with liquid or semisolid material
_____	15. comedo	o.	any small, solid elevation on the skin

Correct the Spelling

The terms in the left column have been spelled incorrectly. Write in the correct spelling in the space provided.

1. erithemma _____
2. peritis _____
3. absess _____
4. ertikaria _____
5. paller _____
6. keeloid _____

Diseases and Disorders of the Integumentary System

Review some of the word parts that specifically apply to the diseases and disorders of the integumentary system that are covered in the following section. Note that the word parts are color-coded to help you identify them: prefixes are yellow, combining forms are red, and suffixes are blue.

Prefix	Definition
ec-	outside, out
par-	alongside, abnormal

Combining Form	Definition
actin/o	radiation
aden/o	gland
albin/o	white
carcin/o	cancer
cellul/o	little cell
chym/o	juice
crypt/o	hidden
derm/o, dermat/o	skin
follicul/o	little follicle
hidr/o	sweat
kerat/o	hard
leuk/o	white
melan/o	black
myc/o	fungus
onych/o	nail
pedicul/o	body louse
scler/o	hard
trich/o	hair
xer/o	dry

Suffix	Definition
-a	singular
-ia	condition of
-ic	pertaining to
-ism	condition or disease
-itis	inflammation
-malacia	softening
-oma	tumor
-osis	condition of
-pathy	disease
-rrhea	discharge

KEY TERMS A–Z

acne
AK nee

pustules & comedones all over skin

5.36 Acne is an uncomfortable condition of the skin resulting from bacterial infection of sebaceous glands and ducts (■ Figure 5.8). The skin disease known as _____ is characterized by the presence of numerous open comedones (blackheads) and closed comedones (whiteheads) in affected parts of the face and may also involve the neck, back, and chest. Acne is the most common skin disease of adolescence, caused by rapid growth of sebaceous glands during this period of life. The term *acne* is derived from a similar Greek word that means "facial eruption."

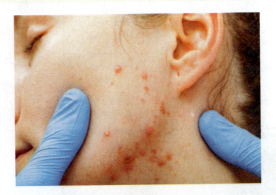

■ **Figure 5.8**
Acne.
Source: Ocskay Bence/Shutterstock.

*elder people after alot of
sun exposure - precancer*

actinic keratosis
ak TIN ik * kair ah TOH siss

5.37 Actinic keratosis is a precancerous condition of the skin caused by exposure to sunlight. It forms skin lesions resulting from overgrowths of the epidermis, usually with scaly surfaces. The term _____ _____ is a constructed word, *actin/ic kerat/osis*, in which *actinic* means "pertaining to radiation" and *keratosis* means "a condition of hard." In general, any form of keratosis produces a sign of scaly skin.

*can't produce
melanin*

albinism
AL bin izm

5.38 A genetic condition characterized by the reduction of the pigment melanin in the skin is known as **albinism**. The term _____ uses the combining form *albin/o*, which is derived from the Latin word for white, *albus*. The constructed word, albin/ism, means "a condition or disease of white." The term **albino** refers to a person afflicted with albinism.

Baldness

alopecia
al oh PEE she ah

5.39 A loss or lack of scalp hair is a clinical sign known as baldness, or **alopecia**. The term *alopecia* is from the Greek word *alopex*, which means "fox," and refers to a form of hair loss (called *mange*) that may be seen in foxes. Alopecia may be a sign of an infection of the scalp, high fever, drug reactions, chemotherapy, or emotional stress. Alternatively, the common appearance of _____ in men, often called **male-pattern baldness**, is the result of a genetically controlled factor that prevents the development of hair follicles in certain areas of the scalp.

burn

*Classified
By:*
*{ - amount of
skin burned
- How deep
burn goes*

5.40 A **burn** is an injury to the skin caused by excessive exposure to fire, electricity, chemicals, or sunlight. The extent of injury caused by the _____ is determined by the amount of surface area damaged, called **total body surface area (TBSA)**, and the **depth** of the damage. A burn becomes life-threatening when a large TBSA has become damaged, exposing the body to infection. The depth of burn classification is illustrated in ■ Figure 5.9.

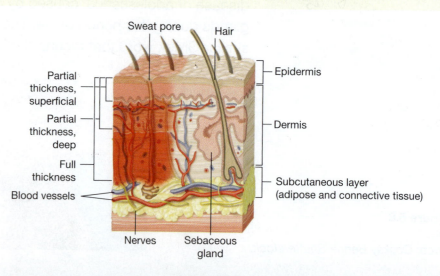

■ **Figure 5.9**
Classification of burn injury by depth in skin.

carbuncle
KAR bung kl

abscess

5.41 A **carbuncle** is a skin infection composed of a cluster of furuncles, or boils (■ Figure 5.10). The most common source of infection is *Staphylococci* bacteria, or "staph." The term _____ is derived from the Latin word *carbo*, which means "live coal" and refers to the hot pain associated with this disease.

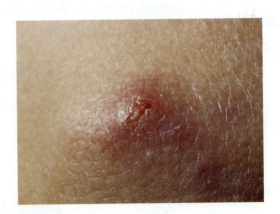

■ **Figure 5.10**
Carbuncle.
*Source: Rob Bouwman/
Shutterstock.*

carcinoma
kar sih NOH mah

Cancerous tumor

most skin cancer tumors are from sun exposure

5.42 Remember that the combining form *carcin/o* means "cancer." When you add the suffix that means "tumor," it forms the word _____. Several forms of cancer, or carcinoma, affect the skin. **Basal cell carcinoma** (■ Figure 5.11) and **squamous cell carcinoma** are tumors arising from the epidermis that usually remain localized, although the lesions do spread and can become serious if they are not treated. Squamous cell carcinomas, in particular, can be dangerous, while the less dangerous basal cell carcinomas are more common. The third major form of skin cancer is **melanoma**, which is described later in Frame 5.51.

Basal cell carcinoma: Begins at the base of the skin, grows slowly, usually doesn't spread, easily removed in Dr's office

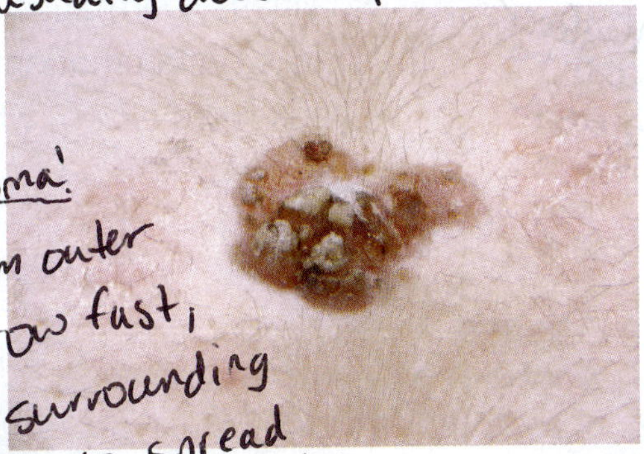

Squamous cell carcinoma: begins with cell from outer layer of skin, grow fast, cause damage to surrounding area, don't tend to spread to entire body, can usually be removed and patient not die.

melanoma: begins in melanocyte, spreads rapidly throughout body & often results in death, prevent sun expo... mostly in light skin people

■ **Figure 5.11**
Basal cell carcinoma.
*Source: Centers for Disease
Control and Prevention.*

[Handwritten notes: infection spreading through deep layers of skin (Stapharious Streptacocous)]

cellulitis
  sell you LYE tiss

[Handwritten note: MRSA = antibiotic resistent stapharious]

5.43 Cellulitis is an inflammation of the connective tissue in the dermis (■ Figure 5.12). It is caused by an infection that spreads from the skin surface or hair follicles to the dermis and sometimes the subcutaneous tissue. It is usually bacterial in origin. The term _____ is a constructed word, cellul/itis, which literally means "inflammation of little cells." The related term used for follicle infection, **folliculitis** (foh LIK yoo LYE tiss), is also a constructed word. It means "inflammation of little follicles."

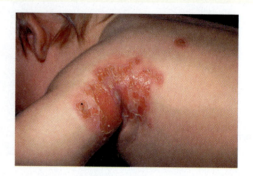

■ Figure 5.12
Cellulitis.
Source: Centers for Disease Control and Prevention.

dermatitis
  der mah TYE tiss

[Handwritten note: skin inflammation]

[Handwritten note: atopic dermatitis: most common]

eczema
  EK zeh mah

[Handwritten note: asthma & hayfever correlation to eczema]

5.44 Dermatitis is a generalized inflammation of the skin, involving edema (Frame 5.15) of the dermis (■ Figure 5.13). In addition to swelling, symptoms may include pruritus (Frame 5.28), urticaria (Frame 5.32), vesicles (Frame 5.34), and wheals (Frame 5.35), or some combination of these. The major types of _____ include **contact dermatitis**, caused by physical contact with a triggering substance such as poison ivy; **seborrheic** (SEB or EE ik) **dermatitis**, which is an inherited form characterized by excessive sebum production; and **actinic dermatitis**, caused by sunlight exposure. **Eczema** is a superficial form of dermatitis and may also be called **atopic dermatitis**. The primary symptoms of _____ include severe, chronic pruritus and deep scaliness. Dermatitis is a constructed word, dermat/itis, which literally means "inflammation of the skin," and eczema is derived from the Greek word *ekzeo*, which means "to boil over."

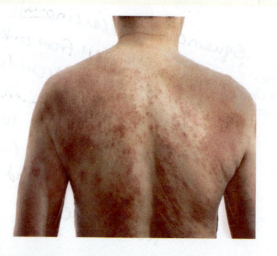

■ Figure 5.13
Dermatitis.
Source: joseph s l tan matt/Shutterstock.

ecchymosis
ek ih MOH siss

[handwritten: bruise]
[handwritten: bruise caused by trauma is a contusion]

5.45 Ecchymosis is a condition of the skin caused by leaking blood vessels in the dermis, producing purplish patches of purpura (Frame 5.29) that are larger in size than petechiae (Frame 5.27). The term _____ is a constructed word, ec/chym/osis, which literally means "condition of juice leaking out." The combining form chym/o comes from the Greek word *chymus*, meaning "juice."

herpes
HER peez

[handwritten: chronic virus]

5.46 A viral skin eruption producing clusters of deep blisters is known as **herpes**. The vesicles (Frame 5.34) appear periodically, affecting the borders between mucous membranes and skin. There are several types of _____, all of which are caused by the herpes simplex virus (HSV). The major types are **oral herpes**, caused by herpes virus type 1 (■ Figure 5.14), and **genital herpes**, caused by herpes virus type 2. Herpes is an infectious disease, transferable when the vesicles burst open and physical contact is made between the carrier and another person. In the absence of lesions, it may also be transferable by body fluid contact.

[handwritten: Shingles = herpes zoster, it's the chicken pox virus]

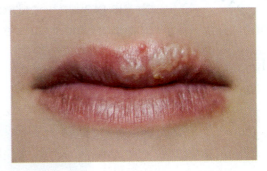

■ **Figure 5.14**
Herpes. The blisters often last for several days to a week and form in response to periodic outbreaks of the virus.
Source: Sergii Chepulskyi/ Shutterstock.

hyperhidrosis
HIGH per high DROH sis

[handwritten: excessive sweating condition]
[handwritten: (low blood sugar, nervous disorder, thyroid disease]

5.47 Sweating (perspiration) is a normal response by the skin's sweat glands to cool the body when you are hot, physically active, or nervous. In the condition **hyperhidrosis**, the individual sweats often and more than a normal amount. It is a constructed term, written hyper/hidr/osis, which literally means "condition of excessive sweat" because hidr/o is the combining form for "sweat." The condition of _____ may be caused by a nervous disorder, low blood sugar, or a thyroid disease.

[handwritten: mosquitos strep bacteria - need antibiotics]

[handwritten: Can lead to kidney failure]

impetigo
imp eh TYE goh

[handwritten: golden crust]

5.48 Impetigo is a contagious skin infection (■ Figure 5.15). Similar to oral herpes due to the development of small vesicles (Frame 5.34) usually forming around the lips, it is often caused by bacteria that enter a break in the skin (such as an animal or insect bite) and is characterized by the presence of golden crusts following the rupture of the vesicles. The term _____ is a Latin word meaning "scabby eruption."

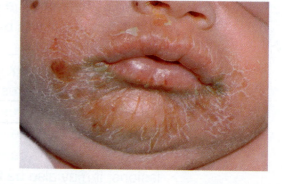

■ **Figure 5.15**
Impetigo. Note the presence of yellow crusts, which distinguishes this condition from the blisters in oral herpes (Figure 5.14).
Source: Mediscan/Alamy Stock Photo.

[handwritten: skin & lymphatic cancer common with HIV]

Kaposi sarcoma
KAP oh see * sar KOH mah

5.49 Kaposi sarcoma is a form of skin cancer arising from the connective tissue of the dermis (■ Figure 5.16). It is indicated by the presence of brown or purple patches on the skin and appears among some elderly patients. _____ _____ is also a common condition associated with HIV/AIDS.

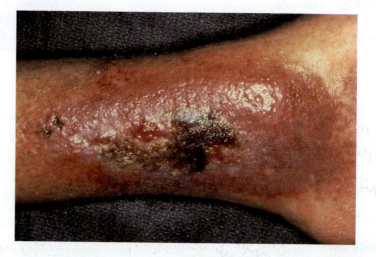

■ **Figure 5.16**
Kaposi sarcoma on the skin of the ankle.
Source: Centers for Disease Control and Prevention.

leukoderma
loo koh DER mah

5.50 As some people age, their skin becomes lighter in color due to reduced activity of the pigment-producing cells in the skin, the melanocytes. This condition is called **leukoderma**. The term _____ is a constructed word, leuk/o/derm/a, which literally means "white skin."

5.51 The most life-threatening skin cancer is **malignant melanoma**, which is shown in ■ Figure 5.17. It arises from the cells normally providing the pigment **melanin** (MELL ah nin) to the skin, called **melanocytes** (mell AN oh sites). _____ is a constructed term, melan/oma, which literally means "black tumor." Once established in the skin, the tumor grows rapidly and metastasizes (goes elsewhere in the body). About one-half of cases arise from nevi (moles).

melanoma

mell ah NOH mah

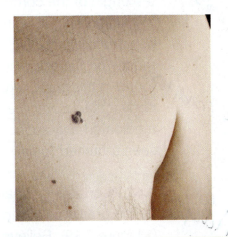

■ **Figure 5.17**
Melanoma. The telltale signs of this form of skin cancer include a change in size or color of a nevus and, as seen in this specimen, irregular borders.
Source: Librakv/Shutterstock.

ingrown nail

onychocryptosis

ON ih koh krip TOH siss

5.52 The combining form for nail is onych/o and is used in the construction of terms relating to nail diseases. In general, a disease of the nail is an **onychopathy** (ON ih KOHP a thee). In the nail condition called **onychocryptosis**, a nail becomes buried in the skin due to abnormal growth. It is commonly called an **ingrown nail**. The term _____ is a constructed word, onych/o/crypt/osis, and means "condition of hidden nail."

soft nails

onychomalacia

ON ih koh mah LAY she ah

5.53 In the condition **onychomalacia**, the nails are abnormally soft. The condition may be a result of calcium or vitamin D deficiency or a fungal infection (described in Frame 5.54). The term _____ is a constructed word, onych/o/malacia, which means "softening of the nail."

onychomycosis

ON ih koh my KOH siss

fungal infection of nails

5.54 The condition _____ is a fungal infection of one or more nails (■ Figure 5.18). Notice that the word root for fungus, myc, is included in this constructed term, onych/o/myc/osis, to form its meaning into "condition of nail fungus."

■ **Figure 5.18**
Onychomycosis.
Source: Australis Photography/ Shutterstock.

(handwritten note) infection beside the nail — usually from a hang nail

paronychia
pair oh NIK ee ah

5.55 In **paronychia**, the prefix *par-*, which means "alongside, abnormal," is included to build the term. Thus, the constructed word par/onych/ia means "condition of alongside the nail." As you might guess, _____ is an infection around the nail.

(handwritten note) parasites

pediculosis
peh dik yoo LOH siss

(handwritten note) lice condition

5.56 The Latin word for a parasitic body louse is *pediculus*, which is the origin of the combining form of *pedicul/o*. When this combining form is combined with the suffix for "condition of," it forms the constructed word _____. **Pediculosis** occurs mostly on the scalp, where it is called *head lice*, but it may also be found in the pubic region (called *pubic lice*) and other parts of the body (called *body lice*). Pediculosis can be treated effectively with medicated shampoo. The small eggs laid by lice can sometimes be seen attached to hair shafts and are called **nits**.

(handwritten note) Silvery color scales itchy thought to be genetic

psoriasis
soh RYE ah siss

5.57 Psoriasis is a painful, chronic disease of the skin characterized by the presence of red lesions covered with silvery epidermal scales (■ Figure 5.19). Believed to be an autoimmune disease of the skin in which the body's own white blood cells attack healthy cells, _____ is a Greek word meaning "to itch" and is spelled exactly like the clinical term.

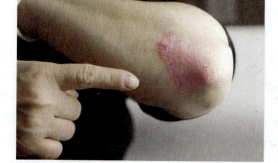

■ **Figure 5.19**
Psoriasis.
Source: Hriana/Shutterstock.

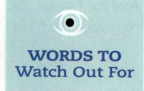

WORDS TO
Watch Out For

Psoriasis

Psoriasis is a very commonly misspelled term. It is one of the medical terms that is spelled with a silent *p* (terms with the word root *psych* are the others). One way to remember to include the *p* is to think of the **p**atches of red lesions that characterize this condition.

[handwritten: tiny mites that burrow under the skin]

scabies
SKAY bees

[handwritten: parasites]

[handwritten: between fingers wrist, abdomen } starts in these areas]

5.58 The condition **scabies** is a skin eruption caused by the female itch mite, which burrows into the skin to extract blood (■ Figure 5.20). From the Latin word *scabere* that means "scratch," _____ produces the symptoms of dermatitis (Frame 5.44), such as erythema (Frame 5.16), swelling or edema (Frame 5.15), and pruritus (Frame 5.28).

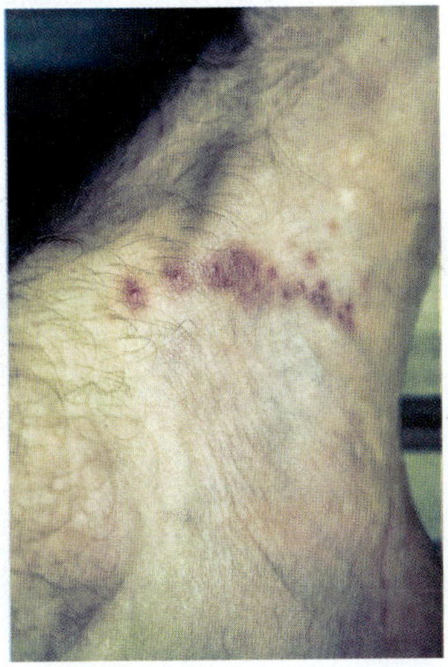

■ **Figure 5.20**
Scabies.
Source: Jaroslav Moravcik/ Shutterstock.

scleroderma
sklair oh DER mah

5.59 Scleroderma uses the combining form *scler/o*, which means "hard." It is an abnormal thickening or hardness of the skin, caused by overproduction of collagen in the dermis. The term _____ is a constructed word, *scler/o/derm/a*, which means "skin hardness."

systemic lupus erythematosus
sis TEM ik * LOO pus *
air ih them ah TOH siss

[handwritten: lupus]

5.60 Systemic lupus erythematosus, abbreviated **SLE**, is a chronic, progressive disease of connective tissue in many organs including the skin. The early stages of _____ _____ _____, commonly referred to as just **lupus**, are marked by red patches on the skin of the face and joint pain.

? Did You **KNOW**

LUPUS
The Latin word for wolf is *lupus*. The disease lupus was named by the appearance of the reddish face rash that reminded early physicians of the face of a wolf.

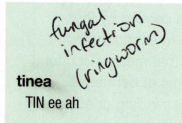

tinea
TIN ee ah

5.61 Tinea is a fungal infection of the skin. It is often called **ringworm** because of the ring-shaped pattern on the skin that forms in response to the fungi (■ Figure 5.21). In fact, the term _____ is the Latin word for worm or larval moth. The three major forms of tinea are **tinea capitis**, which forms on the scalp and can lead to alopecia (Frame 5.39); **tinea pedis**, which forms on the feet and is also known as athlete's foot; and **tinea corporis**, which may occur elsewhere on the body.

(handwritten note: fungal infection (ringworm))

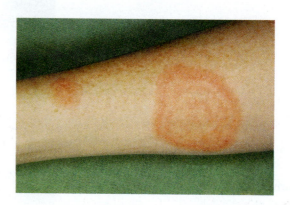

■ **Figure 5.21**
Tinea. Although it is a fungal infection, tinea is often called *ringworm*.
Source: Mediscan/Alamy Stock Photo.

(handwritten note: hair fungus)

trichomycosis
TRIK oh my KOH siss

5.62 A general term for a disease affecting the hair is **trichopathy** (trye KOH path ee), which connects the combining form for hair (*trich/o*) and the suffix for disease (*-pathy*). The condition **trichomycosis** is a fungal infection of hair. In this constructed term, trich/o/myc/osis, the combining form for *hair* and the word root for *fungus* are combined to form the term _____.

xeroderma
zee roh DER mah

5.63 The combining form *xer/o* means "dry"; when this is combined with the word root that means "skin," it forms the word _____. Not surprisingly, the disease **xeroderma** is characterized by abnormally dry skin. It is caused by hyposecretion (abnormally low secretion) of the oil glands and is an inherited condition. It is a constructed term, xer/o/derm/a, which literally means "dry skin."

PRACTICE: Diseases and Disorders of the Integumentary System

The Right Match

Match the term on the left with the correct definition on the right.

_____ 1. tinea

_____ 2. acne

_____ 3. burn

_____ 4. herpes

_____ 5. alopecia

_____ 6. impetigo

_____ 7. scabies

_____ 8. psoriasis

a. results from bacterial infection of sebaceous glands and ducts

b. autoimmune disease of the skin characterized by red lesions covered with silvery epidermal scales

c. baldness

d. contagious bacterial skin infection with a yellowish crust

e. caused by excessive exposure to fire, electricity, chemicals, or sunlight

f. skin eruption caused by the female itch mite

g. viral skin eruption that produces clusters of deep blisters

h. fungal infection of the skin

Break the Chain

Analyze these medical terms:

   a) Separate each term into its word parts; each word part is labeled for you (**p** = prefix, **r** = root, **cf** = combining form, and **s** = suffix).

   b) For the Bonus Question, write the requested word part or definition in the blank that follows.

The first set has been completed for you as an example.

1. a)   dermatitis   ___**dermat/itis**___
                                        r   s

    b) *Bonus Question:* What is the definition of the suffix? ___**inflammation**_____

2. a)   melanoma   _____/_____
                                        r   s

    b) *Bonus Question:* What is the definition of the suffix? _____

3. a)   onychomycosis   _____/___/_____/_____
                                        cf   r   s

    b) *Bonus Question:* What is the definition of the *second* word root? _____

4. a)   pediculosis   _____/_____
                                        r   s

    b) *Bonus Question:* What is the definition of the suffix? _____

5. a)   scleroderma   _____/___/_____/_____
                                        cf   r   s

    b) *Bonus Question:* What is the definition of the combining form? _____

6. a)   trichomycosis   _____/___/_____/_____
                                        cf   r   s

    b) *Bonus Question:* What is the definition of the *combining* form? _____

7. a) cellulitis _____/_____
                        r   s

    b) *Bonus Question:* What is the definition of the suffix? _____

8. a) leukoderma _____/___/_____/_____
                        cf   r   s

    b) *Bonus Question:* What is the definition of the *second* word root? _____

Treatments, Procedures, and Devices of the Integumentary System

Review some of the word parts that specifically apply to the treatments, procedures, and devices of the integumentary system that are covered in the following section. Note that the word parts are color-coded to help you identify them: prefixes are yellow, combining forms are red, and suffixes are blue.

Combining Form	Definition
abras/o	to rub away
aut/o	self
derm/o, dermat/o	skin
rhytid/o	wrinkle

Suffix	Definition
-ectomy	surgical excision, removal
-ion	process
-plasty	surgical repair
-tome	cutting instrument

KEY TERMS A–Z

biopsy
BYE op see

5.64 A **biopsy** is a minor surgery involving the removal of tissue for evaluation. Abbreviated **bx** or **Bx**, a _____ is usually a necessary step toward making a diagnosis of a suspected tumor of the skin.

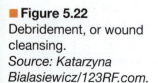
Wound cleansing

debridement
de-BREED-ment

5.65 Wounds are often complicated by physical contact with a dirty object, including the ground. To clean the wound, a procedure called **debridement** is often used (■ Figure 5.22). A French word meaning "unbridled," _____ involves excision (surgical removal) of foreign matter and unwanted tissue.

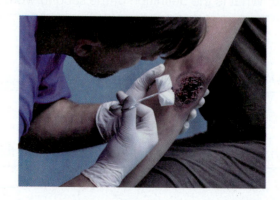

■ **Figure 5.22**
Debridement, or wound cleansing.
Source: Katarzyna Bialasiewicz/123RF.com.

dermabrasion
DERM ah BRAY zhun

5.66 Remember that the combining form *derm/o* means "skin." When combined with the suffix that means "process" and the combining form that means "to rub away," *abras/o*, it forms the word _____. **Dermabrasion** is a form of **cosmetic surgery**, in which the skin is surgically changed to improve appearance. During dermabrasion, abrasives similar to sandpaper are used to remove unwanted scars and other elevations and may also be used to remove tattoos. Alternatives to dermabrasion include **chemical peels**, in which a chemical agent is used to remove the outer epidermal layers to treat acne, wrinkles, and sun-damaged skin.

Skin graft from one own self

dermatoheteroplasty graft from someone else

dermatoautoplasty
DER mah toh AW toh
PLASS tee

5.67 Some burns and similar injuries cause extensive damage to a large area of skin, challenging the normal healing process. In these cases, the surgical procedure of **dermatoautoplasty** may be used to improve healing. This is a constructed term that can be written as dermat/o/aut/o/plasty. In this term, note the combining form that means "self," *aut/o*. This surgery involves using the patient's own skin as a graft, usually after it has grown in a media solution. _____ is also called an **autograft**. Alternatively, a skin graft from another person may be used. This procedure is called **dermatoheteroplasty** (DER mah toh HETT er oh PLASS tee), or **allograft**. During both procedures, an instrument

knife to cut skin, or area of skin supplied by a particular spinal nerve

dermatome
DER mah tohm

called a **dermatome** (DER mah tohm) is used to cut thin slices of skin for grafting. A _____ may also be used to excise small skin lesions. Recall that the suffix *-tome* means "cutting instrument."

Surgical repair- skin graft

dermatoplasty
DER mah toh plass tee

5.68 The general term for a surgical procedure of the skin is **dermatoplasty**. This term uses the combining form that means "skin" with the suffix *-plasty*, which means "surgical repair." In _____, skin tissue is transplanted to the body surface.

emollient
ee MALL ee ant

5.69 An _____ is a chemical agent that softens or smooths the skin. Topical and oral **antibiotics** (ahn tye bye OT iks) are used to manage infections, such as acne and carbuncles. **Retinoids** (RET ih noydz) may also be used to manage certain forms of acne because they cause the upper layers of the epidermis to slough away. Acne and related disorders may also be treated by **ultraviolet light therapy**, which causes a similar effect on the epidermis.

Chemical peel, acne med- toxic

Antibiotics only for bacteria

surgical repair [handwritten]

rhytidectomy
rit ih DEK toh mee

surgical removal of wrinkle [handwritten]

5.70 Plastic surgery is a popular form of skin treatment that is used for skin repair following a major injury, correction of a congenital defect, or cosmetic improvement. Several of the terms related to plastic surgery use the combining form *rhytid/o*, which means "wrinkle." Plastic surgeries that are primarily cosmetic include **rhytidoplasty** (RIT ih doh PLASS tee), which is the surgical repair of skin wrinkles (■ Figure 5.23); _____, during which wrinkles are surgically removed; and **liposuction** (LIE poh suk shun), which is the removal of subcutaneous fat (fat immediately deep to the skin) by insertion of a device that applies a vacuum to pull the fat tissue out of the body.

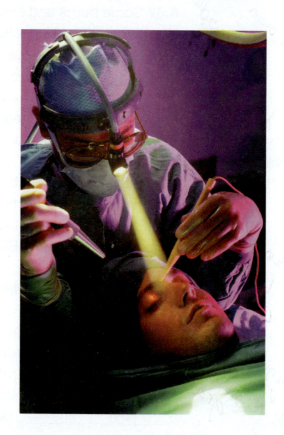

■ Figure 5.23
Rhytidoplasty. This is a common form of plastic surgery in which the skin is pulled and sutured to decrease skin wrinkles.
Source: Kim Steele/Photodisc/ Getty Images.

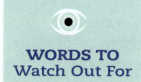

WORDS TO Watch Out For

The *Y* in Rhytid

It may be tempting to spell the term *rhytidectomy* with an *i* instead of a *y*. One way to remember to use a *y* is to think of the word *elderly*. As you've learned, the word root *rhytid* means "wrinkle." Elderly people commonly have wrinkles, and the word *elderly* ends with a *y*.

PRACTICE: Treatments, Procedures, and Devices of the Integumentary System

The Right Match

Match the term on the left with the correct definition on the right.

_____ 1. biopsy	a. chemical agent that softens or smooths the skin
_____ 2. emollient	b. wound-cleaning procedure
_____ 3. debridement	c. surgically changing the skin to improve appearance
_____ 4. cosmetic surgery	d. surgery that uses a patient's own skin as a graft
_____ 5. autograft	e. the removal of tissue for evaluation

Linkup

Link the word parts in the list to create the terms that match the definitions. You may use word parts more than once. Remember to add in combining vowels when needed—and that some terms do not use any combining vowel. The first one is completed for you as an example.

Combining Form	Suffix
abras/o	-ectomy
aut/o	-ion
derm/o, dermat/o	-plasty
rhytid/o	-tome

Definition   **Term**

1. use of abrasives to remove unwanted scars and tattoos   *dermabrasion*
2. surgical repair of skin wrinkles   _____
3. surgical repair of the skin   _____
4. surgery that involves the use of the patient's own skin to improve healing   _____
5. an instrument that is used to cut thin slices of skin for grafting   _____

Abbreviations of the Integumentary System

The abbreviations that are associated with the integumentary system are summarized here. Study these abbreviations and review them in the exercise that follows.

Abbreviation	Definition	Abbreviation	Definition
BCC	basal cell carcinoma	SLE *LUPUS*	systemic lupus erythematosus
bx, Bx	biopsy	SqCCa	squamous cell carcinoma
HSV	herpes simplex virus	TBSA	total body surface area

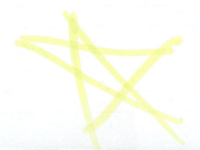

PRACTICE: Abbreviations

Fill in the blanks with the abbreviation or the complete medical term.

Abbreviation	Medical Term
1. _____	biopsy
2. BCC	_____
3. _____	systemic lupus erythematosus
4. SqCCa	_____
5. _____	total body surface area
6. HSV	_____

CHAPTER REVIEW

Word Building

Construct medical terms from the following meanings. The first question has been completed for you as an example.

1. literally means "black tumor"   melan**oma**_____

2. inflammation of connective tissue   _____itis

3. disease of the nail   _____pathy

4. fungal infection of a nail   onycho_____

5. abnormally dry skin   _____derma

6. a skin wound caused by scraping   abras_____

7. an infection arising from a follicle   _____itis

8. disease that affects the hair   tricho_____

9. blisters that later form a yellowish crust   _____igo

10. a small, solid circumscribed skin elevation   nev_____

11. a discolored flat spot   _____ule

12. derived from the Latin word "to soften"   emoll_____

Define the Combining Form

In the space provided, write the definition of the combining form, followed by one example of the combining form used to build a medical term in Chapter 5.

	Definition	Use in a Term
1. derm/o	_____	_____
2. follicul/o	_____	_____
3. actin/o	_____	_____
4. kerat/o	_____	_____
5. melan/o	_____	_____
6. trich/o	_____	_____
7. onych/o	_____	_____

Complete the Labels

Complete the blank labels in ■ Figure 5.24 by writing the labels in the space provided.

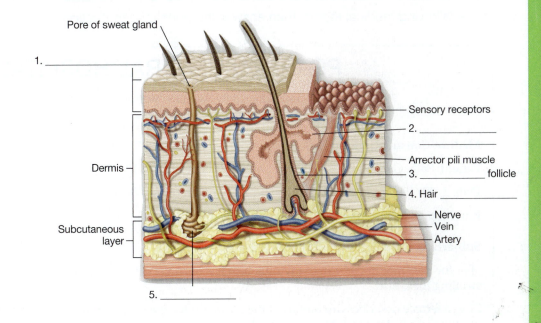

Pore of sweat gland

1. _____

Sensory receptors

2. _____
   _____

Arrector pili muscle

3. _____ follicle

4. Hair _____

Nerve
Vein
Artery

Dermis

Subcutaneous layer

5. _____

■ **Figure 5.24**
Anatomy of the skin.

1. _____
2. _____
3. _____
4. _____
5. _____

MyLab Medical Terminology™

MyLab Medical Terminology is a premium online homework management system that includes a host of features to help you study. Registered users will find:

- A multitude of quizzes and activities built within the MyLab platform
- Powerful tools that track and analyze your results—allowing you to create a personalized learning experience
- Videos and audio pronunciations to help enrich your progress
- Streaming lesson presentations (Guided Lectures) and self-paced learning modules
- A space where you and your instructors can view and manage your assignments

MEDICAL REPORT EXERCISES

Sally Garcia

Read the following medical report, then answer the questions that follow.

PGH

PEARSON GENERAL HOSPITAL

5500 University Avenue, Metropolis, New York
Phone: (211) 594-4000 • Fax (211) 594-4001

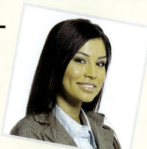

Medical Consultation: Dermatology   **Date:** 07/15/2017

Patient: Sally Garcia   **Patient ID:** 123456

Dob: 3/20/1996   **Age:** 21   **Sex:** Female   **Allergies:** NKDA

Provider: Jane K. Hernandez, MD

Subjective:

"For the past month the skin of my right arm has been very itchy, and sometimes painful. I have noticed swelling there also."

21 y/o female describes discomfort of the right arm for the past month. About a month ago, she began working in a factory warehouse where she reports exposure to dust and high humidity. She reports that chemicals had been used in the workplace, but she does not know what chemicals. She indicated no relevant family history issues of the skin.

Objective:

Vital Signs: T: 98.6°F; **P:** 78; **R:** 20; **BP:** 118/77

Ht: 5′5″

Wt: 123 lb

General Appearance: No obvious signs of physical stress noted, such as edema, pallor, or diaphoresis.

Except for right arm, skin appears healthy. Skin of right arm shows some erythema and edema, and formation of scar tissue is evident. There is a 3 cm × 1 cm keloid on the lateral aspect of right arm.

Heart: Rate at 78 bpm, with no abnormal sounds.

Lungs: CTA

AbD: Bowel sounds normal all four quadrants.

MS: Joints and muscle symmetric. No swelling, masses, or deformity.

Assessment:

Contact dermatitis of right arm.

Plan:

1. Treat dermatitis with topical 2% cortisone. Advise patient to refrain from scratching the site.

2. Schedule follow-up appointment in 2 weeks. If inflammation persists, antibiotic ointment to be administered.

Photo Source: Imging/Shutterstock.

Comprehension Questions

1. What is the probable cause of the scars on her arm? _____

    _____

    _____

2. If the symptom of pruritus returns after the initial treatment, how might the formation of new scar tissue be prevented? _____

    _____

    _____

3. Why do you think antibiotic therapy is included in the follow-up treatment if the condition persists?

    _____

    _____

Case Study Questions

The following case study provides further discussion regarding the patient in the medical report. Fill in the blanks with the correct terms. Choose your answers from the following list of terms. (Note that some terms may be used more than once.)

actinic keratosis	ulcers	pruritus	emollients
dermatitis	biopsy	vesicles	
keloids	dermatology	cicatrices	

At the (a) _____ clinic where patients with skin ailments are referred, Sally Garcia,

a patient with an unusual skin condition, was observed. The skin condition included a generalized skin

inflammation, or (b) _____, which included abnormal redness, swelling, and pain.

Skin damage caused by sunlight, a precancerous condition known as (c) _____

_____, was ruled out as a diagnosis, along with all known forms of skin cancer. Rather,

an allergic agent was the likely cause. After several days of general inflammation, fluid-filled skin elevations,

or (d) _____, appeared. The elevations gave the patient symptoms of itching or

(e) _____. Scratching the elevations produced open sores, or (f) _____,

which upon healing left scars, or (g) _____. In some areas, the scar tissue became

overgrown, forming (h) _____. Treatment included the application of topical ointments,

or (i) _____, and antibiotic treatments were prescribed during follow-up.

Patricia Velasquez

For a greater challenge, read the following medical report and answer the questions that follow.

PGH   **PEARSON GENERAL HOSPITAL**

5500 University Avenue, Metropolis, New York
Phone: (211) 594-4000 • Fax (211) 594-4001

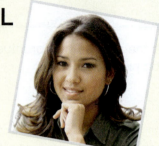

Medical Consultation: Dermatology   **Date:** 05/30/2017

Patient: Patricia Velasquez   **Patient ID:** 123456

Dob: 1/15/1990   **Age:** 27   **Sex:** Female   **Allergies:** NKDA

Provider: Robert M. O'Brady, MD

Subjective:

"The skin on the top of my right shoulder is sensitive to the touch and hurts when I put on clothes."

27 y/o female complains of skin sensitivity and pain at the top of her right shoulder. She has spent a lot of time outdoors since childhood due to her interest in competitive swimming and diving. She knows of no history of skin disease in her immediate family.

Objective:

Vital Signs: T: 98.8°F; **P:** 75; **R:** 19; **BP:** 116/75

Ht: 5'3"

Wt: 110 lb

General Appearance: No obvious signs of physical stress noted, such as edema, pallor, or diaphoresis.

Skin tone is healthy. Numerous freckles and nevi are present, and at the top of the right shoulder is a single nevus larger than others that is not circumscribed and surrounded with erythema. The nevus measures 0.9 cm dia.

Heart: Rate at 75 bpm, with no abnormal sounds.

Lungs: CTA

AbD: Bowel sounds normal all four quadrants.

MS: Joints and muscle symmetric, with very little SC fat. No swelling, masses, or deformity.

Assessment:

Possible melanoma on right shoulder.

Plan:

Outpatient excision of mass approved by patient, with lidocaine injection and removal with #8 scalpel.

Biopsy sent to lab for analysis.

Photo Source: ESB Basic/Shutterstock.

Comprehension Questions

1. What patient behaviors support the initial diagnosis? _____

_____

_____

2. What is a common word for nevus? _____

_____

_____

3. Do you think antibiotic therapy should be included in the treatment? _____

_____

_____

Case Study Questions

The following case study provides further discussion regarding the patient in the medical report. Recall the terms from this chapter to fill in the blanks with the correct terms.

Patricia Velasquez, a 25-year-old female, had trained for competitive swimming and diving since the age

of 12 years. According to her mother, Patricia has had no prior medical concerns and was given the usual

vaccinations as a young child. Several months before Patricia's visit to her personal physician, she had been

complaining of a nagging irritation on the skin of her right shoulder. Because, at first, she believed the skin

irritation to be a minor response to a new skin lotion, or (j) _____, she delayed consulting

a physician. When her mother noticed the mole, or (k) _____, on Patricia's right shoulder

had changed in shape and become darker, she decided to make an appointment. After a physical exam

with otherwise negative findings, her personal physician observed the mole and referred her immediately to

a skin specialist, or (l) _____. Upon observing the nevus, which had increased in size from

0.5 cm to 0.9 cm since her prior appointment only 3 weeks earlier, the skin specialist recorded the lesion as

a possible form of skin cancer arising from pigment-producing skin cells, called (m) _____.

He determined that an immediate course of action was necessary and asked for Patricia's approval to remove

the suspected tumor as an outpatient treatment in his office. Patricia agreed, and the specialist performed

the minor surgery within minutes. The specimen was sent to the lab for analysis as part of the biopsy

procedure, abbreviated (n) _____. Because of the large incision necessary, a skin repair

procedure, (o) _____, was performed to aid healing and prevent the formation of a scar,

or (p) _____. Although the lab reported that the specimen was positive for melanoma, the

specimen did not show evidence of metastasis, so no further cancer treatments were deemed necessary.

Chapter 6

The Skeletal and Muscular Systems

Learning Objectives

After completing this chapter, you will be able to:

6.1 Define and spell the word parts used to create medical terms for the skeletal and muscular systems.

6.2 Break down and define common medical terms used for symptoms, diseases, disorders, procedures, treatments, and devices associated with the skeletal and muscular systems.

6.3 Build medical terms from word parts associated with the skeletal and muscular systems.

6.4 Pronounce and spell common medical terms associated with the skeletal and muscular systems.

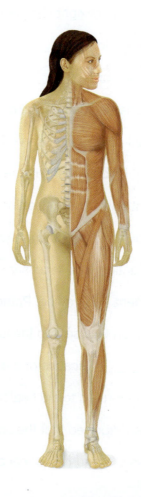

Anatomy and Physiology Terms

The following table provides the combining forms that commonly apply to the anatomy and physiology of the skeletal and muscular systems. Note that the combining forms are colored red to help you identify them when you see them again later in the chapter.

Combining Form	Definition
arthr/o	joint
articul/o	joint
burs/o	purse or sac, bursa
carp/o	wrist
chondr/o	cartilage
condyl/o	knuckle of a joint
cost/o	rib
cran/o, crani/o	skull, cranium
fasci/o	fascia
femor/o	thigh, femur
fibr/o	fiber
fibul/o	fibula
ili/o	flank, hip, groin, ilium of the pelvis
ischi/o	haunch, hip joint, ischium
menisc/o	meniscus
muscul/o	muscle
my/o, myos/o	muscle
myel/o	bone marrow

Combining Form	Definition
orth/o	straight
oste/o	bone
pariet/o	wall
patell/o	patella
ped/o	child
petr/o	stone
phalang/o	phalanges
phys/o	growth
pub/o	pubis
radi/o	radius
sacr/o	sacred, sacrum
skelet/o	skeleton
spondyl/o	vertebra
stern/o	chest, sternum
synov/o, synovi/o	synovial
tars/o	tarsal bone
ten/o, tendon/o	stretch, tendon
vertebr/o	vertebra

musculoskeletal

MUS kyoo loh SKEHL eh tahl

movement

6.1 The skeletal and muscular systems are combined in this chapter because their organs, bones, and muscles are closely connected. Together they form the _____ **system**. Notice how this constructed term is assembled with four word parts: muscul/o/ skelet/al. As you know, the bones and muscles work together to support the body and produce body _____. In fact, nearly every one of the 206 bones in your body receives an attachment to one or more muscles.

Support
movement } purpose/function of MS system
Heat

muscle

bones

6.2 Each bone is an organ, composed of mainly connective tissue receiving blood vessels, lymphatics, and nerves. Bones support and protect soft internal organs, store mineral salts including calcium and phosphorus, and produce blood cells within the red bone marrow. They also serve as an attachment site for muscles. Joints are organs of the musculoskeletal system too and include the knee, elbow, shoulder, hip, and anywhere else in the body where two opposing bones meet. Each _____ is an organ also, composed mainly of skeletal muscle tissue and connective tissue. Muscles are attached to bones by way of tough, dense bands of connective tissue called **tendons**. As a muscle shortens in length by contraction, it pulls on the tendons attaching to _____ to produce body movement. The range of motion (ROM) produced by the muscle contraction is mainly determined by the type of joint between the opposing bones. The joints of the body allowing the greatest ROM, such as the shoulder and knee, are known as *synovial joints* because they are filled with a shock-absorbing fluid called *synovial fluid*. **Ligaments**, like tendons, are also bands of dense connective tissue, but they extend from bone to bone to stabilize and strengthen joints. For example, the anterior cruciate ligament (ACL) is a ligament that stabilizes the knee joint.

6.3 Review the anatomy of the musculoskeletal system by studying ■ Figures 6.1 through 6.3.

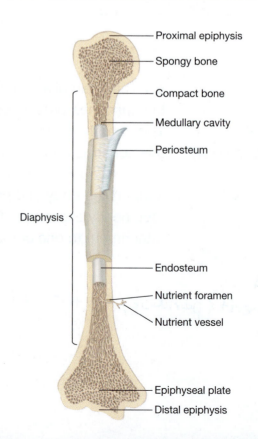

Proximal epiphysis

Spongy bone

Compact bone

Medullary cavity

Periosteum

Diaphysis

Endosteum

Nutrient foramen

Nutrient vessel

Epiphyseal plate

Distal epiphysis

■ **Figure 6.1**
Parts of a bone.

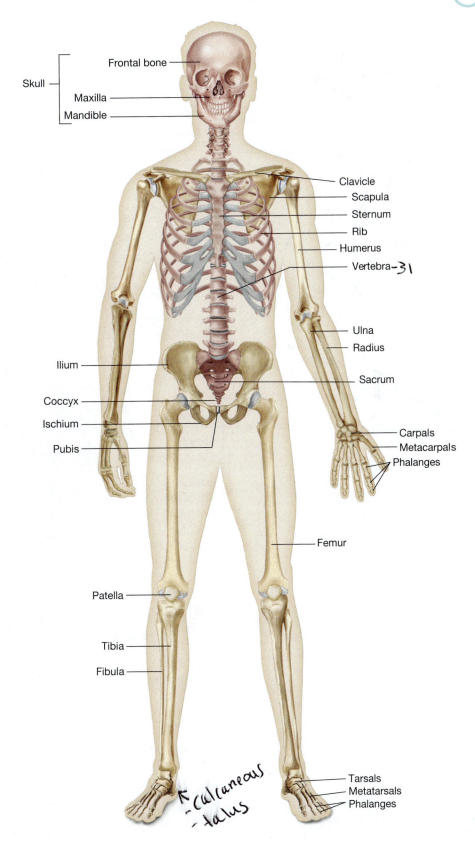

Figure 6.2
The bones of the skeleton.
The skeleton, anterior view.

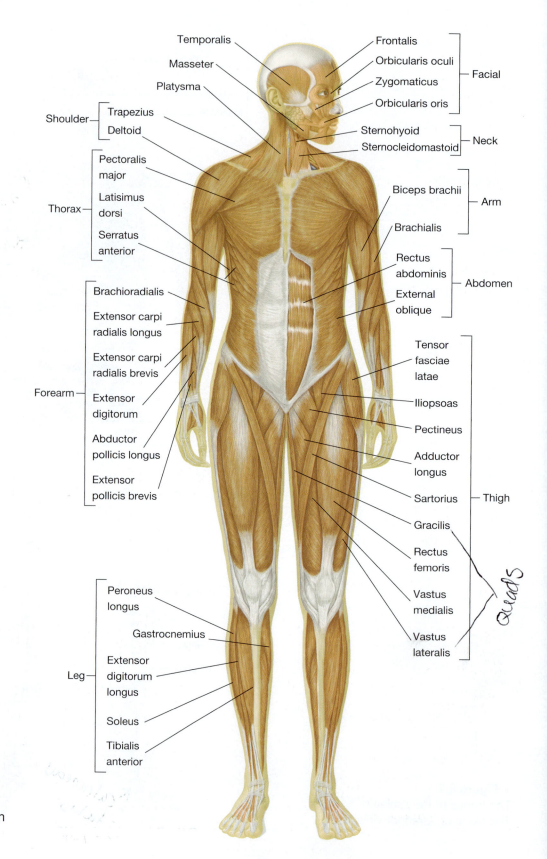

Temporalis
Masseter
Platysma
Shoulder — Trapezius
Deltoid
Thorax — Pectoralis major
Latisimus dorsi
Serratus anterior
Forearm — Brachioradialis
Extensor carpi radialis longus
Extensor carpi radialis brevis
Extensor digitorum
Abductor pollicis longus
Extensor pollicis brevis
Leg — Peroneus longus
Gastrocnemius
Extensor digitorum longus
Soleus
Tibialis anterior

Frontalis
Orbicularis oculi — Facial
Zygomaticus
Orbicularis oris
Sternohyoid — Neck
Sternocleidomastoid
Biceps brachii — Arm
Brachialis
Rectus abdominis — Abdomen
External oblique
Tensor fasciae latae
Iliopsoas
Pectineus
Adductor longus
Sartorius — Thigh
Gracilis
Rectus femoris
Vastus medialis
Vastus lateralis

Quads

■ **Figure 6.3**
The major muscles of the human body, anterior view.

Medical Terms of the Skeletal and Muscular Systems

orthopedic
OR thoh PEE dik

orthopedist
(OR thoh PEE dist)

6.4 The diseases of the skeletal and muscular systems are often the result of physical injury but can also be caused by infections, tumor development, endocrine disease, and inherited disorders. The branch of medicine focusing on these diseases is known as **orthopedics**, which is commonly abbreviated to **ortho**. The term _____ is a constructed word: orth/o/ped/ic. It includes the combining form orth/o, which is derived from the Greek word orthos and means "straight," and the word root ped, which is also from the Greek language and means "child." A physician specializing in this field of medicine is called an _____.

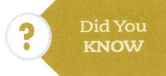

? **Did You KNOW**

ORTHOPEDICS
The term orthopedics was first coined in 1740 by French physician Nicholas Andry, who combined the two Greek word parts orthos ("straight") and ped ("child") into the term orthopedie ("straightening a child") to describe his medical practice of treating the broken limbs of children. The anglicized version of this term, orthopedic, entered worldwide medical use in 1840.

muscular
MUS kyoo lar

6.5 In the following sections, we review the prefixes, combining forms, and suffixes that combine to build the medical terms of the skeletal and _____ systems.

Signs and Symptoms of the Skeletal and Muscular Systems

Here are the word parts that specifically apply to the signs and symptoms of the skeletal and muscular systems that are covered in the following section. Note that the word parts are color-coded to help you identify them: prefixes are yellow, combining forms are red, and suffixes are blue.

Prefix	Definition
a-	without, absence of
brady-	slow
dys-	bad, abnormal, painful, difficult
hyper-	excessive, abnormally high, above

Combining Form	Definition
arthr/o	joint
kinesi/o	motion
my/o	muscle
tax/o	reaction to a stimulus, movement
ten/o	stretch, tendon
troph/o	development

Suffix	Definition
-a	singular
-algia	condition of pain
-dynia	condition of pain
-ia	condition of
-y	process of

KEY TERMS A–Z

arthralgia
ahr THRAL jee ah

[handwritten: Joint pain]

ataxia
ah TAK see ah

[handwritten: Jerky, uncoordinated muscle movement]

atrophy
AT roh fee

[handwritten: without development]

bradykinesia
BRAD ee kih NEE see ah

[handwritten: Condition of Slow movement]

decalcification
DEE kal sih fih KAY shun

6.6 Referring to the preceding word parts table, notice that the suffix -*algia* means "condition of pain." Add that to a combining form that means "joint," and it forms the word that means "condition of joint pain," or _____. This is often the first symptom of joint or bone disease. **Arthralgia** is also a common complaint following injury to a joint. The constructed form of this word is arthr/algia.

6.7 The word root *tax* means "reaction to a stimulus." By adding the prefix *a-* ("without"), the meaning of the term becomes negative. When the suffix -*ia* ("condition of") is added, it forms the word _____, which is the inability to coordinate muscles during a voluntary activity. **Ataxia** is a sign of a nervous system disorder, often inherited, that results in a loss of muscle coordination. The constructed form of this word is a/tax/ia.

6.8 Stabilizing a broken limb by casting it in plaster is a common treatment for bone fractures. It prohibits movement of the limb to promote the healing process. Unfortunately, the lack of movement leads to a reduction in muscle strength due to disuse, a sign of reduced muscle size known as **atrophy**. The muscle reduction is reversible when healing is complete and muscle activity is restored. Similar to the term *ataxia*, the term _____ also uses the prefix *a-* to make the meaning of the word root negative. The word root *troph* means "development" and -*y* means "process of." The three word parts that form the word can be written as a/troph/y.

6.9 An abnormally slow movement is a clinical sign of an underlying bone, muscle, or nervous disorder. It is known as _____, which literally means "condition of slow motion." This term is a constructed word that can be written as brady/kines/ia, in which *brady-* means "slow," *kinesi* is the word root that means "motion," and the suffix -*ia* means "condition of." (Note that the *i* at the end of the word root is dropped when using a suffix that begins with an *i*.)

6.10 The abnormal reduction of calcium in bone is a clinical sign known as **decalcification**, which is often caused by a hormonal disorder upsetting the calcium balance between the bloodstream and bone. In many patients, _____ can be treated with a combination of hormonal therapy, a diet rich in calcium and vitamin D, and mild exercise.

dyskinesia
diss kih NEE see ah

difficult movement

6.11 Difficulty in movement is a common sign of a musculoskeletal disorder. Remember from the term *bradykinesia* that the word root *kinesi* means "motion" and the suffix *-ia* means "condition of." When the prefix *dys-* is added, it forms the word _____, which literally means "condition of bad, abnormal, painful, or difficult motion." The constructed form of **dyskinesia** can be written as dys/kines/ia.

dystrophy
DISS troh fee

6.12 A general symptom of progressive muscle weakness that results from a genetic mutation is often called a _____, which literally means "process of (*-y*) bad, abnormal, painful, or difficult (*dys-*) development (*troph*)." It is a constructed term that can be written as dys/troph/y. The progressive muscle weakness is a common symptom of nine known forms of the disease, most of which appear during early childhood and are collectively called **muscular dystrophies**.

hypertrophy
high PER troh fee

overgrowth

6.13 The sign of excessive muscle growth or development is known as _____. Although it is an abnormality, it is often induced by exercise enthusiasts by adding tension to weight-training activities. Muscular hypertrophy is produced by the addition of protein to muscle fibers, which is stimulated by strenuous muscle activity. The constructed form of this word is hyper/troph/y, in which *hyper-* means "excessive," *troph* means "development," and *-y* means "process of."

muscle pain

myalgia
my AL jee ah

6.14 During strenuous exercise, muscle cell activity may exceed the capacity of the cell to obtain and use oxygen during metabolism. When this occurs, the resulting "oxygen debt" will cause the cell to metabolize without oxygen (called *anaerobic respiration*), resulting in the buildup of lactic acid in the muscle tissue. Because lactic acid causes muscle pain, a common symptom of strenuous exercise is _____, which literally means "condition of muscle (*myo*) pain (*-algia*)." Its constructed form is my/algia. This form of **myalgia** is temporary, lasting about one day. Chronic forms of myalgia usually suggest an underlying musculoskeletal disease.

tenodynia
TEN oh DINN ee ah

tendon pain

6.15 Tendon pain, or **tenodynia**, is a common symptom of "weekend athletes": people who work inactive jobs during the workweek and become very active on their days off. The symptom of _____ usually indicates minor injury to one or more tendons, often lasting weeks or months. The suffix *-dynia* means "condition of pain," and *ten/o* means "stretch, tendon." The constructed form of this term is ten/o/dynia. If tenodynia is intense, it may indicate tearing of the tendons, which requires medical intervention. Remember that another suffix with the meaning of "condition of pain" is *-algia*.

PRACTICE: Signs and Symptoms of the Skeletal and Muscular Systems

Break the Chain

Analyze these medical terms:

a) Separate each term into its word parts; each word part is labeled for you (**p** = prefix, **r** = root, **cf** = combining form, and **s** = suffix).

b) For the Bonus Question, write the requested definition in the blank that follows.

The first set has been completed for you as an example.

1. a) arthralgia   _arthr/algia_
                                  r   s

   b) *Bonus Question*: What is the definition of the suffix? **_condition of pain_**

2. a) ataxia   _____ / _____ / _____
                                  p   r   s

   b) *Bonus Question*: What is the definition of the word root? _____

3. a) atrophy   _____ / _____ / _____
                                  p   r   s

   b) *Bonus Question*: What is the definition of the word root? _____

4. a) bradykinesia   _____ / _____ / _____
                                  p   r   s

   b) *Bonus Question*: What is the definition of the prefix? _____

5. a) dyskinesia   _____ / _____ / _____
                                  p   r   s

   b) *Bonus Question*: What is the definition of the word root? _____

6. a) dystrophy   _____ / _____ / _____
                                  p   r   s

   b) *Bonus Question*: What is the definition of the suffix? _____

7. a) hypertrophy   _____ / _____ / _____
                                  p   r   s

   b) *Bonus Question*: What is the definition of the prefix? _____

8. a) myalgia   _____ / _____
                                  r   s

   b) *Bonus Question*: What is the definition of the word root? _____

9. a) tenodynia   _____ / _ / _____
                                  cf   s

   b) *Bonus Question*: What is the definition of the suffix? _____

Diseases and Disorders of the Skeletal and Muscular Systems

Here are the word parts that commonly apply to the diseases and disorders of the skeletal and muscular systems and are covered in the following section. Note that the word parts are color-coded to help you identify them: prefixes are yellow, combining forms are red, and suffixes are blue.

Prefix	Definition
a-	without, absence of
epi-	upon, over, above, on top
para-	alongside, abnormal
poly-	excessive, over, many
quadri-	four

Combining Form	Definition
ankyl/o	crooked
arthr/o	joint
burs/o	purse or sac, bursa
carcin/o	cancer
carp/o	wrist
chondr/o	cartilage
condyl/o	knuckle of a joint
fibr/o	fiber
kyph/o	hump
leuk/o	white
lith/o	stone
lord/o	bent forward
menisc/o	meniscus
my/o, myos/o	muscle
myel/o	bone marrow
oste/o	bone
por/o	hole
sarc/o	flesh, meat
scoli/o	curved
spondyl/o	vertebra
synov/o, synovi/o	synovial
ten/o, tendon/o	stretch, tendon

Suffix	Definition
-algia	condition of pain
-asthenia	weakness
-cele	hernia, swelling, protrusion
-emia	condition of blood
-genesis	origin, cause
-itis	inflammation
-malacia	softening
-oma	tumor
-osis	condition of
-plasia	formation, growth
-plegia	paralysis
-ptosis	drooping

KEY TERMS A–Z

achondroplasia
ah kon droh PLAY zee ah

without cartilage formation (dwarfism)

6.16 Dwarfism is a condition characterized by abnormally short limbs and stature. A disease that causes dwarfism is _____. The term combines the prefix *a-* ("without, absence of"), the combining form *chondr/o* ("cartilage"), and the suffix *-plasia* ("formation, growth") to form the meaning "without cartilage formation." The constructed form of this term is a/chondr/o/plasia. About 80% of the cases of **achondroplasia** are caused by a random mutation of genes before birth, and the remaining 20% of cases are inherited. In either type, the condition involves the abnormal lack of growth of the skeleton, mainly long bones, resulting in a short and disproportional body form. See ■ Figure 6.4.

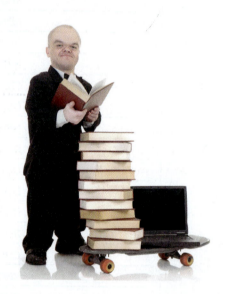

■ **Figure 6.4**
Achondroplasia. The individual in this photograph has the reduced limb development that typifies this cause of dwarfism.
Source: Sam100/Shutterstock.

ankylosis
an kill OH siss

stiff or abnormally crooked joints or bones

6.17 In the disease that literally means "condition of crooked," _____, joints are abnormally stiff and movement is difficult. **Ankylosis** is the abnormal adhesion of two bones, which damages the joint structure between them. When the condition affects two or more bones of the vertebral column to cause a rigid spine, it is called **ankylosing spondylitis (AS)**, in which spondylitis means "inflammation of vertebrae" (■ Figure 6.5). The constructed form of the term *ankylosis* is ankyl/osis, and *spondylitis* is spondyl/itis.

Spine without ankylosing spondylitis

Spine with ankylosing spondylitis

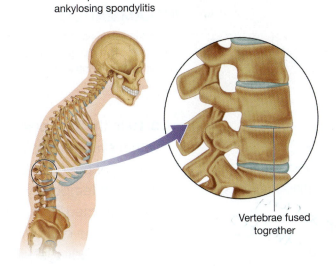

Vertebrae fused togrether

■ Figure 6.5
Ankylosing spondylitis. Side view of two subjects, in which a normal spine is compared to a spine with this condition. The inset shows a magnified view of the fusion that has occurred between adjacent vertebrae, which causes the loss of flexibility and posture.

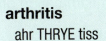

arthritis
ahr THRYE tiss

6.18 The general disorder resulting in inflammation and degeneration of a joint is known as _____. It literally means "joint inflammation," which is easy to see in the constructed form of the term, arthr/itis, in which *arthr* means "joint" and the suffix *-itis* means "inflammation." There are two major forms of arthritis, each with a different cause. **Osteoarthritis (OA)** is a common condition as people age, in which the joint structures become worn over time and are gradually replaced by bone. See ■ Figure 6.6. **Rheumatoid arthritis (RA)** is an autoimmune disease, in which joint structures become eroded by the action of the body's own white blood cells.

Septic Arthritis:
Joint is infected
w/ bacteria

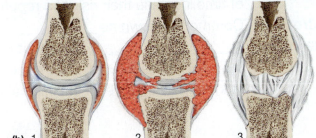

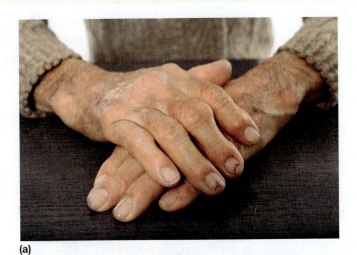

■ Figure 6.6
Arthritis. (a) Photograph of osteoarthritis within the joints of the fingers. (b) Progressive changes of rheumatoid arthritis: (1) inflammation of synovial membrane; (2) progressive inflammation and beginning of cartilage destruction; (3) complete loss of synovial membrane; and (4) complete joint loss.
Photo Source: Catalin Petolea/ Shutterstock.

(a)

(b) 1   2   3   4

? Did You KNOW

INFLAMMATION

The suffix *-itis* is used frequently in this chapter and means "inflammation." The Latin word *inflammatio* is the origin of this term, which literally means "to ignite" or "set ablaze." Because the symptoms of inflammation are heat, swelling, redness, and pain, this term is aptly named!

arthrochondritis
AHR throh kon DRY tiss

temporary arthritis

6.19 In the joint disease **arthrochondritis**, the articular cartilage within synovial joints undergoes inflammation, resulting in joint pain during movements. Unlike arthritis, _____ is usually a temporary condition caused by a localized infection. As a constructed term, it can be written arthr/o/chondr/itis by putting together the combining form *arthr/o* ("joint") with the word root *chondr* ("cartilage") and the suffix *-itis* ("inflammation").

bunion
BUN yun

Chronic inflammation & swelling of the Joint

6.20 A **bunion** is an abnormal enlargement of the joint at the base of the big toe. A _____ is caused by an inflammation of a bursa near the big toe.

? Did You KNOW

BUNION

The term *bunion* is derived from the Old French word *buigne*, which means "a swelling caused by a blow to the head." However, the modern meaning is limited to a swelling of the big toe.

bursitis
ber SIGH tiss

6.21 Remember that the suffix *-itis* means "inflammation," and the word root *burs* means "purse or sac," referring to a fluid-filled sac or bursa that cushions certain joints. So the inflammation of a bursa is known as _____. The constructed form of this term is burs/itis.

bursolith
BER soh lith

6.22 A calcium deposit within a bursa is known as a **bursolith**. The diagnosis of a _____ is confirmed with an x-ray, and it is often surgically removed. The word root *lith* is derived from the Greek word *lithos*, which means "a stone." The constructed form of this term is burs/o/lith. (Note that no suffix is used in this term.)

carpal tunnel syndrome
KAR pahl * TUN ul * SIN drohm

6.23 People working at computer stations for extended periods of time increase their risk of a repetitive stress injury of the wrist. Commonly known as _____ _____ _____, or **CTS**, it is characterized by inflammation of the wrist (tenosynovitis; see Frame 6.57) that causes pressure against the median nerve, resulting in local pain and restricted movement.

carpoptosis
KAR pop TOH siss

Wrist drooping

6.24 Also known as "wrist drop," the condition **carpoptosis** is a weakness of the wrist resulting in difficulty supporting the hand. _____ is a constructed term: carp/o/ptosis. It literally means "drooping of the wrist" (-*ptosis* is the suffix that means "drooping," and the combining form *carp/o* means "wrist").

cramps

6.25 Prolonged, involuntary muscular contractions cause pain wherever they occur, often striking the stomach wall or thigh muscles after strenuous exercise. The painful contractions are called _____.

DJD

Cartilage in joint degrades

6.26 A general term describing a disease of joints in which the cartilage undergoes degeneration is called **degenerative joint disease**, abbreviated _____. This type of disease is progressive, becoming worse in time. During the process of joint degeneration, the articular cartilage degrades and is often replaced with bone. Arthritis (see Frame 6.18) is the most common form of DJD.

Duchenne muscular dystrophy
doo SHEN * MUS kyoo lar * DIS troh fee

most common form affects boys more

6.27 Children are occasionally born with a disease causing skeletal muscle degeneration, resulting in progressive muscle weakness and deterioration. Abbreviated **DMD**, it is called **Duchenne muscular dystrophy**. Although it is the most intensively researched of the nine forms of muscular dystrophy (see Frame 6.12), a cure for _____ _____ _____ is yet to be found.

epicondylitis
ep ih kon dih LYE tiss

tennis elbow

6.28 When the suffix that means "inflammation" is combined with the word root *condyl* ("knuckle of a joint") and the prefix *epi-* ("upon, over, above, on top"), it forms the term _____. The epicondyles are small bony elevations on the humerus near the elbow joint. In epicondylitis, this area of the elbow becomes inflamed, usually due to an injury. The constructed form of this term is epi/condyl/itis.

fibromyalgia
FIE broh my AHL jee ah

fibers & muscle pain

6.29 A disease of unknown origin that produces widespread pain of musculoskeletal structures of the limbs, face, and trunk is known as **fibromyalgia**. This term is constructed with the combining form *fibr/o*, the word root *my*, and the suffix -*algia*, which together mean "condition of pain of the fibers and muscles." _____ can be written as the constructed form fibr/o/my/algia. Also known as **fibromyalgia syndrome**, there is some evidence that it may be a form of autoimmune disease, possibly triggered by infections or injury.

fracture
FRAK sher

6.30 The clinical term for a break in a bone is _____.
The most common fractures are simple, or closed, in which the
fracture is not visible from the skin, and open, or compound, in
which parts of the fractured bone visibly penetrate through the
skin to cause bleeding. Open fractures carry a much higher risk of
infection. Other types of fractures are described in Table 6.1 ■.

Table 6.1 ■ Common Bone Fractures

Type of Fracture	Definition	Illustration	Type of Fracture	Definition	Illustration
Colles' (KOH leez)	A break in the distal part of the radius, common in children		greenstick	A slight break in a bone that appears as a slight fissure in an x-ray exam	
comminuted	A break or breaks resulting in fragmentation of the bone		spiral	A spiral-shaped break, often caused by twisting stresses along the shaft	
oblique	A break along an oblique angle of the bone shaft		compression	A crushed break in a vertebra often due to an impact or fall	
transverse	A break along a transverse plane of the bone shaft		pathological	A fracture caused by another disease process that weakens the bone	

gout
GOWT

6.31 In **gout**, a person experiences sharp pain in the joints of the toes, especially the big toe. See ■ Figure 6.7. The pain of _____ is often exacerbated by a diet high in protein because the disorder is caused by an abnormal accumulation of uric acid crystals in the joints, which are waste products of protein metabolism. It is a form of arthritis because of the injury it causes to the joints. It is sometimes called *gouty arthritis*. Roughly 8 million people are currently diagnosed with gout in the United States, most of whom are men.

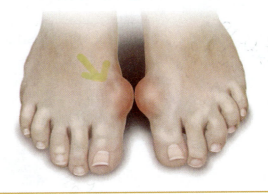

■ **Figure 6.7**
Gout. Also known as gouty arthritis, it often strikes the big toe, as seen in this illustration.

? Did You **KNOW**

GOUT
The term *gout* is derived from the Latin word *gutta*, which means "a drop." The foot pain that characterizes gout was thought to be caused by a body fluid dripping internally onto the joint. It was a malady common to European aristocracy before the 20th century, made worse by poor dietary habits that included diets high in protein and low in fresh vegetables and fruits.

herniated disk
HER nee ay ted * disk

gel comes out

6.32 The rupture of an intervertebral disk, which is a joint between two adjacent vertebrae of the spine, is called a **herniated disk**. It causes pressure against spinal nerves or the spinal cord to produce back pain. A _____ _____ is a back injury often caused by a sudden movement or an attempt to lift a heavy object. See ■ Figure 6.8.

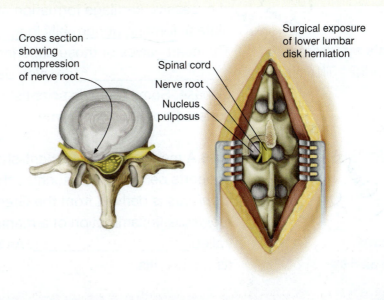

Cross section showing compression of nerve root

Surgical exposure of lower lumbar disk herniation

Spinal cord
Nerve root
Nucleus pulposus

■ **Figure 6.8**
Herniated disk. A herniated disk is a protrusion of the disk's gelatinous center, called the *nucleus pulposus*, which often pushes into the spinal cord or spinal nerves to cause pain and loss of movement (left illustration). The illustration on the right shows the back surgery necessary to access the injury.

kyphosis
kih FOH siss

humpback

lordosis
lor DOH siss

sway back

scoliosis
SKOH lee OH siss

side to side curve

6.33 Spinal curvatures are normal and help us to stand erect. However, some individuals suffer from a deformity of the spine that alters the normal curves. The three primary spinal deformities are **kyphosis**, **lordosis**, and **scoliosis**. A _____ occurs when the upper thoracic curve bends posteriorly, causing an abnormal hump at the upper back (*kyph* means "hump") that often accompanies osteoporosis (see Frame 6.45). A _____ is an exaggerated anterior spinal curve in the lumbar area (*lord* means "bent forward").
A _____ is a lateral curvature of the spine with a congenital origin, usually in the thoracic or lumbar regions (*scoli* means "curved"). See ■ Figure 6.9. All three terms for abnormal spinal curvatures are constructed terms. For example, scoliosis can be written as scoli/osis.

■ **Figure 6.9**
Spinal disfigurements. Kyphosis, or humpback, in which the upper thoracic curve bends posteriorly; lordosis, an exaggerated anterior curve in the lumbar region; and scoliosis, a lateral curvature.

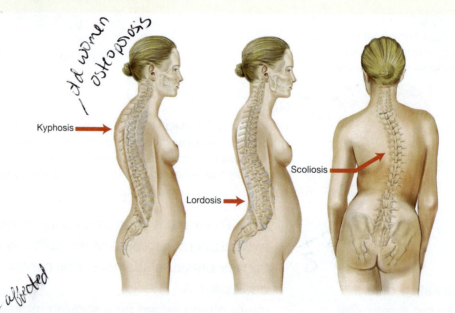

old women osteoporosis

Kyphosis

Lordosis

Scoliosis

Marfan's syndrome
mahr FAHNZ * SIN drohm

eyes are affected
heart
aorta

6.34 The congenital disease called **Marfan's syndrome** results in excessive cartilage formation at the epiphyseal plates (growth plates), forming abnormally long limbs and a tall, thin body form. The heart valves of those suffering from _____ _____ are also deformed, resulting in valvular heart disease. Some forensic scientists have argued that Abraham Lincoln suffered from this syndrome.

meniscitis
MEN ih SIGH tiss

inflammation of the knee cartilage

6.35 A meniscus is a crescent-shaped band of cartilage that supports certain joints, such as the knee and shoulder. The term *meniscus* is derived from the Greek word for "crescent moon," *meniskos*. Inflammation of a meniscus results in joint pain and is called _____. As a constructed term, it is written as menisc/itis.

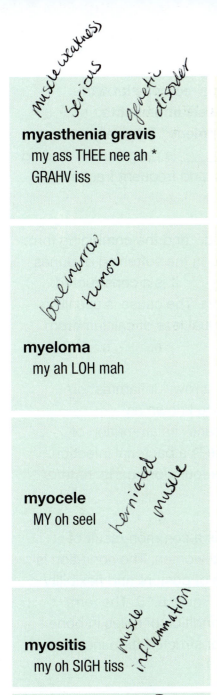

myasthenia gravis
my ass THEE nee ah *
GRAHV iss

muscle weakness
serious
genetic disorder

6.36 Myasthenia gravis is characterized by a progressive failure of muscles to respond to nerve stimulation. The term _____ _____ means "serious muscle weakness." The word *gravis* means "serious," and you may recognize *myasthenia*, which means "muscle weakness," as a constructed term: my/asthenia.

myeloma
my ah LOH mah

bone marrow
tumor

6.37 The red bone marrow is the site of blood cell formation. A malignant tumor associated with this tissue is a *myeloma*, sometimes called *multiple myeloma* or *plasma-cell myeloma*. It arises when a type of white blood cell, called a *plasma cell*, undergoes mutations to form a tumor that first appears in red bone marrow. The term _____ literally means "tumor of bone marrow," in which the root word *myel/o* means "bone marrow" and the suffix *-oma* means "tumor." The constructed form is myel/oma.

myocele
MY oh seel

herniated muscle

6.38 A muscle is surrounded by a layer of tough connective tissue, known as *fascia*. An injury to a muscle may cause the muscle to tear through the fascia, causing a protrusion. This condition is known as a **myocele**. The constructed form of the term _____ is my/o/cele, which is composed of the combining form for muscle, *my/o*, and the suffix *-cele*, which means "hernia, swelling, protrusion."

myositis
my oh SIGH tiss

muscle inflammation

6.39 A common result of muscle injury is a local inflammation known as **myositis**. Combining *myos* (which means "muscle") and *-itis* ("inflammation"), the constructed form of _____ is myos/itis.

osteitis
OSS tee EYE tiss

inflammation of the bone

6.40 When injured or exposed to infection, bone tissue often responds with inflammation. This condition, which combines the suffix that means "inflammation" and *oste*, the word root meaning "bone," is known as _____, which literally means "inflammation of bone." The constructed form is oste/itis.

osteitis deformans
OSS tee EYE tiss * day FOR
manz

bone overgrowth
pagets

6.41 Also called **Paget disease**, osteitis deformans results in bone deformities due to a failure of bone remodeling, which is a balance between bone loss and bone deposition. Common symptoms of _____ _____ include severe bone pain and frequent fractures. Recent evidence suggests this disease may be caused by a combination of environmental and genetic factors. It strikes roughly 1% of the adult population in the United States, mainly men over age 40.

osteogenesis imperfecta

OSS tee oh JEN eh siss * im per FEK tah

[handwritten: weak bones genetic]

6.42 An inherited disease resulting in impaired bone growth and fragile bones is known as **osteogenesis imperfecta**. The term means "imperfect bone development." Tragically, _____ _____ is progressive, leading to severe bone pain, skeletal deformities, and frequent fractures.

osteomalacia

OSS tee oh mah LAY she ah

[handwritten: Bone softening]

6.43 The suffix *-malacia* means "softening," and the combining form *oste/o* means "bone." A disease resulting in the softening of bones is generally known as _____. It is a constructed term with three word parts: oste/o/malacia. The cause is usually a hormonal imbalance, resulting in the gradual loss of calcium from bone tissue.

osteomyelitis

OSS tee oh my eh LYE tiss

[handwritten: Bone & bone marrow inflammation Bacterial infection]

6.44 The word root *myel* means "bone marrow." Inflammation of the red bone marrow is a painful disease known as _____, which literally means "inflammation of bone marrow and bone." The usual cause is a bacterial infection. **Osteomyelitis** is a constructed term with four word parts: oste/o/myel/itis.

osteoporosis

OSS tee oh por ROH siss

[handwritten: bone full of holes]

6.45 The abnormal loss of bone density is a common result of aging, especially among postmenopausal women. The condition is called **osteoporosis** and results in a loss of posture and flexibility and an increased risk of fractures. See ■ Figure 6.10. The term _____ literally means "condition of holes in bone." (The word root *por* means "hole.") The constructed term includes four word parts: oste/o/por/osis.

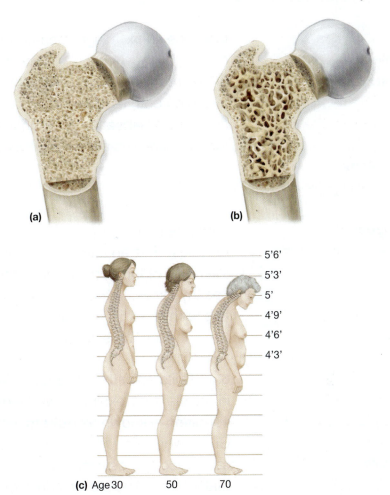

Figure 6.10
Osteoporosis. (a) A section through normal spongy bone. (b) A section through a bone with osteoporosis reveals a reduction of bone spicules and additional space. (c) Spinal curvatures resulting from osteoporosis of the vertebral column with advancing age.

osteosarcoma
OSS tee oh sar KOH mah

- hits teenagers
- amputation

6.46 An **osteosarcoma** (■ Figure 6.11) is bone cancer arising from connective tissue, usually within the bone itself. It is an aggressive form of cancer, striking mostly the young and middle teens. The constructed form of _____ is oste/o/sarc/oma. A second form of malignant bone cancer arises from the cells of the red bone marrow and is called **leukemia** (loo KEE mee ah). This term literally means "condition of white blood," named because of the high levels of deformed white blood cells in a blood sample that are a diagnostic of the disease. Leukemia is described further in Chapter 7.

Figure 6.11
Osteosarcoma. X-ray of the leg revealing an internal osteosarcoma just below the knee joint on the tibia.
Source: Wonderisland/Shutterstock.

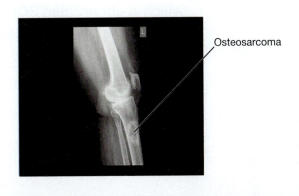

Osteosarcoma

paraplegia PAR ah PLEE jee ah **quadriplegia** KWAHD rih PLEE jee ah	**6.47** The suffix *-plegia* means "paralysis." One form of paralysis is _____, in which there is a loss of sensation or voluntary movement of the area of the body below the hips, including both legs. In another form of paralysis, all four limbs are without sensation or voluntary movement. The term for this form of paralysis utilizes a prefix that means "four" and is called _____.
polymyositis PAHL ee my oh SYE tiss	**6.48** The term _____ means "inflammation of many muscles." It is an autoimmune disease because the inflammation is the result of the body's own white blood cells attacking otherwise healthy tissue, in this case muscle tissue. The constructed form of this term is poly/myos/itis, in which the prefix *poly-* means "many," *myos* means "muscle," and the suffix *-itis* means "inflammation."
rickets RIHK ehts	**6.49** Children with a long-term deficiency of vitamin D or calcium in the diet may exhibit bowed legs and growth retardation. The condition is known as **rickets**, which is a modern version of the Greek word *rhakitis* that means "spine." Most _____ cases occur in developing countries because of widespread malnutrition. The skeletal deformities result from insufficient levels of vitamin D, calcium, or both in the bloodstream that lead to bone softening. When bone softening occurs in adults, it is called *osteomalacia* (Frame 6.43).
rotator cuff injury	**6.50** The rotator cuff is a combination of four muscles and their tendons that surround and stabilize the shoulder joint: teres minor, supraspinatus, infraspinatus, and subscapularis. A trauma to the shoulder can tear one or more tendons and muscles, resulting in a _____ _____ _____ that can cause local inflammation, pain, and joint dislocation.
spinal cord injury	**6.51** A trauma to the vertebral column may result in _____ _____ _____, which is abbreviated **SCI**. If severe, the injury can cause paralysis of areas of the body below the vertebral level of the injury.

spondylarthritis
SPON dill ahr THRYE tiss

arthritis of backbone

6.52 The clinical term that is formed by combining the suffix meaning "inflammation," the word root *arthr*, meaning "joint," and the word root *spondyl*, meaning "vertebra" is _____, which means "inflammation of joints of vertebrae." It is a general term for inflammatory diseases of the joints and their associated tendons and ligaments. Because the most common source of inflammation occurs in intervertebral joints, the most common symptom is low back pain. Ankylosing spondylitis, described in Frame 6.17, is an example of **spondylarthritis**. The constructed form of this term is spondyl/arthr/itis.

sprain

6.53 A _____ is a tear of collagen fibers within a ligament. See ■ Figure 6.12. It is usually caused by stretching the ligament beyond its normal range without warming up or slowly stretching before exercise.

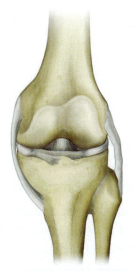
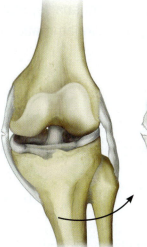
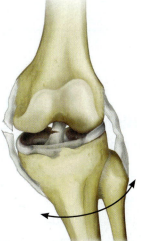

First-degree sprain
Localized joint pain and tenderness, but no joint laxity.

Second-degree sprain
Detectable joint laxity, plus localized pain and tenderness.

Third-degree sprain
Complete disruption of ligaments and gross joint instability.

■ **Figure 6.12**
Sprain. A sprain involves damage to one or more ligaments and is categorized into three degrees of injury as shown.

strain

damage to fibers in the muscle

6.54 Similar to a sprain but involving a muscle, a _____ is usually caused by stretching a muscle beyond its normal range. Muscle tissue tearing and the resulting capillary damage often cause a bruise.

temporomandibular joint disease TEMP or oh man DIH byoo lahr * JOYNT * dis EEZ	**6.55** The temporomandibular joint is the junction of the mandible and the temporal bone, which allows the lower jaw to move when speaking and chewing. A disease of this joint is known as _____ _____ _____, or **TMJ**, and results in frequent dislocations that make it difficult and painful to move the jaw during speaking and chewing.
tendonitis TEN dunn EYE tiss	**6.56** Inflammation of a tendon is a common sports injury and is known as _____. An example occurs when damage is caused by throwing a ball without warming up, which is known as **rotator cuff tendonitis**. *Tendonitis* is a constructed term, written as tendon/itis.
tenosynovitis TEN oh sin oh VYE tiss	**6.57** A form of tendonitis that includes inflammation of the synovial membrane surrounding the joint is known as _____. This term has four word parts: ten/o/synov/itis, in which *ten/o* means "stretch, tendon," *synov* means "synovial," and *-itis* means "inflammation."

PRACTICE: Diseases and Disorders of the Skeletal and Muscular Systems

The Right Match

Match the term on the left with the correct definition on the right.

_____ 1. Pott's

_____ 2. gout

_____ 3. bunion

_____ 4. Duchenne muscular dystrophy

_____ 5. cramps

_____ 6. sprain

_____ 7. fracture

_____ 8. strain

_____ 9. comminuted

_____ 10. rotator cuff injury

a. an abnormal enlargement of the joint at the base of the big toe

b. a condition that causes skeletal muscle degeneration, which results in progressive muscle weakness and deterioration; abbreviated DMD

c. prolonged, involuntary muscular contractions

d. a trauma that causes tearing of tendons and/or muscles of the shoulder

e. caused by an abnormal accumulation of uric acid crystals in the joints; usually affects the big toe joints

f. an injury that results from stretching a muscle beyond its normal range

g. a type of fracture that involves a break resulting in fragmentation of the bone

h. a tear of collagen fibers within a ligament

i. a type of fracture that involves a break at the ankle that affects both bones of the leg

j. clinical term for a break in the bone

Linkup

Link the word parts in the list to create the terms that match the definitions. You may use word parts more than once. Remember to add combining vowels when needed and that some terms do not use any combining vowel. The first one is completed as an example.

Prefix	Combining Form	Suffix
epi-	arthr/o	-asthenia
poly-	burs/o	-itis
	condyl/o	-malacia
	lith/o	-osis
	lord/o	
	menisc/o	
	my/o, myos/o	
	oste/o	
	synov/o	
	ten/o	

Definition

		Term
1.	weakness in the muscles	*myasthenia*
2.	inflammation of many muscles simultaneously	
3.	a spine deformity with an anterior curve of the spine	
4.	inflammation of bony elevations (epicondyles) near the elbow joint	
5.	inflammation and degeneration of a joint	
6.	a gradual and painful softening of bones	
7.	inflammation of a bursa	
8.	inflammation of bone tissue	
9.	a calcium deposit or stone within a bursa	
10.	inflammation of a meniscus	
11.	form of tendonitis that also involves inflammation of the synovial membrane	

Treatments, Procedures, and Devices of the Skeletal and Muscular Systems

Here are the word parts that commonly apply to the treatments, procedures, and devices associated with the skeletal and muscular systems and are covered in the following section. Note that the word parts are color-coded to help you identify them: combining forms are red and suffixes are blue.

Combining Form	Definition
arthr/o	joint
burs/o	purse or sac, bursa
chir/o	hand
chondr/o	cartilage
cost/o	rib
crani/o	skull, cranium
electr/o	electricity
fasci/o	fascia
lamin/o	thin, lamina
my/o	muscle
orth/o	straight
oste/o	bone
pod/o	foot
spondyl/o	vertebra
syn/o	connect
ten/o	stretch, tendon
vertebr/o	vertebra

Suffix	Definition
-centesis	surgical puncture
-clasia, -clasis	break apart
-desis	surgical fixation, fusion
-ectomy	surgical excision, removal
-gram	a record or image
-graphy	recording process
-iatry	treatment, specialty
-ist	one who specializes
-lysis	loosen, dissolve
-pathy	disease
-plasty	surgical repair
-rrhaphy	suturing
-scope	instrument used for viewing
-scopy	process of viewing
-tic	pertaining to
-tomy	incision, to cut

KEY TERMS A–Z

remove fluid from joint

arthrocentesis

AHR throh sen TEE siss

6.58 The suffix *-centesis* means "surgical puncture," and the combining form *arthr/o* means "joint." Many joint injuries result in the condition of inflammation, which may slow healing and lead to additional complications. In the procedure known as _____, excess fluids are **aspirated**, or withdrawn by suction, through a surgical puncture into the synovial cavity of the joint. See ■ Figure 6.13. This constructed term includes three word parts: arthr/o/centesis.

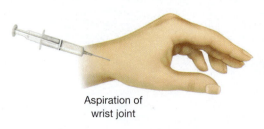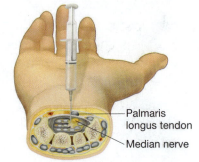

■ **Figure 6.13**
Arthrocentesis. The aspiration of fluid is a common treatment for joint injuries resulting in inflammation, such as carpal tunnel syndrome (CTS), shown in this illustration.

Aspiration of wrist joint

Palmaris longus tendon

Median nerve

arthroclasia

ahr throh KLAY see ah

Break joint during surgery to get it moving again

6.59 Occasionally, an abnormally stiff joint must be broken during surgery to increase the **range of motion**, or **ROM**. This procedure is called _____, in which the suffix *-clasia* means "break apart." After **arthroclasia**, it is common to undergo ROM exercises to increase muscle strength and joint mobility. Arthroclasia is a constructed term with three word parts: arthr/o/clasia.

arthrodesis

ahr throh DEE siss

6.60 The suffix *-desis* means "surgical fixation, fusion." Thus, the term _____ means "surgical fixation of a joint." The constructed form of this term is arthr/o/desis.

X ray of joint

arthrogram

AHR throh gram

6.61 Prior to joint surgery, it is common to obtain an x-ray of the joint after injection of contrast media, air, or both to highlight the synovial joint. The image is printed on a film or recorded digitally and is called an _____ because the suffix *-gram* means "a record or image" (■ Figure 6.14). The constructed form of this term is arthr/o/gram.

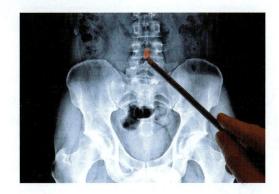

■ **Figure 6.14**
Arthrogram. X-ray of the lower back and pelvis that reveals inflammation (in red) of an intervertebral disc.
Source: Tlegend/Shutterstock.

arthrolysis

ahr THROL oh siss

dissolved & suctioned out

6.62 The suffix *-lysis* means "loosen, dissolve." During an _____, a joint is loosened of abnormal restrictions, such as calcium deposits and bursoliths (see Frame 6.22). The constructed form of this term is arthr/o/lysis.

arthroplasty

AHR throh PLASS tee

Joint repair

6.63 The suffix *-plasty* means "surgical repair." The goal of an _____ procedure is to repair a joint. A **complete arthroplasty** refers to a joint replacement, the most common of which is a knee replacement. The constructed form of this term is arthr/o/plasty.

arthroscopy

ahr THROSS koh pee

6.64 An endoscopic visual examination of a joint cavity uses an instrument that integrates fiber optics, live-action photography, and computer enhancement, known as an **arthroscope**. The viewing process is called _____. When arthroscopy is part of a surgery, the procedure is called **arthroscopic surgery**. See ■ Figure 6.15.

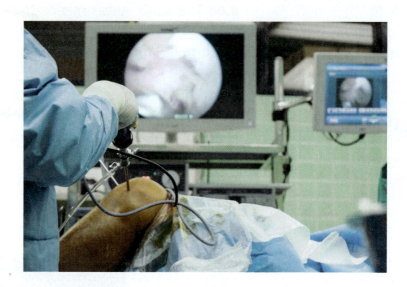

■ **Figure 6.15**
Arthroscopic surgery. In this photograph, the knee joint is undergoing surgery with a specialized endoscope called an _arthroscope_ in the procedure known as _arthroscopic knee surgery_.
Source: Samrith Na Lumpoon/ Shutterstock.

arthrotomy

ahr THROTT oh mee

cutting into joint

6.65 The suffix _-tomy_ means "incision, to cut." A surgical incision into the synovial cavity of a joint is known as _____. The constructed form of the term is arthr/o/tomy.

bursectomy

ber SEK toh mee

surgical removal of bursa

6.66 A surgery involving the removal of a bursa from a joint is known as a _____. The constructed form of the term is burs/ectomy, in which _burs_ means "purse or sac" and _-ectomy_ means "surgical excision or removal."

chiropractic

KIGH roh PRAK tik

6.67 The field of therapy that is centered on manipulation of bones and joints, most commonly the vertebral column, is known as _____. A practitioner of this therapy is called a **chiropractor** (KIGH roh prak tor). The term _chiropractor_ is constructed from the combining form _chir/o_, which means "hand," and the suffix _-practic_, which means "one who practices."

chondrectomy
kon DREK toh mee

removal of cartilage (handwritten)

6.68 Surgical excision, or removal, of the cartilage associated with a joint is a common procedure known as _____. The surgery commonly uses arthroscopy to reduce the size of the incision and improve the surgeon's view. *Chondrectomy* is a constructed term that can be written as chondr/ectomy to reveal its two word parts: *chondr*, which means "cartilage," and *-ectomy*, which means "surgical excision or removal."

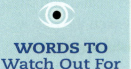

WORDS TO Watch Out For

-ectomy or *-tomy*?

These two suffixes look very similar, but how do you tell them apart? One easy way is to remember that *-ectomy* means "**e**xcision" (see how they both start with an *e*?). The suffix *-tomy* means "incision" or "to cut," and this meaning does not start with an *e*.

---

chondroplasty
KON droh plass tee

6.69 The suffix *-plasty* means "surgical repair." Surgical repair of cartilage associated with a joint is known as _____. The constructed form of the term is chondr/o/plasty.

costectomy
koss TEK toh mee

6.70 A surgery involving the removal of a rib (the combining form is *cost/o*) is known as a _____.

cranioplasty
KRAY nee oh plass tee

surgical repair of skull (handwritten)

6.71 When one or more bones of the cranium (*crani/o*) undergo repair during surgery (*-plasty*), the procedure is called _____. The constructed term for this procedure is crani/o/plasty.

craniotomy
KRAY nee OTT oh mee

cut into skull (handwritten)

6.72 To perform surgery of the brain, a **craniotomy** is required, during which the surgeon enters the cranial cavity by cutting an opening through the cranium. The constructed form of _____ is written as crani/o/tomy, in which the combining form *crani/o* means "skull, cranium" and the suffix *-tomy* means "incision, to cut."

diskectomy
disk EK toh mee

6.73 A surgical procedure that is used frequently to reduce the pain of a herniated disk by surgically removing the intervertebral disk is a _____. It may also be called a **spinal fusion** when the adjacent vertebrae are fused together following the removal of the disk. An alternate term for spinal fusion is **spondylosyndesis** (SPON dih loh sin DEE siss), which literally means "surgical fixation to connect vertebrae." This constructed term includes four word parts: spondyl/o/syn/desis, in which the combining form *spondyl/o* means "vertebra," *syn* means "connect," and the suffix *-desis* means "surgical fixation, fusion." Also performed to treat a herniated disk is a **laminectomy** (lahm ih NEK toh mee), during which the part of a vertebra known as the lamina is surgically removed to relieve pressure on the spinal cord.

electromyography
ee LEK troh my OG rah fee

6.74 The strength of a muscle contraction can be measured and recorded by a procedure called **electromyography (EMG)**. It utilizes an instrument that electrically stimulates a muscle, and the resulting contraction is recorded and analyzed on a computer. In this term, *electr/o* means "electricity," *my/o* means "muscle," and *-graphy* means "recording process." _____ includes five word parts: electr/o/my/o/graphy (■ Figure 6.16).

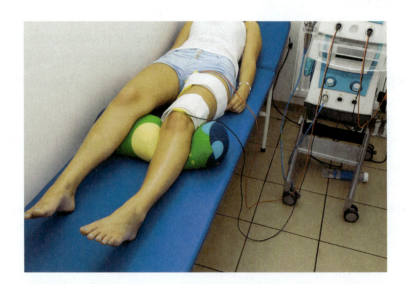

■ **Figure 6.16**
Electromyography. Photograph of a patient undergoing electrical muscle stimulation and analysis for muscle function testing. *Source: Photoshooter2015/ Shutterstock.*

fasciotomy
FASH ee OTT oh mee

6.75 A surgical incision into the connective tissue sheath surrounding a muscle, called *fascia*, is known as a _____. The constructed form of this term is fasci/o/tomy.

closed fracture reduction

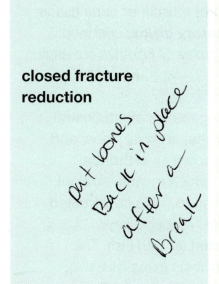

put bones Back in place after a Break

6.76 Orthopedic surgeons, or orthopedists, treat fractures by aligning the broken bones to their normal positions in a procedure known as **reduction** (■ Figure 6.17), which means "bringing back to normal". Manipulating the bone without surgery during reduction is known as _____ _____ _____. If surgical intervention is needed to align and stabilize the broken area, the procedure is called **open fracture reduction**. During this procedure, pins, screws, rods, or plates may be inserted to stabilize the alignment, known as **internal fixation**. In **external fixation**, metal rods and pins are attached from outside the skin surface. External fixation carries the advantage of avoiding the use of a plaster cast for immobilization. If the normal healing process is impeded, **bone grafting** or **electrical bone stimulation** may be applied to stimulate the healing process.

■ **Figure 6.17**
Fracture reduction. X-ray of two lower legs, right (R) and left (L), following orthopedic surgery. The right tibia and fibula, both with a simple fracture, have been treated through closed fracture reduction by placing the limb within a plaster cast to immobilize it. The left tibia and fibula have a more severe injury, both with a compound comminuted fracture. As a result, an open fracture reduction has been performed to connect the shattered bones with metal pins to an external metal rod (white), in the procedure called *external fixation*.
Source: Jarva Jar/Shutterstock.

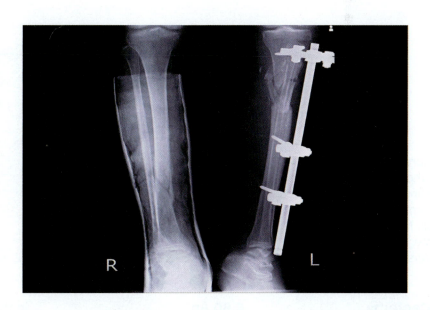

myoplasty
  MY oh plass tee

myorrhaphy
  my OR ah fee

6.77 The combining form *my/o* means "muscle." A muscle can tear during a serious injury and require surgical intervention to promote healing. During a _____, a muscle undergoes surgical repair (the suffix *-plasty* means "repair"). The constructed form of the term is *my/o/plasty*. The repair often includes suturing the torn ends together in a procedure known as _____. The constructed form of the term is *my/o/rrhaphy*, in which the suffix *-rrhaphy* means "suturing."

NSAIDs *ibuprofin*

6.78 The most common pharmacological treatment for any condition, including inflammation or pain of muscle or bone tissue, is the use of **nonsteroidal anti-inflammatory drugs**, commonly abbreviated _____. Examples of NSAIDs are aspirin and ibuprofen.

orthotics
or THOTT iks

6.79 The field of medical support involving the construction and fitting of orthopedic appliances, such as lifts, artificial limbs, and retraction devices, to assist a patient is known as **orthotics**. Formed from the combining form *orth/o*, which means "straight," and the suffix *-tic*, which means "pertaining to," this constructed term includes three word parts: orth/o/tics. A specialist in _____ is called an **orthotist** (or THOTT ist). The medical term for an artificial limb is **prosthesis** (pross THEE siss), which literally means "to place in addition" (■ Figure 6.18).

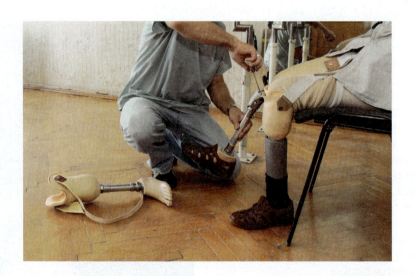

■ **Figure 6.18**
An orthotics lab. An orthotist is adjusting a prosthetic device on a patient who lost both legs to enable him to walk again.
Source: Mykola Komarovskyy/ Shutterstock.

ostectomy
oss TEK toh mee

6.80 An _____ is the surgical removal, or excision, of bone tissue. It is performed to remove unwanted bony formations. The constructed form of this term is ost/ectomy, in which the suffix meaning "surgical excision or removal" is added to the word root for bone (*ost*).

osteoclasis
OSS tee oh KLAY siss

6.81 In some cases, it becomes necessary to break a bone purposely to correct a defect or an improperly healed fracture. Formed by adding the suffix *-clasis*, meaning "break apart," to the combining form for bone (*oste/o*), the name of the procedure is _____. It is a constructed term: oste/o/clasis.

osteopathy
OSS tee OPP ah thee

6.82 A medical field that emphasizes the relationship between the musculoskeletal system and overall health with an emphasis on body alignment and nutrition is called **osteopathy**. The constructed form is oste/o/pathy. A physician trained in _____ is known as an **osteopath** or **osteopathic surgeon** and is symbolized by the abbreviation **DO** (Doctor of Osteopathy).

osteoplasty
OSS tee oh plass tee

6.83 The surgical repair of bone is a general procedure known as _____. This term is formed by adding the suffix *-plasty* ("surgical repair") to the combining form oste/o ("bone"). The constructed form is oste/o/plasty.

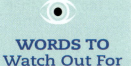

WORDS TO Watch Out For

-pathy or *-plasty*?

These two suffixes look very similar, but how do you tell them apart? The suffix *-pathy* means "disease," whereas the meaning of the suffix *-plasty* is "surgical repair." One easy way to tell them apart is to think of the sound of *-plasty*: it sounds like "plaster," which is a home product that is used to repair walls.

---

podiatry
poh DYE ah tree

6.84 The Greek word for foot is *podos*. When the combining form of this Greek word (*pod/o*) is combined with the suffix *-iatry*, which means "treatment or specialty," the result is the constructed term _____, which is the specialty that focuses on foot health. A healthcare professional trained in this field is called a **podiatrist** (poh DYE ah trist).

RICE

6.85 A very common treatment for most internal injuries of the musculoskeletal system, such as sprains (Frame 6.53) and strains (Frame 6.54), is often called by its popular acronym, **RICE**. The meaning of _____ is **r**est, **i**ce compresses, **c**ompression of the injury site, and **e**levation of the injured limb.

tenomyoplasty
TEN oh MY oh plass tee

6.86 Some injuries involve damage to both the muscle and its associated tendon. The surgical procedure involving the repair of both muscle and tendon is called a _____. This constructed term is shown as ten/o/my/o/plasty to reveal its word parts: the combining forms *ten/o*, meaning "stretch, tendon," and *my/o*, meaning "muscle," and the suffix *-plasty*, meaning "surgical repair."

tenorrhaphy
ten OR ah fee

6.87 Stepping into a hole and falling can cause a serious injury to the calcaneal tendon of the ankle. This tendon, also known as the *Achilles tendon*, attaches the powerful calf muscles to the large heel bone (calcaneus). If it tears, mobility of the affected leg becomes impossible until surgical intervention corrects the injury. The surgery is called a _____ and involves the suturing of a tendon to close a tear. This constructed term is ten/o/rrhaphy to reveal its word parts. In this term, the suffix -*rrhaphy*, which means "suturing," is added to the combining form that means "stretch, tendon."

tenotomy
ten OTT oh mee

6.88 A tenorrhaphy often includes the _____ procedure, during which one or more incisions are made into a tendon. Also a constructed term, it is written as ten/o/tomy, using the combining form that means "stretch, tendon" and the suffix that means "incision, to cut."

vertebroplasty
VERT eh broh plass tee

6.89 A surgical procedure that repairs damaged or diseased vertebrae is called a _____. Adding the combining form that means "vertebra" with the suffix that means "surgical repair" creates this constructed term. It includes three word parts: vertebr/o/plasty.

PRACTICE: Treatments, Procedures, and Devices of the Skeletal and Muscular Systems

The Right Match

Match the term on the left with the correct definition on the right.

_____ 1. reduction

_____ 2. aspiration

_____ 3. arthrocentesis

_____ 4. nonsteroidal anti-inflammatory drugs

_____ 5. spinal fusion

_____ 6. arthroscopy

_____ 7. chondroplasty

_____ 8. tenorrhaphy

_____ 9. podiatry

_____ 10. arthrogram

a. the most common pharmacological treatment for inflammation or pain of muscle or bone tissue

b. a procedure in which adjacent vertebrae are fused together following a diskectomy

c. withdrawing by suction

d. a procedure in which excess fluids are aspirated through a surgical puncture in the joint

e. a procedure that aligns broken bones to their normal positions

f. an x-ray image of a joint

g. healthcare specialty that focuses on foot health

h. an endoscopic visual examination of a joint cavity

i. surgical repair of cartilage

j. a surgery that sutures a tear in a tendon

Break the Chain

Analyze these medical terms:

a) Separate each term into its word parts; each word part is labeled for you (**p** = prefix, **r** = root, **cf** = combining form, and **s** = suffix).

b) For the Bonus Question, write the requested word part or definition in the blank that follows.

1. a) arthrodesis _____/___/_____
                        cf   s

    b) *Bonus Question*: What is the definition of the suffix? _____

2. a) chondrectomy _____/_____
                            r   s

    b) *Bonus Question*: What is the definition of the word root? _____

3. a) craniotomy _____/___/_____
                        cf   s

    b) *Bonus Question*: Does this term contain a prefix? _____

4. a) laminectomy _____/_____
                            r   s

    b) *Bonus Question*: What is the definition of the suffix? _____

5. a) electromyography _____/___/_____/___/_____
                               cf   cf   s

    b) *Bonus Question*: What is the definition of the second combining form? _____

6. a) orthotics _____/___/_____
                        cf   s

    b) *Bonus Question*: What is the definition of the combining form? _____

7. a) osteoclasis _____/___/_____
                         cf   s

    b) *Bonus Question*: What is the definition of the suffix? _____

8. a) tenomyoplasty _____/___/_____/___/_____
                            cf   cf   s

    b) *Bonus Question*: What is the definition of the suffix? _____

9. a) osteoplasty _____/___/_____
                         cf   s

    b) *Bonus Question*: What is the definition of the combining form? _____

Abbreviations of the Skeletal and Muscular Systems

The abbreviations that are associated with the skeletal and muscular systems are summarized here. Study these abbreviations and review them in the exercise that follows.

Abbreviation	Definition
ACL	anterior cruciate ligament, a ligament that stabilizes the knee joint
AS	ankylosing spondylitis
CTS	carpal tunnel syndrome
DJD	degenerative joint disease
DMD	Duchenne muscular dystrophy
DO	physician specializing in osteopathy
EMG	electromyography
HNP	herniated nucleus pulposus, a herniated intervertebral disk
MG	myasthenia gravis
NSAIDs	nonsteroidal anti-inflammatory drugs

Abbreviation	Definition
OA	osteoarthritis
ortho	orthopedics
RA	rheumatoid arthritis
RICE	rest, ice, compression, elevation
ROM	range of motion
SCI	spinal cord injury
THR	total hip replacement
TKA	total knee arthroplasty
TKR	total knee replacement
TMJ	temporomandibular joint disease
Vertebrae	
C1 through C7	the seven cervical vertebrae
T1 through T12	the twelve thoracic vertebrae
L1 through L5	the five lumbar vertebrae

PRACTICE: Abbreviations

Fill in the blanks with the abbreviation or the complete medical term.

Abbreviation	Medical Term
1. _____	spinal cord injury
2. TKA	_____
3. _____	rheumatoid arthritis
4. DMD	_____
5. _____	herniated nucleus pulposus
6. EMG	_____
7. _____	anterior cruciate ligament
8. THR	_____
9. _____	the five lumbar vertebrae
10. CTS	_____
11. _____	range of motion
12. OA	_____
13. _____	total knee replacement
14. T1–T12	_____
15. _____	degenerative joint disease
16. TMJ	_____
17. _____	myasthenia gravis
18. AS	_____

CHAPTER REVIEW

Word Building _____

Construct medical terms from the following meanings. The first question has been completed for you as an example.

1. a gradual and painful softening of bone   osteo***malacia***_____

2. abnormal loss of bone density   osteo_____

3. paralysis of lower body, including both legs   _____plegia

4. abnormal lateral curve of the spine   scoli_____

5. inflammation of a tendon and synovial membrane   teno_____

6. x-ray image of a joint   arthro_____

7. inflammation of a meniscus   _____itis

8. surgical incision into a joint   arthro_____

9. muscular weakness   my_____

10. protrusion of muscle through its fascia   myo_____

11. a repetitive stress injury of the wrist   _____tunnel syndrome

12. a therapy in which a joint is loosened of its restrictions   arthro_____

13. a viral infection of bone that accelerates bone loss   _____'s disease

14. a rupture of an intervertebral disk   _____ disk

15. surgical repair of a joint   arthro_____

16. pain in a tendon   teno_____

17. a calcium deposit within a bursa   burso_____

18. abnormal condition of joint stiffness   _____osis

Define the Combining Form _____

In the space provided, write the definition of the combining form, followed by one example of the combining form used to build a medical term in Chapter 6.

	Definition	**Use in a Term**
1. ankyl/o	_____	_____
2. arthr/o	_____	_____
3. burs/o	_____	_____
4. spondyl/o	_____	_____
5. myel/o	_____	_____
6. oste/o	_____	_____
7. chondr/o	_____	_____
8. synovi/o	_____	_____

Complete the Labels

Complete the blank labels in ■ Figures 6.19, 6.20, and 6.21 by writing the labels in the spaces provided.

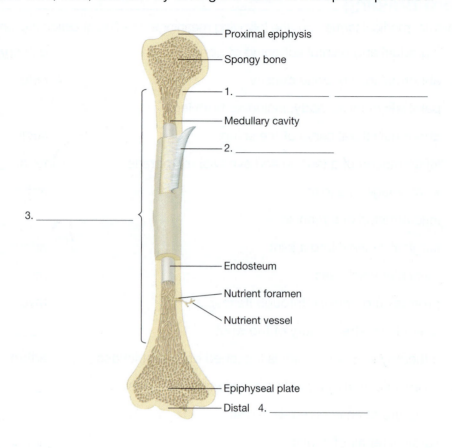

- Proximal epiphysis
- Spongy bone
- 1. _____ _____
- Medullary cavity
- 2. _____
- 3. _____
- Endosteum
- Nutrient foramen
- Nutrient vessel
- Epiphyseal plate
- Distal 4. _____

■ **Figure 6.19**
Parts of a bone.

1. _____

2. _____

3. _____

4. _____

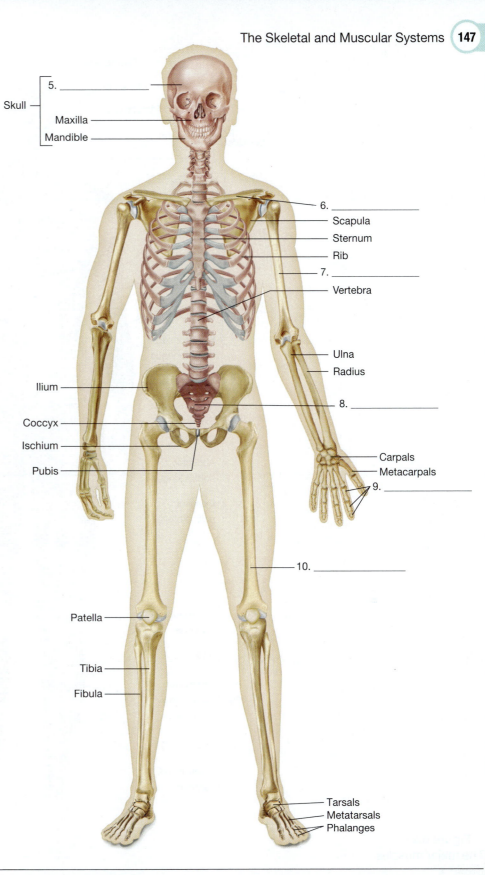

5. _____
Skull
Maxilla ————
Mandible ————

6. _____
Scapula
Sternum
Rib
7. _____
Vertebra

Ulna
Radius

8. _____

Carpals
Metacarpals
9. _____

Ilium ————

Coccyx ————
Ischium ————
Pubis ————

10. _____

Patella ————

Tibia ————

Fibula ————

Tarsals
Metatarsals
Phalanges

■ **Figure 6.20**
The bones of the skeleton.

5. _____

6. _____

7. _____

8. _____

9. _____

10. _____

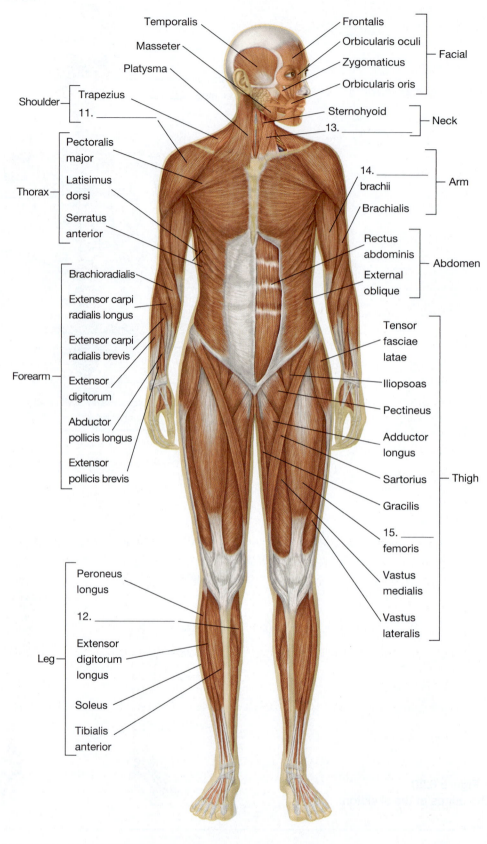

Temporalis
Masseter
Platysma
Frontalis
Orbicularis oculi
Zygomaticus
Orbicularis oris
— Facial

Shoulder — Trapezius
11. _____

Sternohyoid
13. _____
— Neck

Thorax — Pectoralis major
Latisimus dorsi
Serratus anterior

14. _____ brachii
Brachialis
— Arm

Rectus abdominis
External oblique
— Abdomen

Forearm — Brachioradialis
Extensor carpi radialis longus
Extensor carpi radialis brevis
Extensor digitorum
Abductor pollicis longus
Extensor pollicis brevis

Tensor fasciae latae
Iliopsoas
Pectineus
Adductor longus
Sartorius
Gracilis
15. _____ femoris
Vastus medialis
Vastus lateralis
— Thigh

Leg — Peroneus longus
12. _____
Extensor digitorum longus
Soleus
Tibialis anterior

■ **Figure 6.21**
The major muscles.

11. _____

12. _____

13. _____

14. _____

15. _____

MEDICAL REPORT EXERCISES

Jorge Johnson

Read the following medical report, then answer the questions that follow.

PEARSON GENERAL HOSPITAL

PGH

5500 University Avenue, Metropolis, New York
Phone: (211) 594-4000 • Fax (211) 594-4001

Medical Consultation: Orthopedics

Patient: Jorge Johnson

Dob: 5/20/1982   **Age**: 35   **Sex**: Male

Provider: Jonathon McIntyre, MD

Date: 09/11/2017

Patient ID: 123456

Allergies: NKDA

Subjective:

"My right ankle hurts a lot, even when I am lying down. I twisted it while playing touch football just 10 hours ago."

35 y/o male. The patient is in great discomfort. Swelling of the right ankle is apparent, and some bleeding is present at the injury site.

Objective:

Vital Signs: **T**: 98.6°F; **P**: 82; **R**: 25; **BP**: 138/95

Ht: 6'2"

Wt: 203 lb

General Appearance: Physical stress is noted by diaphoresis, heavy breathing, facial expression of discomfort, edema of the right ankle. Break in the skin at the right ankle with minor bleeding.

Heart: Rate at 82 bpm, with no abnormal sounds.

Lungs: Clear without signs of disease.

AbD: Bowel sounds normal all four quadrants.

MS: Joints and muscles symmetric. No swelling, masses, or deformity in areas other than right ankle.

Assessment:

Compound Pott's fracture at the distal end of r. tibia and fibula with tendonitis of Achilles tendon.

Plan:

Apply RICE STAT. X-ray right ankle. If confirmed, prep for ortho surgery to remove bone fragments and realign fracture. Close and cast injury in plaster, with follow-up in 2 weeks.

Photo Source: Monkey Business Images/Shutterstock.

Comprehension Questions

1. What is the evidence supporting a diagnosis of a compound fracture? _____

_____

_____

2. Why are x-rays required before treatment can begin? _____

_____

_____

3. In what area of the body might a Pott's fracture occur? _____

_____

_____

Case Study Questions

The following case study provides further discussion regarding the patient in the medical report. Fill in the blanks with the correct terms. Choose your answers from the list of terms that precedes the case study. (Note that some terms may be used more than once.)

compound	myositis	Pott's
myalgia	polymyositis	tendonitis

A 35-year-old patient named Jorge Johnson received injuries during a weekend touch football game in

the park. Upon his arrival at emergency, he presented an open, or (a) _____, fracture of

the distal end of the right tibia and fibula, pain, and discoloration of the ankle that suggested damage to

a tendon, or (b) _____, and muscle tenderness or (c) _____ that suggested

damaged muscle fibers, or (d) _____, and inflammation of all muscles of the right lower

extremity, or (e) _____. An x-ray examination revealed a fracture at the right ankle, called

a (f) _____ fracture, with associated inflammation of the Achilles tendon, or generalized

(g) _____.

Debra Simpson

For a greater challenge, read the following medical report and answer the critical thinking questions that follow.

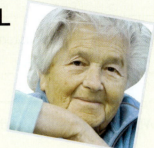

PEARSON GENERAL HOSPITAL

5500 University Avenue, Metropolis, New York
Phone: (211) 594-4000 • Fax (211) 594-4001

Medical Consultation: Orthopedics

Date: 09/19/2017

Patient: Debra Simpson

Patient ID: 123456

Dob: 8/10/1934   **Age**: 85   **Sex**: Female

Allergies: NKDA

Provider: Paula S. Medina, MD

Subjective:

"I have a lot of trouble moving: walking, climbing into and out of bed, reaching for cans out of my cabinet. I can't stand straight anymore without pain. My hands hurt most of the time, sometimes worse when it's cold out."

85 y/o widowed patient lives alone, with three children living within 50 miles. She says this is her first visit to a medical institution in 25 years. Her discomfort is apparent in her face and voice. She keeps as active as possible, although recently she has stopped her daily walks due to the pain.

Objective:

Vital Signs: **T**: 97.6°F; **P**: 80; **R**: 23; **BP**: 145/102

Ht: 5'3"

Wt: 129 lb

General Appearance: Skin pallor with numerous pigmented patches, eyes clear, stooped posture with kyphosis, walks with shuffling gait, low energy, voice faint and crackling.

Heart: Rate at 80 bpm, with no abnormal sounds.

Lungs: Clear without signs of disease.

AbD: Bowel sounds normal all four quadrants.

MS: Joints and muscles symmetric for her age. Swelling and erythema at the joints of hands and feet, especially at carpometacarpal and metacarpophalangeal joints.

Assessment:

Osteoporosis, osteoarthritis

Plan:

HRT with calcium/vit D supplements. Recommend NSAIDs to help manage the OA.

Photo Source: Absolut/Shutterstock.

Comprehension Questions

1. What is the diagnosis? _____

   _____

   _____

2. What term is abbreviated OA? _____

   _____

   _____

3. What is the meaning of the term *osteoporosis*? _____

   _____

   _____

Case Study Questions
The following case study provides further discussion regarding the patient in the medical report.
Recall the terms from this chapter to fill in the blanks with the correct terms.

Debra Simpson, an 85-year-old female, was initially seen by her personal general practitioner when she

complained of difficulty in movement, or (h) _____, and joint pain, or (i) _____,

of both wrists. The GP referred her to (j) _____ due to an abnormal bent-over posture,

called a (k) _____, the presence of a minor back hump, or (l) _____,

and x-ray exams that indicated a loss of bone density. Based on these findings, the initial diagnosis was

(m) _____. The orthopedist also reported advanced joint degeneration in her carpometacarpal

and metacarpophalangeal joints that was diagnosed as (n) _____ due to her advanced age.

Treatments were prescribed to include hormone therapy with calcium supplements, mild exercise for the bone

loss, and NSAIDs for OA management.

MyLab Medical Terminology™

MyLab Medical Terminology is a premium online homework management system that includes a host of features to help you study. Registered users will find:

- A multitude of quizzes and activities built within the MyLab platform
- Powerful tools that track and analyze your results—allowing you to create a personalized learning experience
- Videos and audio pronunciations to help enrich your progress
- Streaming lesson presentations (Guided Lectures) and self-paced learning modules
- A space where you and your instructors can view and manage your assignments

Chapter 7

Blood, the Lymphatic System, and Immunology

 ## Learning Objectives

After completing this chapter, you will be able to:

7.1 Define and spell the word parts used to create terms for the blood, the lymphatic system, and immunology.

7.2 Break down and define common medical terms used for symptoms, diseases, disorders, procedures, and treatments associated with the blood, the lymphatic system, and immunology.

7.3 Build medical terms from the word parts associated with the blood, the lymphatic system, and immunology.

7.4 Pronounce and spell common medical terms associated with the blood, the lymphatic system, and immunology.

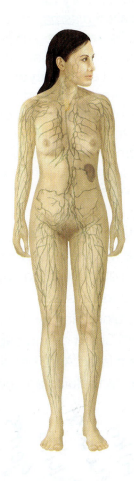

Anatomy and Physiology Terms

The following table provides the combining forms that commonly apply to the anatomy and physiology of the blood, the lymphatic system, and immunology. Note that the combining forms are colored red to help you identify them when you see them later in the chapter.

Combining Form	Definition	Combining Form	Definition
aden/o	gland	lymph/o	clear water or fluid
bacteri/o	bacteria	path/o	disease
blast/o	germ, bud, developing cell	splen/o	spleen
erythr/o	red	thromb/o	clot
hem/o, hemat/o	blood	thym/o	wartlike, thymus gland
immun/o	exempt, immunity	tox/o	poison
leuk/o	white		

blood

blood & lymph carry white blood cells

7.1 Although the blood is a tissue that is part of the cardiovascular system, the blood is also closely associated with another system, the lymphatic system. Therefore, the blood and lymphatic system are combined in this chapter. In the human body, blood is normally found only within the heart and blood vessels of the cardiovascular system. As _____ courses through these organs, it performs its primary function of transport. Blood includes a watery medium, called *plasma,* which carries within its current two major types of cells: red blood cells (RBCs), which transport oxygen, and white blood cells (WBCs), which combat infection. Red blood cells are also called **erythrocytes**, which mean "red cells." Similarly, white blood cells are also called **leukocytes**, which mean "white cells." Fragments of cells are also present in blood. Called **platelets**, they trigger the formation of blood clots to reduce blood loss following an injury. Another type of body fluid, known as *lymph*, also transports substances throughout the body, but this fluid is found only within lymphatic vessels.

lymph

lymph flows back to the ♡

7.2 Lymphatic vessels and _____ are important parts of the lymphatic system, along with the lymph nodes, spleen, and thymus gland. Lymph carries the components of immunity, such as white blood cells and the products they use to fight infection. Amazingly, blood and lymph are intertwined because lymph is formed from blood during capillary exchange and rejoins the bloodstream later. And, because both blood and lymph carry white blood cells, both fluids are involved in the fight against infection.

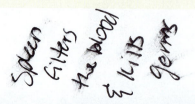
Spleen filters the blood & kills germs

transport

protection

7.3 The primary function of blood is the _____ of substances throughout the body. Vital substances carried by the blood include oxygen, carbon dioxide, hormones, enzymes, nutrients, and waste materials. The blood also protects against infectious disease and helps regulate body temperature. The primary function of the lymphatic system is _____ from infectious disease. It also recycles fluids from the extracellular environment to the bloodstream.

7.4 Review the anatomy of the blood and lymphatic system by studying ■ Figure 7.1 and ■ Figure 7.2.

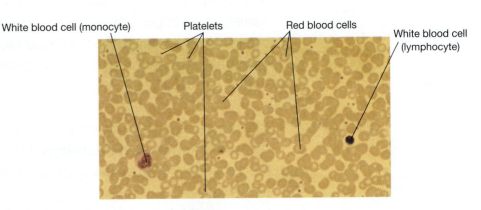

White blood cell (monocyte) Platelets Red blood cells White blood cell (lymphocyte)

■ **Figure 7.1**
A blood smear. The smear reveals representative cells from each formed element group: red blood cells, platelets, and two white blood cells (shown is a lymphocyte and a monocyte).

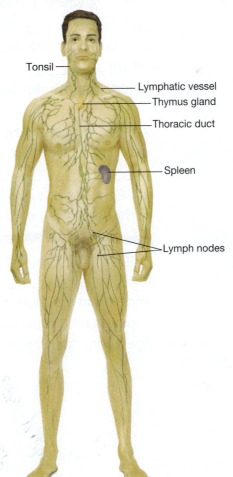

Tonsil

Lymphatic vessel
Thymus gland
Thoracic duct

Spleen

Lymph nodes

■ **Figure 7.2**
The lymphatic system. Lymphatic vessels, major lymph nodes, and lymphatic organs. The direction of lymph flow is toward the heart.

Medical Terms of the Blood, the Lymphatic System, and Immunology

transport

diagnostic

7.5 Because blood is a vital fluid, making sure it is healthy is an important part of healthcare management. Like any other tissue, blood can become diseased from any one of several sources, including inherited abnormalities, infection, or tumor development. The loss of blood itself can become a life-threatening situation if intervention is not provided in time, due to its important function as a _____ medium for gases, enzymes, nutrients, hormones, blood cells, and other substances. Fortunately, blood serves as an important diagnostic tool. Because blood can be conveniently removed from a blood vessel and analyzed, it is an important avenue for testing body chemistry as well as blood cells during a _____ evaluation.

hemat/o/logy

hematologist

7.6 The general field of medicine focusing on blood-related disease is known as **hematology** (HEE mah TAHL oh jee). You should recognize this term as being constructed of three word parts and shown as _____/_____/_____. It includes the combining form *hemat/o*, which is derived from the Greek word for blood, *haima*, and the suffix *-logy* that means "study or science of." A physician specializing in the treatment of disease associated with blood is called a _____ (HEE mah TAHL oh jist) or, alternatively, a **hematopathologist** (hee MAH toh path AHL oh jist).

infection

lymph

7.7 The lymphatic system has dual functions: filtering and recycling of fluid to the bloodstream and battling against _____. A disease of the lymphatic system can affect either function, or perhaps both. Also, because the lymphatic system components are distributed throughout the body, a lymphatic disease can spread quickly to distant areas of the body. In fact, metastasizing cancer cells often use the low-pressure current of the _____ to travel from one area of the body to another. In addition to tumors, lymphatic disease also includes infections that may overwhelm the immune response and inherited conditions that result in deficiencies in immune protection.

immun/o/logy

bacteriology

7.8 Our understanding of infectious disease has grown rapidly during the past 50 years, due mainly to new information coming from research labs. The field of medicine that treats this form of disease is generally called **immunology** (IM yoo NAHL oh jee) or, at some hospitals, **infectious disease**. The term *immunology* refers to the body's ability to defend against infection and includes a variety of mechanisms. This is a constructed term, written as _____/_____/_____, where *immun/o* is a combining form derived from the Latin word *immunis*, which means "exempt or immunity," and *-logy* is the often-used suffix that means "study or science of." Subspecialties in the field of infectious disease include **virology** (vih RAHL oh jee; study of viruses) and _____ (bak TEER ee AHL oh jee; study of bacteria).

lymphatic
lim FAT ik

7.9 In the following sections, we review the prefixes, combining forms, and suffixes that combine to build the medical terms of the blood, the _____ system, and immunology.

Signs and Symptoms of the Blood, the Lymphatic System, and Immunology

Here are the word parts that commonly apply to the signs and symptoms of the blood, the lymphatic system, and immunology that are covered in the following section. Note that the word parts are color-coded to help you identify them: prefixes are yellow, combining forms are red, and suffixes are blue.

Prefix	Definition
an-	without, absence of
iso-	equal
macro-	large
poly-	excessive, over, many

Combining Form	Definition
bacteri/o	bacteria
cyt/o	cell
erythr/o	red
hem/o	blood
leuk/o	white
poikil/o	irregular
splen/o	spleen
thromb/o	clot
tox/o	poison

Suffix	Definition
-emia	condition of blood
-ia	condition of
-lysis	loosen, dissolve
-megaly	abnormally large
-osis	condition of
-penia	abnormal reduction in number, deficiency
-rrhage	abnormal discharge

KEY TERMS A–Z

anisocytosis
an EYE soh sigh TOH siss

7.10 The presence of red blood cells of unequal size in a sample of blood is an abnormal finding. It is a sign known as **anisocytosis**. The constructed form of this term is an/iso/cyt/osis, in which *an-* is a prefix that means "without or absence of," *iso-* is a prefix that means "equal," *cyt/o* is the combining form for "cell," and *-osis* means "condition of." Thus, _____ literally means "condition of without equal cells."

bacteremia
  bak ter EE mee ah

7.11 The presence of bacteria in a sample of blood is a sign of an infection and is called **bacteremia**, as shown in ■ Figure 7.3. The constructed form of this term reveals two word parts, bacter/emia. Because the suffix -*emia* means "condition of blood," _____ literally means "condition of bacteria in the blood."

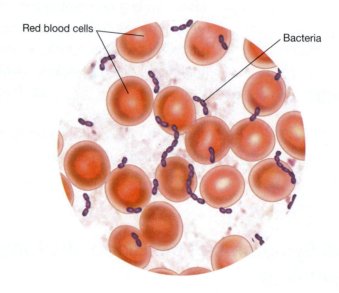

Red blood cells   Bacteria

■ **Figure 7.3**
Bacteremia. Illustration of blood infected with bacteria, as seen through a microscope.

erythropenia
  ee RITH roh PEE nee ah

erythr/o/cyt/o/penia

7.12 The suffix -*penia* means "abnormal reduction in number, deficiency." It is used in the term _____ to describe an abnormally reduced number of red blood cells in a sample of blood. This constructed term is written erythr/o/penia. It is also called **erythrocytopenia**, which is also a constructed term and is written _____/___/___/___/_____.

hemolysis
  hee MALL ih siss

7.13 The rupture of red blood cells may occur if a blood transfusion is not compatible with the recipient's blood, or during a salt imbalance in which more salt is present in the cells than in the plasma. The rupture of the red blood cell membrane is called **hemolysis**. The constructed form of _____ is written hem/o/lysis, which literally means "dissolve blood."

hemorrhage
  HEM eh rihj   *Bleeding rapidly*

7.14 The abnormal loss of blood from circulation is a sign of trauma or illness. It is called _____, which is a constructed term written hem/o/rrhage.

Ct. scan or luxavoscopy to detect internal Hemorrhage

leukopenia
loo koh PEE nee ah

leuk/o/cyt/o/penia

7.15 An abnormally reduced number of white blood cells in a sample of blood is a sign of disease called _____. The constructed form of this term is leuk/o/penia. It is also called **leukocytopenia** (LOO koh SIGH toh PEE nee ah), which is also a constructed term and is written _____/___/____/___/_____.

---

macrocytosis
MAK roh sigh TOH siss *C1*

7.16 The presence of abnormally large red blood cells in a sample of blood is a sign of disease and is called **macrocytosis**. The constructed form of _____ is written macro/cyt/osis, which literally means "condition of large cell."

---

several types of anemia

poikilocytosis
POY kih loh sigh TOH siss
— CBC

7.17 The combining form *poikil/o* means "irregular." Normally, red blood cells are round biconcave disks, but the sign of _____ occurs when more than 10% of the cells have irregular shapes. The constructed form of this term is poikil/o/cyt/osis, which literally means "condition of irregular cell."

---

polycythemia
pall ee sigh THEE mee ah
CBC

too many red blood cells- not delivery enough oxygen

7.18 The prefix *poly-* means "excessive, over, many." When combined with the word roots that mean cell (*cyt*) and blood (*hem*) and the suffix that means "condition of" (*-ia*), the term _____ is formed. This constructed term is written poly/cyt/hem/ia. **Polycythemia** is an abnormal increase in the number of red blood cells in the blood. It results from a genetic mutation within stem cells of the red bone marrow, and may also be called **erythrocytosis** (eh RITH roh sigh TOH siss). This is also a constructed term, written erythr/o/cyt/osis, that literally means "condition of red cell."

---

splenomegaly *enlarged spleen*
splee noh MEG ah lee

7.19 The suffix *-megaly* means "abnormally large." Abnormal enlargement of the spleen is a sign of injury or infection and is called _____. The constructed form is written splen/o/megaly, which literally means "abnormally large spleen."

---

thrombopenia *low platelet count*
throm boh PEE nee ah

not clotting right

thromb/o/cyt/o/penia

7.20 An abnormally reduced number of platelets in a sample of blood is a sign of disease and is called **thrombopenia**. The constructed form of _____ is thromb/o/penia. It is also called **thrombocytopenia** (THROM boh SIGH toh PEE nee ah), which is also a constructed term and is written _____/___/____/___/_____.

---

toxemia
tahk SEE mee ah

7.21 The presence of toxins in the bloodstream is known as _____. The constructed form is tox/emia, which literally means "condition of blood poison."

toxic shock syndrome from staphococus

PRACTICE: Signs and Symptoms of the Blood, the Lymphatic System, and Immunology

The Right Match

Match the term on the left with the correct definition on the right.

_____ 1. anisocytosis   a. presence of bacteria in the blood

_____ 2. bacteremia   b. abnormally reduced number of red blood cells

_____ 3. splenomegaly   c. abnormally large red blood cells

_____ 4. toxemia   d. presence of red blood cells of unequal size

_____ 5. erythropenia   e. abnormal increase in number of red blood cells

_____ 6. macrocytosis   f. irregularly shaped red blood cells

_____ 7. poikilocytosis   g. presence of toxins in the bloodstream

_____ 8. polycythemia   h. abnormal loss of blood from the circulation

_____ 9. hemorrhage   i. abnormal enlargement of the spleen

Break the Chain

Analyze these medical terms:

   a) Separate each term into its word parts; each word part is labeled for you (**p** = prefix, **r** = root, **cf** = combining form, and **s** = suffix).

   b) For the Bonus Question, write the requested definition in the blank that follows.

The first set has been completed as an example.

1. a) polycythemia   _**poly/cyt/hem/ia**_

                                      p   r   r   s

   b) *Bonus Question*: What is the definition of the suffix? _**condition of**_ _____

2. a) thrombopenia   _____/___/_____

                                    cf   s

   b) *Bonus Question*: What is the definition of the combining form? _____

3. a) leukopenia   _____/___/_____

                                    cf   s

   b) *Bonus Question*: What is the definition of the suffix? _____

4. a) hemolysis   _____/___/_____

                                    cf   s

   b) *Bonus Question*: What is the definition of the suffix? _____

5. a) leukocytopenia   _____/___/_____/___/_____

                                    cf   cf   s

   b) *Bonus Question*: What is the definition of the first combining form? _____

Diseases and Disorders of the Blood, the Lymphatic System, and Immunology

Here are the word parts that commonly apply to the diseases and disorders of the blood, the lymphatic system, and immunology that are covered in the following section. Note that the word parts are color-coded to help you identify them: prefixes are yellow, combining forms are red, and suffixes are blue.

Prefix	Definition
an-	without, absence of
ana-	up, toward
mono-	one

Combining Form	Definition
aden/o	gland
aut/o	self
botul/o	sausage
fung/o	fungus
globin/o	protein
hem/o, hemat/o	blood
hydr/o	water
iatr/o	physician
idi/o	individual
immun/o	exempt, or immunity
leuk/o	white
lymph/o	clear water or fluid
necr/o	death
nosocom/o	hospital
nucle/o	kernel, nucleus
path/o	disease
sept/o	putrefying; wall or partition
staphylococc/o	Staphylococcus (bacterium)
streptococc/o	Streptococcus (bacterium)
thym/o	wartlike, thymus gland

Suffix	Definition
-emia	condition of blood
-genic	pertaining to producing, forming
-ial	pertaining to
-ic	pertaining to
-ism	condition or disease
-itis	inflammation
-oma	tumor
-osis	condition of
-pathy	disease
-philia	loving, affinity for
-phobia	fear
-phylaxis	protection
-rrhagic	pertaining to abnormal discharge

KEY TERMS A–Z

AIDS

7.22 The acronym for **acquired immunodeficiency syndrome** is _____. This devastating disease is caused by the **human immunodeficiency virus (HIV)**, which disables the immune response by destroying important white blood cells known as helper T cells. The loss of immune function allows opportunistic diseases to proliferate, such as pneumonia caused by *Pneumocystis jiroveci*, dementia, Kaposi's sarcoma, and many others, any of which eventually cause death if aggressive medical intervention is not provided. There is no cure, although many patients respond well to antiretroviral therapy if it is available. Commonly referred to as H-I-V AIDS (written **HIV/AIDS**), it is the most deadly infectious disease on our planet, with nearly 37 million people infected and over 1 million deaths each year.

allergy
AL er jee

byproduct of the immune system

7.23 An **allergy** is the body's immune response to allergens, which are foreign substances that produce a reaction including immediate inflammation. An _____ may strike in different forms, the most common of which are **allergic rhinitis** (hay fever), which affects the mucous membranes of the nasal cavity and throat, and **allergic dermatitis**, which affects the skin where it has been in physical contact with the allergen (■ Figure 7.4).

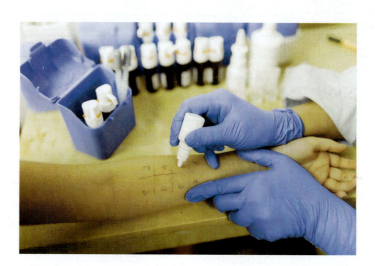

■ **Figure 7.4**
The patient is undergoing an allergy skin test by receiving subdermal inoculations of allergens. Inflammation (redness, swelling, heat, and pain) of the inoculated area is evidence of an allergic reaction.
Source: Gorillaimages/ Shutterstock.

anaphylaxis
AN ah fih LAK siss

7.24 An immediate allergic reaction to a foreign substance that includes rapid inflammation, vasodilation, bronchospasms, shortness of breath, and spasms of the GI tract is called **anaphylaxis**. In severe cases, it can become life-threatening if medical intervention is not available. This term is constructed from the prefix *ana-* that means "up, toward" and the suffix *-phylaxis* that means "protection." Thus, the constructed form of _____ is written ana/phylaxis.

anemia

ah NEE mee ah

[handwritten: blood is unable to carry around enough O₂]

7.25 The prefix *an-* means "without, absence of," and the suffix *-emia* means "condition of blood." Combining these two word parts forms the term **anemia**, which literally means "without blood." The constructed form of this term is written an/emia. _____ is the reduced ability of red blood cells to deliver oxygen to tissues. It may result from a reduced number of normal circulating red blood cells or a reduction in the amount of the oxygen-binding protein in red blood cells called *hemoglobin*. Some common forms of anemia include **aplastic anemia**, *[handwritten: fatal]* in which the red bone marrow fails to produce sufficient numbers of normal blood cells; **iron-deficiency anemia**, caused by a lack of available iron, resulting in the body's inability to make adequate amounts of hemoglobin; **sickle cell anemia**, in which the hemoglobin is defective within cells, resulting in misshaped red blood cells that cause obstructions in blood vessels (■ Figure 7.5); and **pernicious** (per NISH us) **anemia**, caused by a failure to acquire vitamin B$_{12}$ into the bloodstream for its delivery to red bone marrow, which requires it to produce new red blood cells. *[handwritten: from stomach not producing enough acid]*

■ **Figure 7.5**
Sickle cell anemia.
[handwritten: hereditary painful]
(a) Illustration of a blockage in a blood vessel resulting from sickled cells forming a mass, resulting in the reduction of blood flow downstream and the death of tissue (necrosis). (b) Microphotograph of a blood vessel that is blocked by a mass of sickled cells.

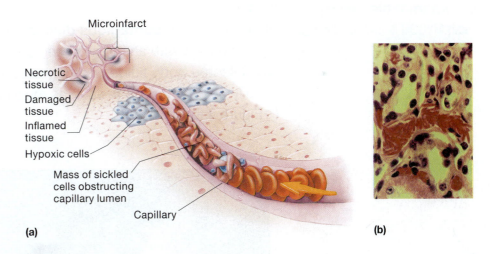

Microinfarct

Necrotic tissue

Damaged tissue

Inflamed tissue

Hypoxic cells

Mass of sickled cells obstructing capillary lumen

Capillary

(a)

(b)

anthrax

AN thraks

[handwritten: deadly infectious — used in bioterrorism — can be saved in powdered form]

7.26 A bacterial disease that has been threatened to be used in **bioterrorism**, which is the application of disease-causing microorganisms (pathogens) to cause harm to a population, is **anthrax**. The spores of the bacteria can survive within a powder that can be distributed through the air, making it very dangerous. If inhaled, _____ is usually fatal. The term is derived from the Greek word *anthrakos*, which means "coal," referring to the blackening effect the infection has on the skin and lungs.

autoimmune disease
au toh im YOON * dis EEZ

7.27 A disease that is caused by a person's own immune response attacking otherwise healthy tissues is called **autoimmune disease**. The term *autoimmune* is a constructed term, written aut/o/immune, and literally means "self-exempt" or "self-immunity." Examples of _____ _____ include rheumatoid arthritis, systemic lupus erythematosus, multiple sclerosis, and psoriasis. The triggering mechanism that results in autoimmune disease is not yet known.

(handwritten notes: Also botox for wrinkles; food poisoning; (improperly canned foods))

botulism
BAHT yoo lizm

7.28 One lethal form of foodborne illness is called **botulism**. This disease was first recorded in Europe in 1735 when villagers died after eating German sausage, thereby earning its name after the Latin word for sausage, *botulus*. It is caused by the ingestion of food contaminated with the neurotoxin produced by the bacterium *Clostridium botulinum*. _____ usually occurs when canned food is not prepared properly and is often fatal because of the extreme toxic nature of the botulism neurotoxin: about one millionth of a gram can kill an adult.

communicable disease
kah MYOON ik ah bul * dis EEZ

7.29 A disease that is capable of transmission from one person to another is called a _____ _____. Also known as a **contagious disease**, it may be transmitted by direct contact with an infected person, indirectly by way of contact with infected body fluids or other materials, or by way of vectors, usually biting arthropods such as mosquitoes, ticks, and fleas (■ Figure 7.6).

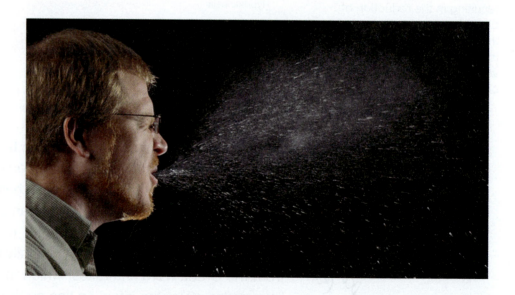

■ **Figure 7.6**
A sneeze is a common source of transmission of a communicable disease. As you can see, it propels infectious material outward for a considerable distance.
Source: Courtesy of Public Health Image Library, Centers For Disease Control and Prevention.

diphtheria

diff THEER ee ah

leathery throat

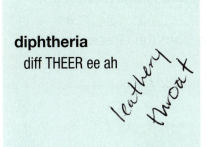

7.30 Diphtheria is an infectious disease resulting in acute inflammation of the mucous membranes, primarily in the mouth and throat. Derived from the Greek word for "leather," _____ is characterized by the formation of an obstructive, leatherlike membrane in the throat. It is illustrated in ■ Figure 7.7. Diphtheria is now a very rare disease in the United States, thanks to a vaccine (often combined with vaccines against tetanus and pertussis, known as DTaP) that has been widely administered to children since the 1960s.

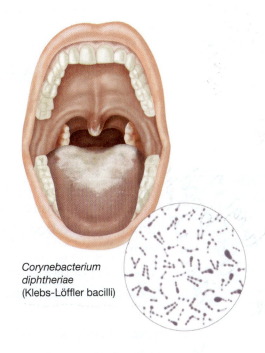

Corynebacterium diphtheriae
(Klebs-Löffler bacilli)

■ **Figure 7.7**
Diphtheria. The bacteria that cause this disease, called *Corynebacterium diphtheriae*, proliferate in the mucous membranes of the throat to establish a leathery, white covering.

? Did You **KNOW**

DIPHTHERIA

Before the availability of the diphtheria vaccine and antibiotics, diphtheria was a life-threatening scourge among children, killing thousands each year in the United States. It is caused by the toxins produced by the bacterium *Corynebacterium diphtheriae*, which produces inflammation of the throat and the formation of a thick secretion. Because the infected throat becomes covered with a leathery membrane, it was named after the Greek word for leather, *diphthera*.

dyscrasia

diss KRAY zee ah

general term for blood disease

7.31 Derived from the Greek word *dyskrasia*, which means "difficult temperament," the clinical term _____ is any abnormal condition of the blood. Apparently, this condition was named after a correlation between a difficult temperament and blood disease was observed.

edema

eh DEE mah

swelling (handwritten)

7.32 The leakage of fluid from the bloodstream into the interstitial space between body cells causes swelling and is one aspect of inflammation. The swelling is called _____, as shown in ■ Figure 7.8. The term is derived from the Greek word *oidema*, which means "swelling."

■ **Figure 7.8**
Edema. The patient's edema of both lower limbs is the result of plasma leaking across damaged blood vessels into the interstitial space, producing swelling and pain.
Source: Valerio Pardi/ Shutterstock.

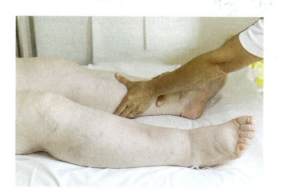

fungemia

fun JEE mee ah

fungi in the blood (found in Aids patients) (handwritten)

7.33 The combining form for fungus is *fung/o*, and the suffix *-emia* means "condition of blood." Putting these word parts together forms the term **fungemia**, which is a fungal infection that spreads throughout the body by way of the bloodstream. As a constructed term, _____ is written *fung/emia* and literally means "condition of blood fungus." Another common term for this infection is **fungal septicemia**.

hematoma

HEE mah TOH mah

large bruise (handwritten)

7.34 When a word root for blood, *hemat/o*, is combined with the suffix that means "tumor" (*-oma*), the term _____ is formed. It is a mass of blood outside blood vessels and confined within an organ or space within the body, usually in a clotted form (■ Figure 7.9). Commonly known as a bruise or a contusion when it is visible through the skin, a hematoma is usually the result of injury or disease. The constructed form of this term is written *hemat/oma*.

■ **Figure 7.9**
Hematoma. A hematoma around the right eye caused by an injury. A hematoma is the result of bleeding below the surface of the skin and is also known as a contusion or bruise when it is visible through the skin.
Source: Molodec/Shutterstock.

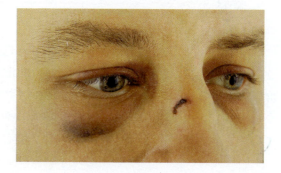

hemoglobinopathy
HEE moh gloh bin AH path ee

disease of hemoglobin

7.35 A general term for a disease that affects hemoglobin within red blood cells is **hemoglobinopathy**. This constructed term contains five word parts, as shown when it is written as hem/o/globin/o/pathy. It literally means "disease of blood protein." Because sickle cell anemia is a disease that affects hemoglobin (Frame 7.25), it is a form of _____.

hemophilia
HEE moh FILL ee ah

need factor 8

7.36 An inherited bleeding disorder that results from defective or missing blood-clotting proteins that are necessary components in the coagulation process is known as **hemophilia**. Because the clotting proteins normally stop the loss of blood after minor injuries, a patient suffering from _____ experiences an abnormal loss of blood with any physical injury. The term is a constructed term, written hem/o/philia, which literally means "love for blood."

hemorrhagic fever
HEM or AJ ik

7.37 An infectious disease that causes internal bleeding, or internal hemorrhage (Frame 7.14), and high fevers is generally known as _____ _____. The disease is often caused by viruses, such as Ebola, and some forms exhibit a high rate of mortality.

iatrogenic disease
EYE ah troh JEN ik * dis EEZ

Common (ex. yeast infection after antibiotics)

7.38 A condition that is caused by a medical treatment is called an **iatrogenic disease**. This constructed term combines the combining form that means "physician," *iatr/o*, with the suffix that means "pertaining to producing, forming," *-genic*. The resulting constructed form is written iatr/o/genic. An example of an _____ _____ is the development of a MRSA infection (Frame 7.58) following a surgical procedure.

idiopathic disease
id ee oh PATH ik * dis EEZ

(ex. scoliosis) unknown cause

7.39 A disease that develops without a known or apparent cause is called an _____ _____. The constructed form of this term is idi/o/path/ic, which literally means "pertaining to individual disease."

immunodeficiency
IM yoo noh dee FISH ehn see

acquired Aids / primary: born with something wrong / w/immune system

7.40 A condition resulting from a defective immune response is called an **immunodeficiency**. It occurs when there are insufficient numbers of functional white blood cells, especially lymphocytes, available to defend the body from sources of infection. A closely related term is **immunocompromised**, which is used to describe a patient suffering from an _____.

immunosuppression
IM yoo noh suh PREH shun

7.41 A reduction of an immune response may be caused by disease or by use of chemical, pharmacological, or immunologic agents. The suppressed status of the immune response that results is called _____.

incompatibility
IN kum PAT ih BILL ih tee

7.42 The combination of two blood types that results in the destruction of red blood cells is called _____. It may occur during a blood transfusion, causing severe consequences, including the possibility of death if the donor blood antibodies attack the recipient's red blood cells.

unexpected
pathogen
in the body

infection
in FEK shun

7.43 A multiplication of disease-causing microorganisms, or pathogens, in the body is called an **infection**. The term is derived from the Latin word *infectus*, which means "to color, stain, or dye," referring to the discoloration of skin during an infection. A disease caused by _____ is called an **infectious disease**. The reaction of the body against an infection is illustrated in ■ Figure 7.10.

■ **Figure 7.10**
Reaction against infection. Pathogens may invade the body by a puncture through the skin. The result of invasion is the proliferation of pathogens within body tissues, or infection. The body responds to the infection by mounting an attack that begins with inflammation, which promotes the movement of phagocytes to the site of the infection. Phagocytes localize the pathogens and destroy them by phagocytosis. Pus is released, which is composed of dead bacteria and phagocytes.

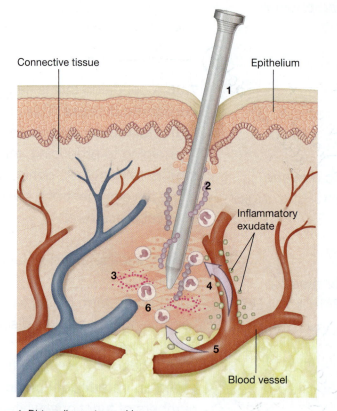

Connective tissue　　　Epithelium

Inflammatory exudate

Blood vessel

1. Dirty nail punctures skin.
2. Bacteria enter and multiply.
3. Injured cells release histamine.
4. Blood vessels dilate and become permeable, releasing inflammatory exudate.
5. Blood flow to the damaged site increases.
6. Neutrophils (polymorphs) move toward bacteria (chemotaxis) and destroy them (phagocytosis).

inflammation
in flah MAY shun

[handwritten: Bodies response to infection]

7.44 The physiological process that serves as the body's initial response to injury and many forms of illness involves the swelling of body tissue. Known as **inflammation**, the swelling results from the movement of plasma from capillaries into the extracellular space to produce edema (Frame 7.32), or fluid accumulation in tissue (see Figure 7.10). The common symptoms of _____ include swelling, redness, heat, and pain. The term *inflammation* is derived from the Latin word *inflammatio*, which means "to ignite" or "to set ablaze."

influenza
in floo EHN zah

[handwritten: flu]

7.45 A viral disease characterized by fever and an acute inflammation of respiratory mucous membranes is called **influenza**. Commonly called "the flu," _____ is highly contagious, and the virus is capable of mutating to escape detection by white blood cells.

leukemia
loo KEE mee ah

[handwritten: Cancer is in Bone marrow (4 types)]

7.46 A form of cancer that literally means "condition of white blood cells" is _____. Leukemia originates from cells within the blood-forming tissue of the red marrow. The constructed form of the term is written leuk/emia. The primary tumor of leukemia spreads throughout the red marrow, transforming the blood-forming tissue into a dysfunctional mass that produces abnormal white blood cells in very large numbers and red blood cells in fewer numbers (■ Figure 7.11). As a result, common symptoms of leukemia include immunodeficiency (Frame 7.40), the development of opportunistic infections, and malaise (low energy) resulting from the reduced production of red blood cells (anemia; Frame 7.25).

■ **Figure 7.11**
Leukemia. Illustration comparing a normal blood smear with a blood smear from a leukemia patient. Notice the reduced red blood cells and increased (abnormal) white blood cells in the leukemia blood.
Source: Alila Medical Media/ Shutterstock.

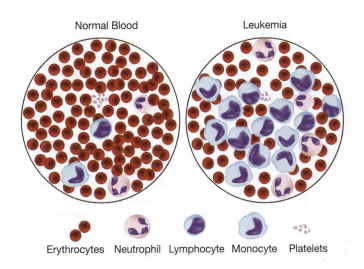

Normal Blood   Leukemia

Erythrocytes   Neutrophil   Lymphocyte   Monocyte   Platelets

lymphadenitis
limm fad eh NYE tiss

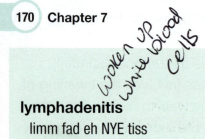

(handwritten: woken up white blood cells)

(handwritten: tumor of lymphnodes (cancer))

lymphoma
limm FOH mah

(handwritten: parasite in red blood cells — killer of children worldwide)

malaria
mah LAIR ee ah

7.47 Inflammation of the lymph nodes is a condition called **lymphadenitis**. The constructed form of this term is lymph/aden/itis. The acute form of _____ is common during infections. The chronic form indicates a more serious disorder may be the cause, such as lymphoma (Frame 7.48).

7.48 The general term for a form of cancer that begins in a type of white blood cell, called a *lymphocyte*, is _____. The constructed form uses the suffix *-oma*, which means "tumor," and is written lymph/oma. There are two main categories of lymphomas, both named after English physician Thomas Hodgkin, who in 1845 first described this cancer of lymphatic tissue with symptoms of swollen lymph nodes and fatigue and the development of numerous infections. The two main categories of lymphoma are **Hodgkin lymphoma**, characterized by its altered lymphocytes called *Reed-Sternberg cells*, and **non-Hodgkin lymphoma (NHL)**, which includes fast-growth and slow-growth forms. Although progress is being made in chemotherapies, lymphomas remain deadly diseases. According to the National Cancer Institute of the National Institutes of Health, in 2016 NHL is expected to cause 72,580 cases and 20,150 deaths, whereas the less-frequent Hodgkin lymphoma is expected to cause 8,500 cases and 1,120 deaths.

7.49 A disease caused by a parasitic protozoan that infects red blood cells and the liver during different parts of its life cycle is called **malaria**. The vector, or carrier, of the protozoan is the *Anopheles* mosquito, and the symptoms of malaria include periodic flare-ups of high fever. The term _____ literally means "bad air," referring to the swampy marshlands where the mosquitoes proliferate to cause higher incidences of the disease.

? Did You KNOW

MALARIA

The term *malaria* is derived from combining the Italian word for bad, *mal*, with that of air, *aria*. It was first used during the Middle Ages, when malaria was believed to have been caused by breathing bad air near swamplands. We now know that this dreaded disease is caused by the bite of an *Anopheles* mosquito carrying the protozoan known as *Plasmodium*. According to the World Health Organization (WHO), in 2015 an estimated 214 million cases of malaria were reported worldwide with 438,000 deaths, making malaria the third deadliest infectious disease in the world. (HIV/AIDS is the deadliest infectious disease, and tuberculosis ranks second.)

7.50 Measles is an acute viral disease that often begins as a fever, followed by the development of a skin rash containing numerous vesicles and often accompanied by a general inflammation of the respiratory tract (■ Figure 7.12). Before the availability of a widely distributed vaccine, _____ killed thousands of children and adults each year in the United States. A clinical synonym is **rubeola**. The word *measles* is derived from the Middle English word *maselen*, which means "many little spots," and *rubeola* is from the Latin word *rubeus*, which means "red."

measles

viral infection

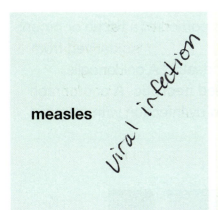

■ **Figure 7.12**
Measles. A photograph of a child stricken with measles, showing the tell-tale sign of the skin rash.
Source: Courtesy of Public Health Image Library, Centers for Disease Control and Prevention.

7.51 A viral disease characterized by enlarged lymph nodes and spleen, atypical lymphocytes, throat pain, pharyngitis, fever, and fatigue is called **mononucleosis**. Also called **infectious mononucleosis**, it is caused by the Epstein-Barr virus and is a communicable disease (■ Figure 7.13). The term _____ is derived from this disease's characteristic feature of the presence of abnormally high numbers of a certain type of white blood cells, called *mononuclear leukocytes*, in a blood sample. The mononuclear leukocytes increase in number to destroy the invading Epstein-Barr virus. The term *mononucleosis* is a constructed term made up of the prefix *mono-*, meaning "one," the word root *nucle*, meaning "kernel, nucleus," and the very common suffix *-osis*, meaning "condition of." It is written as mono/nucle/osis.

mononucleosis

MAHN oh nook lee OH siss

Epstein-Barr virus

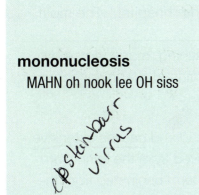

■ **Figure 7.13**
Mononucleosis. Infectious mononucleosis is caused by the Epstein-Barr virus and produces the symptoms of swollen palatine tonsils (pharyngitis), swollen cervical lymph nodes (lymphadenopathy), high fever, fatigue, and a blood sample that reveals large numbers of mononuclear leukocytes.

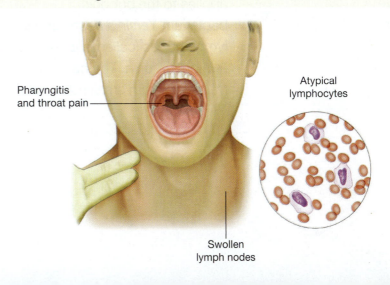

Pharyngitis and throat pain

Atypical lymphocytes

Swollen lymph nodes

necrosis

neh KROH siss

tissue Death

7.52 The death of one or more cells or a portion of a tissue or organ is called **necrosis**. The term _____ is derived from the Greek word *nekrosis*, which means "death." A cell or cells, tissue, or organ that is dead is often called **necrotic**. A photograph of necrosis of a hand, which was caused by infection with plague (Frame 7.54), is shown in ■ Figure 7.14.

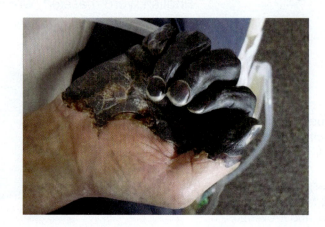

■ **Figure 7.14**
Photograph of the hand of a patient who has tested positive for *Yersinia pestis*, and is thereby diagnosed with bubonic plague. One sign of this dreaded disease is the blackened necrosis of hands and feet. *Source: Courtesy of Public Health Image Library, Centers for Disease Control and Prevention.*

infection acquired in the hospital

nosocomial infection

noh soh KOH mee al * in FEK shun

7.53 An infectious disease that is contracted during a hospital stay is called a **nosocomial infection**. The term *nosocomial* is derived from the Greek word *nosokomeion*, which means "hospital." The most common cause of _____ _____ in recent years has been a lack of handwashing, made worse by the development of antibiotic-resistant strains of *Staphylococcus* (Frame 7.58).

plague

playg

7.54 Any infectious disease that is widespread and causes extensive mortality is called a **plague**. The term is derived from the Latin word *plago*, which means "to strike or beat." The term originated from the first recorded outbreak of bubonic plague in 542 AD. Today, the term still applies to the bubonic _____, which is caused by the bacterium *Yersinia pestis* and is characterized by high fever, enlarged lymph nodes (called *buboes*), skin discoloration, internal hemorrhage, and pneumonia. The bacteria are transmitted by the bite of a flea that may jump from small mammals, such as rats, to humans (Figure 7.14).

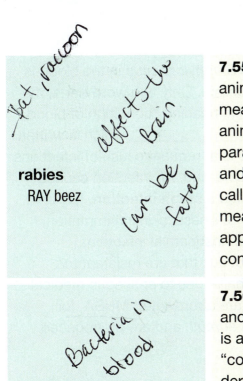

rabies
RAY beez

[handwritten: Fat racoon]
[handwritten: affects the brain]
[handwritten: can be fatal]

septicemia
sep tih SEE mee ah

[handwritten: Bacteria in blood]

smallpox

[handwritten: — gone]

7.55 A viral infection that is spread from the saliva of an infected animal, usually by way of a bite, is known as **rabies**. In Latin, *rabies* means "savage, fierce," which refers to the ferocity of infected animals. The virus acts on the central nervous system to cause paranoia and paralysis and is usually fatal, unless early diagnosis and treatment is provided. _____ has also been called **hydrophobia** (HIGH droh FOH bee ah), which literally means "fear of water" and refers to the symptom of a fear of water appearing during the stage of mental deterioration. *Hydrophobia* is a constructed term, written as hydr/o/phobia.

7.56 A system-wide disease caused by the presence of bacteria and their toxins in the circulating blood is called **septicemia**. This is a constructed term written sept/ic/emia and literally means "condition of putrefying (decaying) blood." The word root, *sept*, is derived from the Greek word *sepsis*, which means "putrefying." If not treated quickly, _____ may progress into a life-threatening systemic inflammatory response, known by its Greek origin as **sepsis**. A person suffering from this condition is referred to as **septic** and requires immediate medical intervention to survive. A septic patient is in danger of developing **septic shock**, which includes a dangerous drop in blood pressure that often leads to death.

7.57 A viral disease caused by the *variola* virus that was the scourge of the human population before its eradication in 1977 is known as **smallpox**. The term was first used around 150 AD to distinguish the disease from syphilis, the "great pox," which at the time was characterized by the formation of large pustules on the skin that exceeded the pustules of smallpox in size and number. The eradication of _____ was the crowning achievement of the World Health Organization, which battled the disease with an aggressive vaccination (Frame 7.89) campaign for about 8 years. Although it is eradicated from the population, reserves of *variola* remain in guarded storage for research purposes.

staphylococcemia
STAFF ih loh kok SEE mee ah

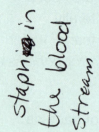

Staph is in the blood stream

7.58 The presence of the bacterium *Staphylococcus* in the blood is a condition known as **staphylococcemia**. Only two word parts, the word root *staphylococc* and the suffix meaning "condition of blood," -*emia*, are used to construct _____, which is written staphylococc/emia. *Staphylococcus* is a frequent cause of infections in wounds, a complication of normal healing. An infection caused by *Staphylococcus* is commonly called a **staph infection**. It is also the most common cause of foodborne illness, skin inflammation, osteomyelitis (infection of bone), and nosocomial infections (Frame 7.53). Varieties of *Staphylococcus* that are resistant to antibiotics are one of the greatest challenges to antiseptic medical procedures. These resistant strains are abbreviated **MRSA**, for methicillin-resistant *Staphylococcus aureus*, and are pronounced "mersa."

streptococcemia
STREP toh kok SEE mee ah

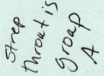

Strep throat is group A

7.59 The presence of the bacterium *Streptococcus* in the blood is known as **streptococcemia**. The constructed term _____ is written streptococc/emia. An infection caused by *Streptococcus* is commonly called a **strep infection**. It frequently begins in the throat as a form of pharyngitis called **strep throat** or in the mouth following a dental procedure and, if not managed, may spread to the bloodstream, which distributes the infection to vital organs.

Can cause Paralysis & death

tetanus
TETT ah nuss

7.60 A disease caused by a powerful neurotoxin released by the common bacterium *Clostridium tetani* is called **tetanus**. The toxin acts on the central nervous system to cause convulsions and spastic paralysis (in which muscles are unable to relax). The term _____ is derived from the Latin word *tetanos*, which means "convulsive tension." Infection can be obtained from a puncture wound that is not properly cleaned, but is easily prevented with periodic vaccination (Frame 7.88). (See Figure 7.10.)

rare tumor of thymus glan

thymoma
thigh MOH mah

7.61 A tumor originating in the thymus gland is called a **thymoma**. The constructed form of _____ uses the word root *thym* and the suffix -*oma* and is written thym/oma.

PRACTICE: Diseases and Disorders of the Blood, the Lymphatic System, and Immunology

The Right Match

Match the term on the left with the correct definition on the right.

_____ 1. sickle cell anemia

_____ 2. rabies

_____ 3. botulism

_____ 4. Hodgkin disease

_____ 5. tetanus

_____ 6. immunodeficiency

_____ 7. fungemia

_____ 8. plague

_____ 9. diphtheria

_____ 10. malaria

a. disease caused by a neurotoxin released by *Clostridium tetani*

b. anemia resulting from defective hemoglobin within cells, resulting in misshaped red blood cells

c. viral infection that is spread from the saliva of an infected animal

d. condition resulting from a defective immune response

e. any infectious disease that is widespread and causes extensive mortality

f. fungal infection that spreads throughout the body by way of the bloodstream

g. a cancer of lymph nodes

h. caused by a neurotoxin produced by *Clostridium botulinum*

i. disease caused by a parasitic protozoan that infects red blood cells and the liver

j. infectious disease resulting in acute inflammation with formation of a leathery membrane in the throat

Linkup

Link the word parts in the list to create the terms that match the definitions. You may use word parts more than once. Remember to add in combining vowels when needed—and that some terms do not use any combining vowel. The first one is completed for you as an example.

Prefix	Combining Form	Suffix
mono-	aden/o	-emia
an-	botul/o	-genic
	globin/o	-ic
	hemat/o	-ism
	hem/o	-itis
	hydr/o	-oma
	iatr/o	-osis
	lymph/o	-pathy
	nucle/o	-philia
	sept/o	-phobia
	thym/o	

Definition

	Term

1. system-wide disease caused by the presence of bacteria and their toxins in the circulating blood — *septicemia* _____
2. tumor originating in the thymus gland _____
3. reduced ability of red blood cells to deliver oxygen to tissues _____
4. poisoning caused by the ingestion of food contaminated with the toxin produced by the bacterium *Clostridium botulinum* _____
5. blood outside the blood vessels and confined within an organ or space within the body, usually in a clotted form _____
6. a condition that is caused by a medical treatment _____
7. an inherited bleeding disorder that results from missing or deficient blood-clotting proteins _____
8. general term for a disease that affects hemoglobin within red blood cells _____
9. inflammation of the lymph nodes _____
10. a viral disease characterized by enlarged lymph nodes, atypical lymphocytes, throat pain, pharyngitis, fever, and fatigue _____
11. another term for rabies that refers to infected animals' inability to drink water due to progressive paralysis _____

Treatments and Procedures of the Blood, the Lymphatic System, and Immunology

Here are the word parts that specifically apply to the treatments and procedures of the blood, the lymphatic system, and immunology that are covered in the following section. Note that the word parts are color-coded to help you identify them: prefixes are yellow, combining forms are red, and suffixes are blue.

Prefix	Definition
anti-	against, opposite of
pro-	before

Combining Form	Definition
aden/o	gland
aut/o	self
bi/o	life
globin/o	protein
hem/o, hemat/o	blood
hom/o	same
immun/o	exempt, immunity
lymph/o	clear water or fluid
splen/o	spleen
thromb/o	clot

Suffix	Definition
-crit	to separate
-ectomy	surgical excision, removal
-logous	pertaining to study
-logy	study or science of
-lysis	loosen, dissolve
-phylaxis	protection
-stasis	standing still
-therapy	treatment
-tic	pertaining to

KEY TERMS A–Z

7.62 A curative treatment involving the use of a substance with known toxicity to bacteria is called **antibiotic therapy**. The constructed form of the term *antibiotic* is written anti/bi/o/tic, which literally means "pertaining to against life." The antibiotic may be obtained from a fungus, usually a mold, or other bacteria. _____ _____ is effective only against bacteria, many types of which are capable of developing resistance, especially when antibiotics are not administered properly.

antibiotic therapy
AN tih bye AHT ik * THAIR ah pee

? Did You KNOW

DISCOVERY OF ANTIBIOTICS

The first antibiotic was discovered in 1928 by Sir Alexander Fleming, who found that a common bread mold (a fungus) could produce toxins capable of killing bacterial colonies (■ Figure 7.15). The *Penicillium* mold produces an antibacterial toxin that is now known as penicillin. In time, the fungal toxins were proven to be effective against many strains of bacteria, and their use as antibiotics has been hailed as the single most important treatment against bacterial infections ever.

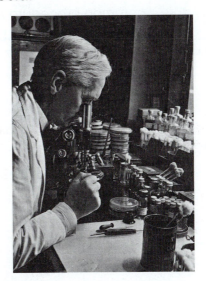

■ **Figure 7.15**
Alexander Fleming photographed in his lab where he observed the natural competition between a fungus and bacteria in 1928, which gave rise to the discovery of antibiotics.
Source: Pictorial Press Ltd./Alamy.

Prevent Clotting

anticoagulant
AN tye koh AG yoo lant

7.63 A chemical agent that delays or prevents the clotting process in blood is called an **anticoagulant**. It is often administered to reduce the likelihood of clot formation after surgery. The most common _____ agent is **warfarin** (Coumadin).

[handwritten: treatment HIV/AIDS]

antiretroviral therapy

AN tye REH troh VYE ral *
THAIR ah pee

7.64 A pharmacological therapy that is useful in battling a class of viruses that tend to mutate quickly, called *retroviruses*, is often called _____ _____. It is used against HIV, the virus that causes AIDS (Frame 7.22). The drugs form a cocktail that includes nucleotide analog reverse transcriptase inhibitors and protease inhibitors, which block HIV replication by a variety of means.

[handwritten: vaccine]

attenuation

ah TEN yoo AY shun

7.65 The process in which pathogens are rendered less virulent, or infectious, prior to their incorporation into a vaccine preparation is called _____. The term is derived from the Latin word *attenuatus*, which means "to make thin."

[handwritten: persons own blood stored in a blood bank]

autologous transfusion

aw TALL oh guss * trans
FYOO zhun

7.66 A transfusion of blood donated by a patient for their personal use is called an **autologous transfusion**. The term includes a constructed form that is written aut/o/logous and means "pertaining to study of self." _____ _____ is a common procedure before surgery to avoid potential incompatibility or contamination of blood (see ■ Figure 7.16).

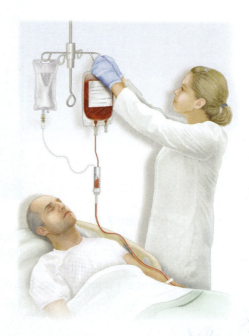

■ **Figure 7.16**
Blood transfusion. A transfusion of one's own blood is called an *autologous transfusion* (see Frame 7.66). A transfusion of donated blood from another person is called a *homologous transfusion* (see Frame 7.78).

blood chemistry

7.67 A test or series of tests on a sample of blood plasma to measure the levels of its composition, including glucose, albumin, triglycerides, pH, cholesterol, and electrolytes is called _____ _____.

blood culture *See if bacteria are present in the blood*	**7.68** A clinical test to determine infection in the blood is called a _____ _____. It is performed by placing a sample of blood in a nutrient-rich liquid medium in an effort to grow populations of bacteria for analysis.
blood transfusions *- surgery, injury, illness*	**7.69** The introduction of blood, blood products, or a blood substitute into a patient's circulation to restore blood volume to normal levels is called **blood transfusion**. The two main types of _____ _____ are **autologous transfusion** (Frame 7.66) and **homologous transfusion** (Frame 7.78). (See Figure 7.16.)
bone marrow transplant *Severe immune deficiency*	**7.70** A common procedure to treat leukemia (Frame 7.46), or injury resulting from radiation therapy or chemotherapy, is a _____ _____ _____. It involves the removal of a sample from a compatible donor, usually from red marrow in the pelvis, and its inoculation into the recipient's red marrow (■ Figure 7.17).

Fleming found penicillian from moldy bread

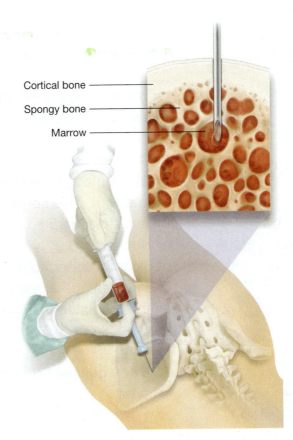

Cortical bone
Spongy bone
Marrow

■ **Figure 7.17**
Bone marrow transplant. A bone marrow transplant is usually extracted from red bone marrow within a donor's pelvis with a syringe, and then inoculated into the recipient's red bone marrow.

coagulation time
koh ahg yoo LAY shun

7.71 A timed blood test to determine the time required for a blood clot to form is called **coagulation time**. One form of this _____ _____ test, called **prothrombin time (PT)**, measures the time required for prothrombin, a precursor blood-clotting protein, to form thrombin. Thrombin then acts on the blood protein fibrinogen to form fibrin, a threadlike protein that coagulates blood. This procedure is often used to monitor the effects of anticoagulants (Frame 7.63). Another type of test is used to evaluate clotting ability and is called **partial thromboplastin time (PTT)**.

complete blood count

7.72 A common laboratory test that evaluates a sample of blood to provide diagnostic information about a patient's general health is abbreviated **CBC**, which means **complete blood count**. A

_____ _____ _____

includes several specific tests, including hematocrit (Frame 7.74), hemoglobin (Frame 7.76), red blood count (Frame 7.85), and white blood count. Sometimes a platelet count (PLT) is also included (Frame 7.83).

differential count

7.73 A microscopic count of the number of each type of white blood cell in a sample of blood is called _____ _____. The procedure uses staining techniques to highlight the features of white blood cells, allowing the hematologist to distinguish between the types.

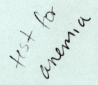
test for anemia

hematocrit
hee MAT oh krit

7.74 A procedure included in a complete blood count that measures the percentage of red blood cells in a volume of blood is called **hematocrit**. This constructed term includes the suffix *-crit*, which means "to separate," and is written hemat/o/crit. Abbreviated **HCT** or **Hct**, a _____ is obtained by centrifuging a sample of blood to separate the cells from plasma in the centrifuge tube. The percentage of red blood cells is then calculated and recorded as the "hematocrit." The normal range in males is 38.8–50%, and in females, 34.9–44.5%.

hematology
HEE mah TALL oh jee

7.75 The general field of medicine focusing on blood-related disease is called _____. The constructed form of this term is hemat/o/logy.

hemoglobin
HEE moh gloh binn

[handwritten: contains iron] [handwritten: protien inside red blood cells that carries O2]

7.76 A procedure included in a complete blood count that measures the level of hemoglobin in red blood cells (in grams) is simply called _____ and is abbreviated **HGB** or **Hgb**. Any level below normal is diagnosed as a form of anemia (Frame 7.25).

hemostasis
HEE moh STAY siss

[handwritten: stopping Bleeding]

7.77 The stoppage of bleeding is a physiological process known as **hemostasis**. It literally means "standing still blood." The constructed form of _____ is written hem/o/stasis.

homologous transfusion
hoh MALL oh guss * trans FYOO zhun

[handwritten: Blood transfusion from Someone else]

7.78 Transfusion of blood that is voluntarily donated by another person is called a _____ _____. The term *homologous* is a constructed term written hom/o/logous and means "pertaining to study of the same." It requires blood-type work called crossmatching to prevent incompatibility (Frame 7.42). (See Figure 7.16.)

immunization
IM yoo nih ZAY shun

7.79 A treatment that establishes immunity against a particular foreign substance that may otherwise cause disease is called _____. The treatment includes inoculation of antigen components that stimulate the patient's immune response to produce memory lymphocytes and antibodies, which will be available in the blood to provide immune protection when a future exposure occurs (■ Figure 7.18).

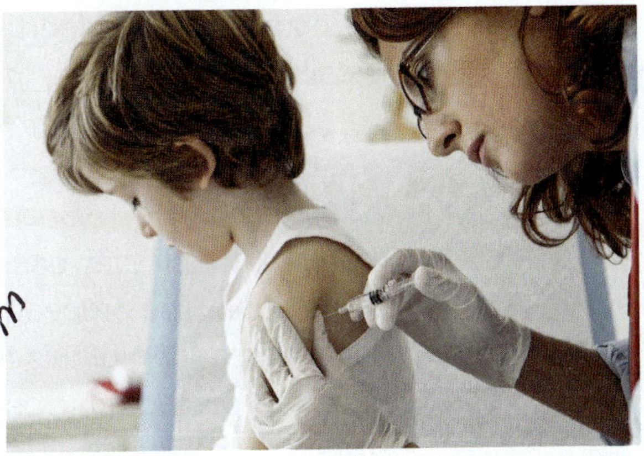

■ **Figure 7.18**
Immunization with a vaccine. A healthcare professional is injecting a vaccine into the patient's arm to provide him with acquired immunity against the influenza virus.
Source: Image Point Fr/ Shutterstock.

immunology
IM yoo NAHL oh jee

[handwritten: deficiencies/diseases of the immune system]

7.80 The science concerned with immunity and allergy is called _____. The constructed form of this term is immun/o/logy.

(handwritten, top left:) treatment for autoimmune diseases — Cancers

immunotherapy
IM yoo noh THAIR ah pee

7.81 The treatment of infectious disease and certain cancers by the administration of pharmacological agents, such as serum, gamma globulin, treated antibodies, activated white blood cells, and suppressive drugs is called _____. This constructed term is written immun/o/therapy.

(handwritten, left:) surgical removal of lymph node

lymphadenectomy
limm fad eh NEK toh mee

7.82 The suffix *-ectomy* means "surgical excision, removal." Placing this suffix at the end of a word root for an organ describes the procedure that surgically removes the organ. For example, the surgical removal of one or more lymph nodes is called _____. The constructed form of this term reveals three word parts, lymph/aden/ectomy.

platelet count

7.83 A laboratory procedure that calculates the number of platelets in a known volume of blood is called a **platelet count**, or **PLT**. A reduced _____ _____ suggests a potential failure of hemostasis (Frame 7.77) because platelets play a major role in blood clot formation and coagulation.

prophylaxis
proh fih LAK siss

(handwritten:) antibiotic

7.84 Any treatment that tends to prevent the onset of an infection or other type of disease is called **prophylaxis**. For example, thoroughly washing your hands is a _____ against spreading an infection with contaminated fingers. The constructed form is written as pro/phylaxis, which literally means "protection before."

red blood count

7.85 A lab test included in a complete blood count that measures the number of red blood cells within a given volume of blood is called a _____ _____ _____, or **RBC**.

splenectomy
splee NEK toh mee

7.86 The surgical removal of the spleen is often necessary if it has ruptured, which may occur during a physical injury to the left side of the trunk. The procedure is called _____. The constructed form of this term is written splen/ectomy. Note that in the term *splenectomy*, one *e* from *spleen* is dropped.

thrombolysis
throm BALL ih siss

(handwritten:) Clot busters

7.87 A treatment that is performed to dissolve an unwanted blood clot, or **thrombus**, is called _____. The constructed form of this term is thromb/o/lysis, which literally means "dissolve clot."

vaccination
VAK sih NAY shun

7.88 The inoculation of a foreign substance that has reduced virulence, or a reduced ability to cause infection, as a means of providing a cure or prophylaxis (Frame 7.84), is called a

_____.

vaccine
vak SEEN

7.89 A preparation that is used to activate an immune response to provide acquired immunity against an infectious agent is called a

_____.

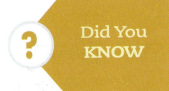

Did You KNOW

VACCINES

Vaccines have been in use since the Middle Ages or possibly earlier, when scrapings from smallpox sores were given to people as prophylaxis against this deadly disease. The use of the term *vaccine* (derived from the Latin word *vaccinus*, which means "relating to a cow") began in 1796, when Edward Jenner published his findings that scrapings of skin pustules from people infected with a similar virus that produced a different disease contracted from milking cows, known as cowpox, provided immunity against the *variola* virus that causes smallpox.

PRACTICE: Treatments and Procedures of the Blood, the Lymphatic System, and Immunology

The Right Match

Match the term on the left with the correct definition on the right.

_____ 1. attenuation
_____ 2. hematocrit
_____ 3. vaccine
_____ 4. immunization
_____ 5. red blood count
_____ 6. prothrombin time
_____ 7. blood chemistry
_____ 8. antiretroviral therapy
_____ 9. prophylaxis
_____ 10. antibiotic therapy

a. measures the number of red blood cells
b. procedure that establishes immunity against a particular antigen
c. process in which pathogens are rendered less virulent, or infectious, prior to their incorporation into a vaccine
d. tests on a sample of plasma to measure the levels of certain chemicals
e. a timed test for coagulation rate
f. measures the percentage of red blood cells in a volume of blood by centrifuging a sample
g. drugs used to battle retroviruses
h. a preventative treatment
i. a therapy against bacterial infections
j. a preparation used to activate an immune response

Break the Chain

Analyze these medical terms:

  a) Separate each term into its word parts; each word part is labeled for you (**p** = prefix, **r** = root, **cf** = combining form, and **s** = suffix).

  b) For the Bonus Question, write the requested definition in the blank that follows.

1. a) immunotherapy   _____ / __ / _____
                                                cf   s

    b) *Bonus Question*: What is the definition of the suffix? _____

2. a) splenectomy   _____ / _____
                                        r   s

    b) *Bonus Question*: What is the definition of the word root? _____

3. a) lymphadenectomy   _____ / _____ / _____
                                        r   r   s

    b) *Bonus Question*: What is the definition of the *second* word root? _____

4. a) immunology   _____ / __ / _____
                                                cf   s

    b) *Bonus Question*: What is the definition of the combining form? _____

5. a) homologous   _____ / __ / _____
                                                cf   s

    b) *Bonus Question*: What is the definition of the combining form? _____

6. a) hematology   _____ / __ / _____
                                                cf   s

    b) *Bonus Question*: What is the definition of the suffix? _____

7. a) autologous   _____ / __ / _____
                                                cf   s

    b) *Bonus Question*: What is the definition of the combining form? _____

8. a) antibiotic   _____ / _____ / __ / _____
                                        p   cf   s

    b) *Bonus Question*: What is the definition of the prefix? _____

9. a) hemostasis   _____ / __ / _____
                                                cf   s

    b) *Bonus Question*: What is the definition of the suffix? _____

10. a) thrombolysis   _____ / __ / _____
                                                cf   s

    b) *Bonus Question*: What is the definition of the suffix? _____

Abbreviations of the Blood, the Lymphatic System, and Immunology

The abbreviations that are associated with the blood, the lymphatic system, and immunology are summarized here. Study these abbreviations and review them in the exercise that follows.

Abbreviation	Definition
AIDS	acquired immunodeficiency syndrome
CBC	complete blood count
HCT, Hct	hematocrit
HGB, Hgb	hemoglobin
HIV	human immunodeficiency virus
MRSA	methicillin-resistant *Staphylococcus aureus*

Abbreviation	Definition
NHL	non-Hodgkin lymphoma
PLT	platelet count
PT	prothrombin time
PTT	partial thromboplastin time
RBC	red blood cell or red blood count
WBC	white blood cell or white blood count

PRACTICE: Abbreviations

Fill in the blanks with the abbreviation or the complete medical term.

Abbreviation

1. _____
2. CBC
3. _____
4. RBC
5. _____
6. PT
7. _____
8. WBC
9. _____
10. HIV
11. _____
12. NHL

Medical Term

acquired immunodeficiency syndrome

_____

platelet count

_____

hemoglobin

_____

partial thromboplastin time

_____

hematocrit

_____

Methicillin-resistant *Staphylococcus aureus*

_____

CHAPTER REVIEW

Word Building

Construct medical terms from the following meanings. (Some are built from word parts, some are not.) The first question has been completed as an example.

1. reduced ability of blood to deliver oxygen   an***emia***_____

2. presence of red blood cells of unequal size   _____cytosis

3. any abnormal condition of the blood   dys_____

4. a serious protozoan infection of red blood cells   _____ aria

5. abnormal reduction of red blood cells   erythro_____

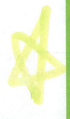

6. inherited defect in blood coagulation   _____philia

7. cancer originating in red bone marrow, producing abnormal   _____emia
   white blood cells

8. abnormally large red blood cells   macro_____

9. condition of staphylococci (bacteria) in the blood   staphylococc_____

10. disease caused by immune reaction against own tissues   _____disease

11. abnormal increase in number of red blood cells   _____ia

12. cancer of lymphatic tissue with Reed-Sternberg cells   _____disease

13. presence of bacteria and toxins in the blood   septic_____

14. inflammation of the lymph nodes   _____itis

Define the Combining Form

In the space provided, write the definition of the combining form, followed by one example of the combining form used to build a medical term in Chapter 7.

	Definition	**Use in a Term**
1. bacteri/o	_____	_____
2. immun/o	_____	_____
3. hem/o, hemat/o	_____	_____
4. erythr/o	_____	_____
5. aden/o	_____	_____
6. lymph/o	_____	_____
7. splen/o	_____	_____
8. tox/o	_____	_____
9. sept/o	_____	_____
10. leuk/o	_____	_____

Complete the Labels

Complete the blank labels in ■ Figures 7.19 and 7.20 by writing the labels in the spaces provided.

1._____   2._____   3._____ _____ _____

Lymphocyte

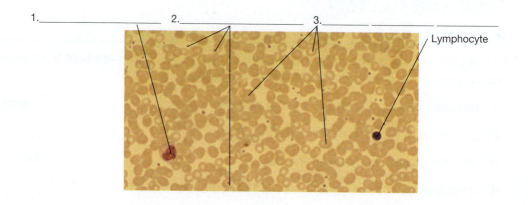

■ **Figure 7.19**
A blood smear.

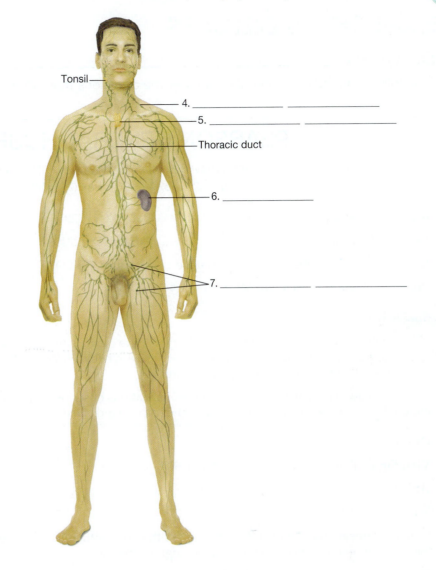

Tonsil

4. _____ _____

5. _____ _____

Thoracic duct

6. _____

7. _____ _____

■ **Figure 7.20**
The lymphatic system.

1. _____

2. _____

3. _____

4. _____

5. _____

6. _____

7. _____

MEDICAL REPORT EXERCISES

Millie Nyugen

Read the following medical report, then answer the questions that follow.

 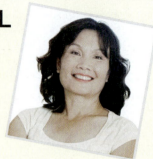

PEARSON GENERAL HOSPITAL

5500 University Avenue, Metropolis, New York
Phone: (211) 594-4000 • Fax (211) 594-4001

Medical Consultation: Hematology   **Date**: 12/17/2016

Patient: Millie Nyugen   **Patient ID**: 123456

Dob: 4/20/1962   **Age**: 54   **Sex**: Female   **Allergies**: NKDA

Provider: Sylvia S. Hernandez, MD

Subjective:

"I have felt warm, tired, and achy for the past few days or so, with headaches at night mostly. During this time I have been taking my temperature and it has been between 99 and 101°F. A few weeks ago I noticed tenderness in both armpits and in the groin area."

54 y/o female Asian patient has no prior hospitalizations or serious complaints. Her demeanor is cheerful, although very concerned about her health. She has also indicated a loss of energy during the past week.

Objective:

Vital Signs: **T**: 101.3°F; **P**: 78; **R**: 16; **BP**: 130/90

Ht: 5'2"

Wt: 110 lb

General Appearance: Pallor and diaphoresis of the skin, with mild edema around the eyes and in the neck. Swollen lymph nodes in cervical, axial, and inguinal regions.

Heart: Rate at 78 bpm, with no abnormal sounds.

Lungs: Clear without signs of disease.

AbD: Bowel sounds normal all four quadrants.

MS: Joints and muscles symmetric. No swelling, masses, or deformity.

Blood: CBC with RBCs normal; WBCs elevated 25%. Blood culture positive for *S. aureus*.

Assessment:

Staphylococcemia

Plan:

Antibiotic therapy with two IV antibiotics to be administered STAT with daily evaluation until blood culture confirms cleared. Follow-up in 2 weeks after discharge.

Photo Source: Monkey Business Images/Shutterstock.

Comprehension Questions

1. What complaints support the diagnosis? _____

   _____

   _____

2. Why do you think antibiotics might fail as a treatment? _____

   _____

   _____

3. What does the term *staphylococcemia* mean? _____

   _____

   _____

Case Study Questions

The following Case Study provides further discussion regarding the patient in the medical report. Fill in the blanks with the correct terms. Choose your answers from the list of terms that precedes the case study. (Note that some terms may be used more than once.)

antibiotic	Hodgkin disease	lymphadenitis	septicemia
blood culture	immunodeficiency	immunotherapy	splenomegaly
differential count	infection	lymphoma	staphylococcemia

A 54-year-old female, Millie Nyugen, was admitted to the infectious disease wing of the clinic after having

been referred by her personal physician, due to a prolonged fever and mild inflammation of the lymph

nodes, called (a) _____, in the neck, armpit, and groin regions. The doctor's initial diagnosis

was an unspecified disease of the lymph nodes, or lymphadenopathy, and she was concerned about a

possible tumor originating in the lymph nodes, or (b) _____, which might include cancer

of the nodes, or (c) _____. Upon more thorough examinations, no evidence of a tumor

was found. However, an abnormal enlargement of the spleen, or (d) _____, was observed.

Blood tests including a(n) (e) _____ were ordered to look for multiplication of pathogens,

or a(n) (f) _____. The tests were positive for bacteria, indicating the patient suffered from

(g) _____, or bacterial infection of the blood. Further tests identified the common bacterium

Staphylococcus as the causative pathogen, providing the diagnosis of (h) _____. The patient

was administered (i) _____ therapy. However, after 2 weeks, the symptoms failed to lessen.

The patient had developed a deficient immune response, or (j) _____. To combat this,

(k) _____ was begun immediately that included antibody treatments in combination with

antibiotic therapy. A complete recovery resulted after 3 months of treatment.

Shane Alexander

For a greater challenge, read the medical report provided and answer the critical thinking questions that follow.

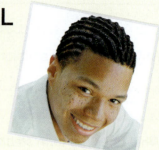

PEARSON GENERAL HOSPITAL

5500 University Avenue, Metropolis, New York
Phone: (211) 594-4000 • Fax (211) 594-4001

Medical Consultation: Infectious Disease   **Date**: 04/11/2017

Patient: Shane Alexander   **Patient ID**: 123456

Dob: 7/10/1999   **Age**: 17   **Sex**: Male   **Allergies**: NKDA

Provider: T.R. McBain, MD

Subjective:

"For the past several months I've felt very tired all the time. I fall asleep easily, and it's hard to get up out of bed in the morning and make it to school. I've been getting sick a lot lately too."

17 y/o male patient appears lethargic, with slow verbal responses to questions. He seems to have a viral cold, and indicates that he's had this cold for weeks. He is very concerned about his lack of energy and states he is getting behind in school. He says he has not yet eaten today and is hungry. The student is a member of a low-income family and states that his diet has been limited lately.

Objective:

Vital Signs: **T**: 100.2°F; **P**: 75; **R**: 18; **BP**: 122/82

Ht: 6'1"

Wt: 167 lb

General Appearance: No obvious signs of physical stress noted, such as edema, pallor, or diaphoresis. Skin appears healthy, with no discoloration.

Heart: Rate at 75 bpm, with no abnormal sounds.

Lungs: Clear without signs of disease.

AbD: Bowel sounds normal all four quadrants.

MS: Joints and muscles symmetric. No swelling, masses, or deformity.

HEENT: Minor erythema and swelling of throat; eyes and ears clear.

Blood: CBC: WBCs normal; RBCs 37%; HCT 35%

Assessment:

Anemia, possibly iron deficient

Plan:

Prescribe iron and folic acid supplements; refer to Social Services to request them to meet with his parents/guardian and discuss dietary requirements for health.

Photo Source: Tracy Whiteside/Shutterstock.

Comprehension Questions

1. Why were dietary supplements administered to the patient? _____

   _____

   _____

2. What is anemia? _____

   _____

   _____

3. How do the patient complaints point to the diagnosis? _____

   _____

   _____

Case Study Questions

The following case study provides further discussion regarding the patient in the medical report. Recall the terms from this chapter to fill in the blanks with the correct terms.

A 17-year-old male named Shane Alexander was seen by his personal physician after complaining of low energy and susceptibility to infections. Prior to seeing the patient, the physician suspected that a nonspecific blood disorder, or (l) _____, was the cause of the symptoms and ordered tests to measure the levels of blood components, known as a (m) _____, including a test for the percentage of red blood cells, called a (n) _____, and a test for the levels of hemoglobin in the blood, called a (o) _____. The tests showed low hemoglobin and low numbers of red blood cells, suggesting a general condition of (p) _____. Dietary supplements of iron and folic acid were administered.

MyLab Medical Terminology™

MyLab Medical Terminology is a premium online homework management system that includes a host of features to help you study. Registered users will find:

- A multitude of quizzes and activities built within the MyLab platform
- Powerful tools that track and analyze your results—allowing you to create a personalized learning experience
- Videos and audio pronunciations to help enrich your progress
- Streaming lesson presentations (Guided Lectures) and self-paced learning modules
- A space where you and your instructors can view and manage your assignments

Chapter 8

The Cardiovascular System

Learning Objectives

After completing this chapter, you will be able to:

8.1 Define and spell the word parts used to create terms for the cardiovascular system.

8.2 Break down and define common medical terms used for symptoms, diseases, disorders, procedures, treatments, and devices associated with the cardiovascular system.

8.3 Build medical terms from the word parts associated with the cardiovascular system.

8.4 Pronounce and spell common medical terms associated with the cardiovascular system.

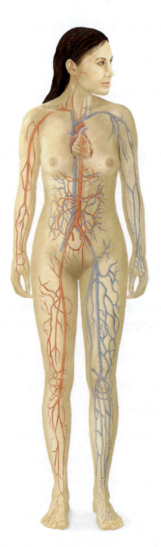

Anatomy and Physiology Terms

The following table provides the combining forms that commonly apply to the anatomy and physiology of the cardiovascular system. Note that the combining forms are colored red to help you identify them when you see them again later in the chapter.

Combining Form	Definition
angi/o	blood vessel
aort/o	aorta
arter/o, arteri/o	artery
atri/o	atrium
cardi/o	heart
coron/o	crown or circle, heart
my/o, myos/o	muscle

Combining Form	Definition
pect/o, pector/o	chest
valvul/o	little valve
vas/o	vessel
vascul/o	little vessel
ven/o	vein
ventricul/o	little belly, ventricle

cardiovascular

kar dee oh VAS kyoo lar

blood

heart

blood vessels

8.1 Every one of the 50 trillion or so cells in your body requires a continuous supply of oxygen and nutrients and an unending removal of waste materials. To meet these demands, the blood carries these materials by way of the body's circulation within a series of closed tubes, called *blood vessels*, pushed along mainly by the movements of the heart. Blood vessels include arteries that carry blood away from the heart, veins that carry blood toward the heart, and microscopic capillaries that bridge arteries and veins, whose thin walls permit the exchange of materials between blood and interstitial fluid. The movement and transport of blood is thereby achieved by the _____ **system**, which consists of the heart and blood vessels, as the word parts that form the term *cardiovascular* suggest. The constructed form is cardi/o/vascul/ar, in which *cardi/o* is a combining form that means "heart," and *vascul* is a word root that means "little vessel." The continuous flow of _____ to all tissues is vital to maintain normal body functions. If the supply of oxygen or nutrients or the removal of carbon dioxide is reduced or cut off, even for a few minutes, the affected cells will die. Thus, a disease of the cardiovascular system can pose life-threatening risks to health and survival.

8.2 The functions of the cardiovascular system may be summarized as:

- Propulsion of blood by the _____
- Transport of blood to all body tissues by the

  _____ _____

- Exchange of materials between the blood and body tissues

8.3 Review the anatomy of the cardiovascular system by studying ■ Figure 8.1 and ■ Figure 8.2.

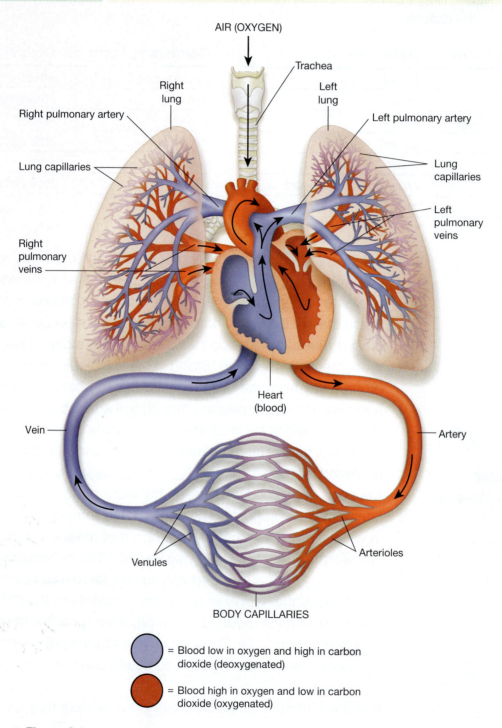

■ **Figure 8.1**
The cardiovascular system. A schematic view of the closed circulation of blood. The heart is sectioned, and the capillaries are enlarged to enable you to see them. The black arrows indicate the direction of blood flow.

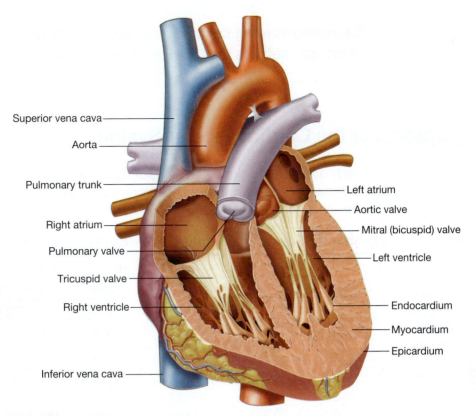

■ Figure 8.2
Internal anatomy of the heart. The heart is sectioned to reveal its internal features.

Medical Terms of the Cardiovascular System

blood	**8.4** Many diseases of the cardiovascular system have a profound effect on the body's overall health. The result of cardiovascular disease is often the reduction or stoppage of blood flow to one or more parts of the body, which results in the death of cells. If _____ flow reduction affects a large area or a critical organ like the brain, kidneys, or heart itself, the resulting cell death can produce a condition that quickly becomes life-threatening.
cardi/o/logy **cardiologist** kar dee AHL oh jist	**8.5** The division of medicine known as **cardiology** (kar dee AHL oh jee) provides clinical treatment for heart disease. *Cardiology* is a constructed term, _____/_____/_____, where the combining form *cardi/o* means "heart" and the suffix *-logy* means "study or science of." A physician specializing in this field is called a **cardiologist**. Generally, a _____ also treats conditions associated with blood vessels because of the close functional relationship between blood vessels and the heart.

cardiovascular

8.6 In the following sections, we review the prefixes, combining forms, and suffixes that combine to build the medical terms of the _____ system.

Signs and Symptoms of the Cardiovascular System

Here are the word parts that commonly apply to the signs and symptoms of the cardiovascular system that are covered in the following section. Note that the word parts are color-coded to help you identify them: prefixes are yellow, combining forms are red, and suffixes are blue.

Prefix	Definition
a-	without, absence of
brady-	slow
dys-	bad, abnormal, painful, difficult
tachy-	rapid, fast

Combining Form	Definition
angi/o	blood vessel
cardi/o	heart
cyan/o	blue
pect/o, pector/o	chest
rhythm/o, rrhythm/o	rhythm
sten/o	narrow

Suffix	Definition
-a	singular
-algia	condition of pain
-dynia	condition of pain
-genic	pertaining to producing, forming
-ia	condition of
-osis	condition of
-plegia	paralysis
-sis	state of
-spasm	sudden involuntary muscle contraction

KEY TERMS A–Z

angina pectoris

an JYE nah * PEK tor iss

Chest pain from C [handwritten]

8.7 The primary symptom of an insufficient supply of oxygen to the heart is chest pain called _____ _____. This Latin term literally means "chest choke." The level of chest pain varies with the patient, varying from a very slight pressure to an overbearing pain that radiates to the shoulders, upper left arm, and back.

angiospasm

AN jee oh spazm

spasm of blood vessel [handwritten]

8.8 The common combining form of "blood vessel" is *angi/o*. Blood vessel disorders include abnormal muscular contractions, or spasms, of the smooth muscles in the vessel walls. This sign is called _____. The constructed form of this term is angi/o/spasm.

angiostenosis
AN jee oh sten OH siss

[handwritten: narrowing of blood vessel from plague]

8.9 Narrowing of a blood vessel is a sign of cardiovascular disease, causing a reduction of blood flow to the part of the body at the receiving end of the narrowed vessel. This sign is called **angiostenosis**. The constructed form of this term is angi/o/sten/osis and includes one combining form: *angi/o*, which means "blood vessel," and the word root *sten*, which means "narrow." Thus, the literal meaning of _____ is "condition of a narrow blood vessel."

arrhythmia
ah RITH mee ah

[handwritten: without normal rythm]

8.10 The prefix *a-* means "without, absence of," and the prefix *dys-* means "bad, abnormal, painful, difficult." In some cases, they may be used interchangeably. For example, a loss of the normal rhythm of the heart is called _____, which means "condition of without rhythm" and is written a/rrhythm/ia. An alternate term for an abnormal heart rhythm is **dysrhythmia**. The constructed form of this term is written dys/rhythm/ia.

WORDS TO Watch Out For

Arrhythmia and *Dysrhythmia*

These two medical terms relating to the abnormal rhythm of the heart are very similar in their meanings, but they have important differences. As you have learned, the prefix *a-* means "without, absence of," and the prefix *dys-* means "bad, abnormal, painful, difficult." Now look closer at the word roots. They are not identical. The term *arrhythmia* ("condition of without rhythm") has an extra *r*. To remember which term is spelled with two *r*s, it might help to think of the expression "without rhyme or reason." A condition of arrhythmia is a heartbeat "*without rhyme or reason*," whereas a condition of dysrhythmia is a heartbeat with an abnormal rhythm. *Arrhythmia* is used much more frequently than *dysrhythmia*.

bradycardia
brad ee KAR dee ah

[handwritten: slow (?) rate]

8.11 The common word root for heart is *cardi*. You will find it used in many terms in this chapter. In the term **bradycardia**, the prefix that means "slow" is used to form the meaning "slow heart." _____ is an abnormally slow heart rate, usually under 60 beats per minute at rest. The normal resting heart rate ranges from 60 to 90 beats per minute.

cardiodynia
kar dee oh DIN ee ah

[handwritten: chest pain]

8.12 The most common term for chest pain is, simply, **chest pain**, abbreviated **CP**. An alternate term may also be used for this symptom. This term, **cardiodynia**, uses the suffix *-dynia*, which means "condition of pain." The constructed form of _____ is cardi/o/dynia.

problem such as pain from C

cardiogenic kar dee oh JENN ik	**8.13** The suffix *-genic* means "pertaining to producing, forming." When combined with the word part for heart, the term _____ is formed. The constructed form of the term is written cardi/o/genic. It refers to a symptom or sign that originates from a condition of the heart. For example, the pain sensation of angina pectoris (Frame 8.7) is a cardiogenic symptom because it is caused by insufficient blood flow to the heart.
cyanosis sigh ah NOH siss	**8.14** A symptom in which a blue tinge is seen in the skin and mucous membranes is called **cyanosis**, which literally means "condition of blue." The constructed form is cyan/osis. _____ is caused by oxygen deficiency in tissues and is a common sign of respiratory failure often caused by cardiovascular disease.
palpitation pal pih TAY shun	**8.15** A symptom of pounding, racing, or skipping of the heartbeat is called _____. The term is derived from the Latin word *palpitatus*, which means "a throbbing."
tachycardia tack ee KAR dee ah	**8.16** The opposite of the prefix *brady-* is the prefix *tachy-*, which means "rapid, fast." A rapid heart rate is called _____. It may be a symptom of heart disease if the heart exceeds 100 beats per minute at rest.
fainting **syncope** SIN koh pee	**8.17** A temporary loss of consciousness and posture is known as **syncope**. Commonly known as "fainting," it is often the result of a temporary reduction of blood flow to the brain. Frequent episodes may be symptoms of a cardiovascular disease. For example, heart disease may cause fainting spells, referred to as cardiogenic _____. The term *syncope* is derived from the Greek word *synkope*, which means "to cut short."

PRACTICE: Signs and Symptoms of the Cardiovascular System

Break the Chain

Analyze these medical terms:

    a) Separate each term into its word parts; each word part is labeled for you. (**p** = prefix, **r** = root, **cf** = combining form, and **s** = suffix).

    b) For the Bonus Question, write the requested definition in the blank that follows.

The first set has been completed for you as an example.

1. a) angiostenosis   _angi/o/sten/osis_
                                     cf   r   s

    b) *Bonus Question*: What is the definition of the suffix? **_condition of_** _____

2. a) bradycardia   _____/_____/_____
                                   p   r   s

    b) *Bonus Question*: What is the definition of the word root? _____

3. a) cardiodynia   _____/___/_____
                                   cf   s

    b) *Bonus Question*: What is the definition of the suffix? _____

4. a) cardiogenic   _____/___/_____
                                   cf   s

    b) *Bonus Question*: What is the definition of the suffix? _____

5. a) cyanosis   _____/_____
                                r   s

    b) *Bonus Question*: What is the definition of the word root? _____

6. a) angiospasm   _____/___/_____
                                    cf   s

    b) *Bonus Question*: What is the definition of the suffix? _____

The Right Match

Match the term on the left with the correct definition on the right.

_____ 1. cyanosis   a. sign or symptom that originates from a condition of the heart

_____ 2. angina pectoris   b. pounding, racing, or skipping of the heartbeat

_____ 3. syncope   c. opposite of bradycardia; fast heartbeat

_____ 4. cardiogenic   d. pain associated with the heart

_____ 5. cardiodynia   e. chest pain or pressure

_____ 6. arrhythmia   f. blue tinge in the skin and mucous membranes

_____ 7. tachycardia   g. fainting

_____ 8. palpitation   h. term that literally means "condition of without rhythm"

Diseases and Disorders of the Cardiovascular System

Here are the word parts that commonly apply to the diseases and disorders of the cardiovascular system that are covered in the following section. Note that the word parts are color-coded to help you identify them: prefixes are yellow, combining forms are red, and suffixes are blue.

Prefix	Definition
endo-	within
epi-	upon, over, above, on top
hyper-	excessive, abnormally high, above
hypo-	deficient, abnormally low, below
peri-	around
poly-	excessive, over, many

Combining Form	Definition
angi/o	blood vessel
aort/o	aorta
arter/o, arteri/o	artery
ather/o	fatty plaque
cardi/o	heart
coron/o	crown or circle, heart
hem/o	blood
isch/o	hold back
my/o	muscle
phleb/o	vein
scler/o	hard
sept/o	putrefying; wall, partition
sten/o	narrow
tampon/o	plug
tens/o	pressure
thromb/o	clot
valvul/o	little valve
varic/o	dilated vein

Suffix	Definition
-ac	pertaining to
-ade	process
-al	pertaining to
-ar	pertaining to
-emia	condition of blood
-ic	pertaining to
-ion	process
-itis	inflammation
-megaly	abnormally large
-oma	tumor
-osis	condition of
-pathy	disease

KEY TERMS A–Z

aneurysm

AN yoo rism

8.18 An abnormal bulging of an arterial wall is called an **aneurysm** and is shown in ■ Figure 8.3. The term is derived from the Greek word *aneurysma*, which means "a widening." An _____ is usually caused by a congenital defect or an acquired weakness of the arterial wall, which worsens in time as blood is pushed against it. The bursting of a large aneurysm is usually life-threatening, resulting in massive hemorrhage.

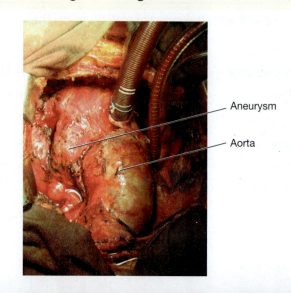

■ Figure 8.3
Aneurysm. Photograph of the aorta, the large blood vessel arising from the heart, with a large bulge, or aneurysm, in its wall (just to the left of the tubing). An aneurysm is caused by a weakened blood vessel wall that is in danger of bursting, which often results in a life-threatening hemorrhage.
Source: Kalewa/Shutterstock.

Aneurysm

Aorta

angiocarditis
AN jee oh kar DYE tiss

8.19 Inflammation of the heart and blood vessels is a disease called **angiocarditis**. It is usually caused by a widespread bacterial infection of the blood, or septicemia (Frame 8.55). The four word parts of _____ are shown when it is written angi/o/card/itis.

angioma
an jee OH mah

benign
tumor of blood vessels
tangled blood vessels

8.20 A term describing a tumor arising from a blood vessel combines the word root for blood vessel, _angi_, with the suffix for tumor, _-oma_, to form _____. This constructed term is written angi/oma. Also known as **hemangioma** (heh MAN jee OH mah), it is a benign clump of endothelium forming a mass. In some cases the mass can obstruct the flow of blood through the vessel. The term _hemangioma_ carries a second meaning of a red or purple birthmark on the skin that does not obstruct blood flow.

aortic insufficiency
ay OR tik * in suf FISH un see

CHF

8.21 The aortic valve is the semilunar valve located at the base of the aorta, which normally prevents blood from returning to the left ventricle. If it fails to close completely during ventricular diastole, blood may return to the left ventricle, causing the left ventricle to work harder. This condition is called **aortic insufficiency**. The long-term result of _____ _____, abbreviated **AI**, is a chronic condition of the heart known as congestive heart failure, which is described in Frame 8.36. An alternate term for AI is **aortic regurgitation**.

aortic stenosis
ay OR tik * sten OH siss

8.22 The word root _sten_ means "narrow." An **aortic stenosis** is a narrowing of the aortic valve, located between the left ventricle and aorta. An _____ _____ causes the left ventricle to work harder than normal. It is usually a more serious condition than aortic insufficiency, although the long-term effect is similar, leading to congestive heart failure (Frame 8.36). It is a constructed term, written aort/ic sten/osis.

aortitis
ay or TYE tiss

not common

8.23 Inflammation of the aorta is called _____. The constructed form of this term is aort/itis. Often caused by a bacterial infection, it can lead to acute aortic insufficiency (Frame 8.21).

arteriopathy
ahr tee ree AH path ee

main cause of high blood pressure

8.24 A general term for a disease of an artery is _____. This constructed term uses the suffix _-pathy_ (meaning "disease") and is written arteri/o/pathy.

arteriosclerosis

ahr TEE ree oh skleh ROH siss

These 2 are used interchangeably

atherosclerosis

ATH er oh skleh ROH siss

8.25 One common form of arteriopathy occurs when an artery wall becomes thickened and loses its elasticity, resulting in a reduced flow of blood to the tissues. The risk of developing this disease, known as **arteriosclerosis**, increases with advanced age. The constructed form of _____ is arteri/o/scler/osis, which literally means "condition of hard artery." If coronary arteries supplying the heart are damaged by this disease, the condition is called **arteriosclerotic heart disease (ASHD)**.

8.26 A term describing a specific form of arteriosclerosis (Frame 8.25), in which one or more fatty plaques form along the inner walls of arteries, uses the combining form that means "fatty plaque," *ather/o*, to form the term _____. The plaques thicken with time, which reduces the flow of blood through the affected vessel (■ Figure 8.4). The constructed form of this term is ather/o/scler/osis, which literally means "condition of hard fatty plaque." A major cause of coronary artery disease (Frame 8.38), **atherosclerosis** poses an immediate threat to life if a plaque disrupts blood flow and releases blood clots, which may trigger an acute myocardial infarction (Frame 8.49).

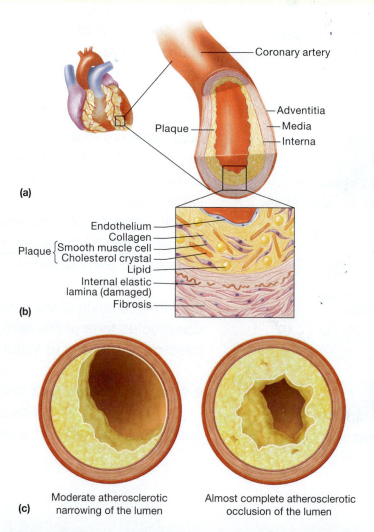

(a)

Coronary artery

Adventitia
Media
Interna

Plaque

Endothelium
Collagen
Plaque { Smooth muscle cell
Cholesterol crystal
Lipid
Internal elastic lamina (damaged)
Fibrosis

(b)

Moderate atherosclerotic narrowing of the lumen

Almost complete atherosclerotic occlusion of the lumen

(c)

■ **Figure 8.4**
Atherosclerosis. (a) A sectioned coronary artery that exhibits an accumulation of fatty plaque, which reduces the internal diameter of the vessel. (b) In this close-up, you can see that the plaque consists of cholesterol, triglycerides, phospholipids, collagen, and smooth muscle cells. (c) Two types and degrees of atherosclerotic narrowing, or stenosis.

atrial septal defect
AY tree al * SEP tal * DEE fekt

8.27 A general condition present at birth that centers on a malfunction of the heart is called a **congenital heart disease**. One form of this disease occurs when an infant's heart allows blood to move between the two atria because of a small opening in the wall separating them. Known as an **atrial septal defect**, it results in a reduction of blood flow to the lungs. As a result, the tissues of an infant with _____ _____ _____ become starved of oxygen. *Atrial* and *septal* are constructed terms, as you can see when they are written as atri/al and sept/al.

atriomegaly
AY tree oh MEG ah lee
atri/o/megaly

8.28 The suffix *-megaly* means "abnormally large." In the condition **atriomegaly**, the atria have become abnormally enlarged or dilated, reducing their ability to push blood into the ventricles. The constructed form of _____ reveals three word parts: _____/_____/_____. It is a form of cardiomegaly (Frame 8.32).

[handwritten: need a pacemaker]

atrioventricular block
AY tree oh ven TRIK yoo lar

8.29 An injury to the atrioventricular node (AV node), which normally receives impulses from the sinoatrial node (SA node) and transmits them to the ventricles to stimulate ventricular contraction, is called an _____ _____, or **AV block**. The injury is usually caused by a myocardial infarction (Frame 8.49), during which the cells of the AV node die due to a loss of blood flow. The term *atrioventricular* is a constructed term: atri/o/ventricul/ar.

cardiac arrest
KAR dee ak * ah REST

[handwritten: heart has stopped, will die in 5 min or less]

8.30 The cessation of heart activity is called _____ _____. As you should know, *cardiac* is a constructed term written cardi/ac. *Arrest* means "stop." In **sudden cardiac arrest**, abbreviated **SCA**, the patient may have little or no warning signs; often the arrest causes death. According to the American Heart Association, more than 320,000 people die from an SCA each year in the United States. Most deaths occur within minutes, primarily due to a sudden loss of blood flow to the brain. The most common cause of SCA is an electrical disturbance to the heart that causes arrhythmia (Frame 8.10), although it may also follow a myocardial infarction, or heart attack (Frame 8.49).

cardiac tamponade
KAR dee ak * tamp oh NAHD

surgical emergency

8.31 Acute compression of the heart due to the accumulation of fluid within the pericardial cavity is known as **cardiac tamponade**. The term is constructed from word parts and is shown as cardi/ac tampon/ade. It literally means "pertaining to heart plug process." _____ _____ is a complication of an inflammatory disease of the pericardium known as *pericarditis* (Frame 8.52).

cardiomegaly
KAR dee oh MEG ah lee

causes ♡ failure

8.32 Recall that the suffix -*megaly* means "abnormally large." The abnormal enlargement of the heart is called _____, which occurs when the heart must work harder than normal to meet the oxygen demands of body cells. The constructed form of this term is cardi/o/megaly.

cardiomyopathy
KAR dee oh my OPP ah thee

most often from viral infection

need ♡ transplant

8.33 A general term for a disease of the myocardium of the heart is **cardiomyopathy**. The constructed form of _____ reveals five word parts: cardi/o/my/o/pathy. The most common causes of cardiomyopathy include coronary artery disease (Frame 8.38), viral or bacterial infection, and stress during pregnancy.

cardiovalvulitis
KAR dee oh val vyoo LYE tiss

8.34 An inflammation of the valves of the heart is called **cardiovalvulitis** (■ Figure 8.5). The constructed form of this term is cardi/o/valvul/itis. As you know, *cardi/o* means "heart," and the suffix -*itis* means "inflammation." The word root *valvul* means "little valve." The most common causes of this disease are bacterial infection, which leads to the deposition of calcium deposits on heart valves (known as *vegetations*), and congenital defects, which result in abnormally shaped valves. _____ is usually diagnosed from the presence of a heart murmur (Frame 8.44), which is a gurgling sound detected during auscultation (Frame 8.68).

■ **Figure 8.5**
Cardiovalvulitis. The human heart has been sectioned to reveal the left ventricle and origin of the aorta, with the aortic valve between them. The yellow growths, called *vegetations*, on the aortic valve have been caused by a *Streptococcus* infection, rendering the valve disfigured and thereby unable to direct the flow of blood properly.
Source: Courtesy of the Public Health Image Library, Centers for Disease Control and Prevention.

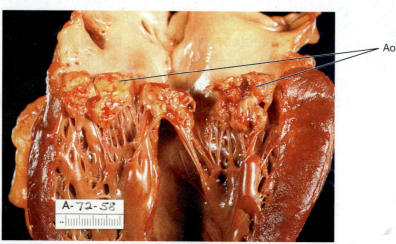

Aortic valve vegetations

8.35 A congenital (present at birth) heart disease affecting the infant's aorta is **coarctation of the aorta**. The term *coarctation* is derived from the Latin word *coarcto*, which means "to press together." _____ of the aorta causes reduced systemic circulation of blood and accumulation of fluid in the lungs and requires surgical repair.

coarctation
 koh ark TAY shun

8.36 A chronic form of heart disease characterized by the failure of the left ventricle to pump enough blood to supply systemic tissues is called **congestive heart failure (CHF)**. Also known as **left-ventricular failure**, the reduced function of the left ventricle characteristic of _____ _____ _____ makes the heart work harder, resulting in cardiomegaly (Frame 8.32), pulmonary congestion (fluid in the lungs), and reduced left-ventricle function that eventually leads to cardiac arrest (Frame 8.30). The primary symptoms of CHF include shortness of breath and fatigue.

congestive heart failure

not enough oxygen

8.37 If a disease of one or both lungs affects blood flow within the lungs, blood may back up in the right ventricle of the heart (the right ventricle normally pumps blood to the lungs). As a result, the right ventricle will be forced to work harder but with less efficiency, which enlarges the heart on the right side. A chronic enlargement and reduced efficiency of the right ventricle resulting from backup of the pulmonary circulation is called **cor pulmonale**. A French word that literally means "heart lung," _____ _____ is also known as **right-ventricular failure**.

cor pulmonale
 kor * pull moh NAY lee

8.38 A general term for a disease that afflicts the coronary arteries supplying the heart is _____ _____ _____ **(CAD)**. The most common form of CAD is atherosclerosis (Frame 8.26). Because the coronary arteries supply the heart with blood, an alternate term to coronary artery disease is **coronary heart disease (CHD)**.

coronary artery disease

coronary occlusion

8.39 *Occlusion* is a general term that means "blockage." A **coronary occlusion** is a blockage within a coronary artery, resulting in a reduced blood flow to an area of the heart muscle. The most common single cause of a _____ _____ is atherosclerosis (Frame 8.26). Atherosclerosis or other diseases may also lead to emboli (drifting blood clots), and a congenital stenosis may also contribute to coronary occlusion.

embolism
EM boh lizm

a solid loose in the blood = clot

8.40 A blockage or occlusion that forms when a blood clot or other foreign particle (including air or fat) moves through the circulation is called an **embolism**. The term is derived from the Greek word *embolisma*, which means "piece or patch." An _____ can produce a severe circulatory restriction when the blood clot or particle, called an **embolus** (plural form is **emboli**), lodges in an artery.

endocarditis
EHN doh kar DYE tiss

8.41 Inflammation of the endocardium, the thin membrane lining the inside walls of the heart chambers, is an acute disease called _____. The constructed form of this term is endo/card/itis. Because the endocardium also covers the heart valves, endocarditis often results in cardiovalvulitis (Frame 8.34). It is usually caused by a bacterial infection.

fibrillation
fih bril AY shun

8.42 A condition of uncoordinated, rapid contractions of the muscle forming the ventricles or atria is called _____. It is a severe form of arrhythmia (Frame 8.10). **Atrial fibrillation (A-fib)** leads to a reduction of blood expelled from the atria and is usually not fatal, although it poses an increased risk of stroke due to blood clots forming in the left atrium that may lodge in the brain. However, **ventricular fibrillation** results in circulatory collapse due to the failure of the ventricles to expel blood. It is often fatal within 5 minutes if medical intervention through CPR (Frame 8.71) or defibrillation (Frame 8.74) is not immediately available.

heart block

8.43 A block or delay of the normal electrical conduction of the heart is called _____ _____. It is often the result of a myocardial infarction (Frame 8.49) that damages the SA node or AV node, which normally manage the rhythmic contractions of the heart.

heart murmur

8.44 An abnormal sound heard during auscultation (Frame 8.68) of the heart is a **heart murmur**. An "innocent" _____ _____ is not associated with a heart condition and is very common, while murmurs that are not innocent suggest heart disease such as cardiovalvulitis (Frame 8.34). A common source of heart murmur is a leaky mitral valve (the atrioventricular valve on the left side), and is known as **mitral valve prolapse (MVP)**. Most people with MVP have an innocent heart murmur, but in some, the prolapse causes regurgitation of blood through the damaged mitral valve into the left atrium and thereby requires medical intervention.

hemorrhoids
HEM oh roydz

Varicose veins in anus

8.45 The presence of dilated, or varicose, veins in the anal region is called _____. The condition produces symptoms of local pain and itching. It usually results from too much pressure on the veins in the anal wall, producing swollen veins within the anal columns (internal hemorrhoids) or near the anal opening (external hemorrhoids).

hypertension
HIGH per TEN shun

damages every organ

8.46 Persistently high blood pressure while at rest is an abnormal condition called _____. This constructed term is written hyper/tens/ion and means "process of abnormally high pressure." It includes **essential hypertension**, in which the condition is not traceable to a single cause, and **secondary hypertension**, in which the high blood pressure is caused by the effects of another disease, such as atherosclerosis or diabetes. Although hypertension usually produces no symptoms, it is one of the most common causes of stroke and kidney failure.

hypotension
HIGH poh TEN shun

Emergency

8.47 A condition of abnormally low blood pressure is called _____, which includes the prefix *hypo-* that means "deficient, abnormally low, below." It is usually an acute reaction to hemorrhage, hypothermia (abnormally low body temperature), or septicemia (Frame 8.55).

ischemia
iss KEE mee ah

lack of O₂ to tissues

8.48 An abnormally low flow of blood to the tissues is the condition known as **ischemia**. The term is a constructed term, isch/emia, which literally means "condition of holding back blood." Coronary _____ is caused by an occlusion, such as atherosclerotic plaque (Frame 8.26), emboli (Frame 8.40), or thrombosis (Frame 8.57), and, because it damages the heart, can lead to a life-threatening myocardial infarction (Frame 8.49).

8.49 Death of a portion of the myocardium is called **myocardial infarction**, abbreviated **MI**. The term *infarction* is derived from the Latin word *infarctus*, which means "stuff into." In medicine, the term is used to describe a death of cells resulting from a sudden loss of blood flow (■ Figure 8.6). The term *myocardial* is constructed from word parts, as shown when it is written as my/o/cardi/al, which means "pertaining to heart muscle." If the _____ _____ affects a large or functionally critical part of the heart, arrhythmia (Frame 8.10), cardiac arrest (Frame 8.30), or both may follow. The common name for an MI is a **heart attack**. According to the American Heart Association, approximately 790,000 individuals experience heart attacks in the United States each year, roughly 25% of which are fatal.

myocardial infarction

my oh KAR dee al * in FARK shun

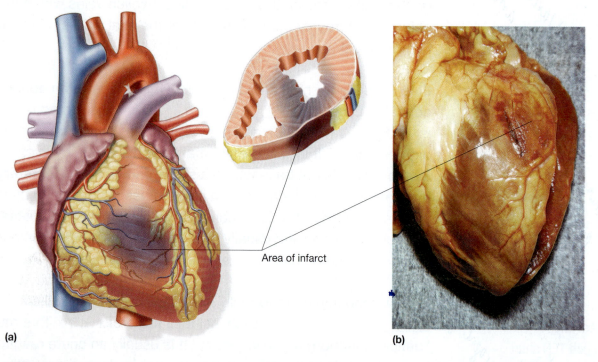

Area of infarct

(a)   (b)

■ **Figure 8.6**
Myocardial infarction. (a) A heart with a myocardial infarction of the ventricle wall, in which cardiac cells have died and surrounding tissues have become damaged. The right image is a section through the heart. (b) Photograph of a human heart (postmortem) to reveal the the dead cardiac tissue (necrosis), which perished due to a sudden loss of blood flow.
Photo Source: Mediscan/Alamy Stock Photo.

myocarditis

my oh kar DYE tiss

Often cant be fixed & needs a transplant

8.50 Inflammation of the myocardium of the heart is an acute condition called _____. The constructed form of this term is my/o/card/itis. Often caused by bacterial infection, it is a form of cardiomyopathy (Frame 8.33).

patent ductus arteriosus
PAY tent * DUCK tuss * ahr tee ree OH siss

8.51 A congenital condition characterized by an opening between the pulmonary artery and the aorta at birth due to a failure of the fetal vessel, called the *ductus arteriosus*, to close is called **patent ductus arteriosus**. The term *patent* means "open." The condition _____ _____ _____ permits the flow of blood from the pulmonary artery to the aorta, which bypasses the pulmonary circulation.

pericarditis
pair ih kar DYE tiss

8.52 Inflammation of the membrane surrounding the heart, the pericardium, is called _____. The constructed form of the term is written peri/card/itis. It is usually caused by bacterial infection and affects both layers of the pericardium (the outer pericardial sac and the inner epicardium).

phlebitis
fleh BYE tiss

8.53 A word root for vein is *phleb*, and it is used in the construction of the term that means "inflammation of a vein." The term is _____, and its constructed form is phleb/itis. In the related condition **thrombophlebitis** (THROM boh fleh BYE tiss), the inflammation of the vein includes an obstruction by a blood clot.

polyarteritis
PALL ee ahr ter EYE tiss

8.54 Simultaneous inflammation of many arteries is a condition known as _____. The constructed form of this term reveals three word parts and is poly/arter/itis.

septicemia
SEP tih SEE mee ah

8.55 A bacterial infection of the bloodstream is called **septicemia**. Because the bacteria are carried throughout the body by way of the infected blood, it becomes widespread and life-threatening quickly. The constructed form of _____ is sept/ic/emia, which literally means "condition of putrefying blood." Recall that **sepsis** is a Greek word that means "putrefying."

tetralogy of Fallot
teh TRALL oh jee * of * fah LOH

8.56 A severe congenital disease in which four defects associated with the heart are present at birth is called **tetralogy of Fallot**. The four defects are pulmonary stenosis (narrowing of the pulmonary valve), ventricular septal defect (Frame 8.59), incorrect position of the aorta, and right-ventricular hypertrophy. As a result of _____ _____ _____, the pulmonary circulation is partially bypassed.

thrombosis throm BOH siss	**8.57** The presence of stationary blood clots within one or more blood vessels is called **thrombosis**. The term is the Greek word for clotting, *thrombosis*. A coronary _____ is often caused by atherosclerosis (Frame 8.26), and its rupture can result in sudden cardiac arrest (Frame 8.30) due to an acute myocardial infarction (Frame 8.49).
varicosis vair ih KOH siss	**8.58** An abnormally dilated vein is called _____, or varicose vein. *Varicosis* is a constructed term, written varic/osis, which literally means "condition of dilated vein." It results when valves within a superficial vein of the leg or elsewhere fail, allowing blood to pool in response to gravitational forces (■ Figure 8.7).

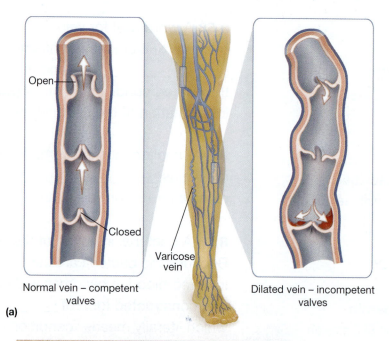

Open

Closed

Varicose vein

Normal vein – competent valves

Dilated vein – incompetent valves

(a)

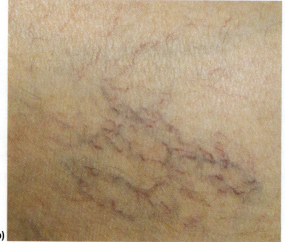

(b)

■ **Figure 8.7**
Varicosis. (a) Varicose veins develop due to the failure of valves in the superficial veins of the leg, which leads to blood accumulation in response to gravity and vein dilation. (b) Photograph of spider veins (small varicose veins) of the leg. *Photo Source: Schankz/ Shutterstock.*

ventricular septal defect

vehn TRIK yoo lar * SEPP tal * DEE fekt

(handwritten: hole in the wall, causes a murmur in baby)

8.59 A congenital disease in which an opening in the septum (*sept/o* in this case means "wall, partition") separating the right and left ventricles is present at birth is called _____ _____ _____, abbreviated **VSD**. The opening allows some blood to flow from the left ventricle to the right ventricle, reducing blood flow to body organs while dangerously increasing blood flow to the lungs.

PRACTICE: Diseases and Disorders of the Cardiovascular System

Linkup

Link the word parts in the list to create the terms that match the definitions. You may use word parts more than once. Remember to add in combining vowels when needed—and that some terms do not use any combining vowel. The first one is completed as an example.

Prefix	Combining Form	Suffix
hyper-	angi/o	-ion
peri-	ather/o	-ism
	cardi/o	-itis
	embol/o	-oma
	my/o	-osis
	scler/o	-pathy
	tens/o	
	thromb/o	
	varic/o	

Definition

1. An occlusion of blood flow
2. A general term for a disease of the myocardium of the heart
3. A specific form of arteriosclerosis in which one or more fatty plaques form along the inner walls of arteries
4. A tumor arising from a blood vessel
5. Inflammation of the membrane surrounding the heart
6. Inflammation of the heart and blood vessels
7. An abnormally dilated vein
8. The presence of a stationary blood clot within a blood vessel
9. Persistently high blood pressure

Term

embolism
_____
_____

_____
_____
_____
_____
_____
_____

The Right Match

Match the term on the left with the correct definition on the right.

_____ 1. aneurysm

_____ 2. cardiac tamponade

_____ 3. cor pulmonale

_____ 4. heart murmur

_____ 5. cardiac arrest

_____ 6. coronary artery disease

_____ 7. coronary occlusion

_____ 8. atrial septal defect

_____ 9. congestive heart failure

_____ 10. heart block

_____ 11. fibrillation

a. a disease of the coronary vessels

b. a congenital heart defect

c. a block of the heart conduction system

d. a blockage in a coronary vessel

e. abnormal bulging of an arterial wall

f. an abnormal sound heard through auscultation

g. cessation of heartbeat

h. uncoordinated, rapid heartbeat

i. literally, "heart lung"

j. left-ventricular failure

k. caused by fluid within the pericardial cavity

Treatments, Procedures, and Devices of the Cardiovascular System

Here are the word parts that commonly apply to the treatments, procedures, and devices associated with the cardiovascular system and are covered in the following section. Note that the word parts are color-coded to help you identify them: prefixes are yellow, combining forms are red, and suffixes are blue.

Prefix	Definition
endo-	within
ultra-	beyond normal

Combining Form	Definition
angi/o	blood vessel
aort/o	aorta
arter/o, arteri/o	artery
cardi/o	heart
coron/o	crown or circle, heart
ech/o	sound
electr/o	electricity
embol/o	plug
man/o	thin, scanty
phleb/o	vein
pulmon/o	lung
son/o	sound
sphygm/o	pulse
thromb/o	clot
valvul/o	little valve

Suffix	Definition
-ac	pertaining to
-ary	pertaining to
-ectomy	surgical excision, removal
-gram	a record or image
-graphy	recording process
-ist	one who specializes
-lytic	pertaining to loosen, dissolve
-meter	measure, measuring instrument
-metry	measurement, process of measuring
-plasty	surgical repair
-rrhaphy	suturing
-scopy	process of viewing
-stomy	surgical creation of an opening
-tomy	incision, to cut

KEY TERMS A–Z

angiography
an jee OG rah fee

8.60 A diagnostic procedure that includes x-ray photography, MRI, or CT scan images of a blood vessel after injection of a contrast medium is called **angiography**. This constructed term is written angi/o/graphy. The image resulting from _____ is called an **angiogram** (AN jee oh gram), which is written angi/o/gram. When the procedure is focused on the heart, it is called **cardiac angiography** or **coronary angiography**.

angioplasty
AN jee oh plass tee

8.61 The surgical repair of a blood vessel is generally known as _____. The constructed form of this term is angi/o/plasty. It includes procedures to reopen blocked vessels, such as **balloon angioplasty**, in which a balloon is inserted into a blocked vessel and inflated (■ Figure 8.8), and **laser angioplasty**, which uses a laser beam to open a blocked artery.

■ **Figure 8.8**
Angioplasty. One popular form is called *balloon angioplasty*, shown here. A balloon catheter is threaded into the blocked artery and positioned into the obstructed area (left). The balloon is then inflated, which presses the plaque against the vessel wall (right). After the balloon catheter is withdrawn, the plaque remains flattened, improving the flow of blood through the vessel.
Source: Pearson Education Inc.

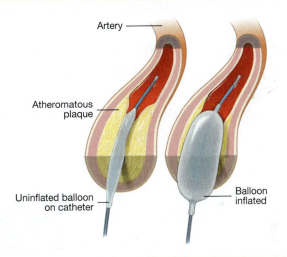

Artery

Atheromatous plaque

Uninflated balloon on catheter

Balloon inflated

angioscopy
AN jee OS koh pee

8.62 The use of a flexible fiber-optic instrument, or endoscope, to observe a diseased blood vessel and to assess any lesions is a procedure called _____. This constructed term is written angi/o/scopy. The endoscope is often a modified instrument, called an **angioscope**, which includes a camera at one end and a video monitor at the opposite end.

angiostomy
an jee OS toh mee

8.63 The suffix *-stomy* means "surgical creation of an opening." The surgical procedure that involves the creation of an opening into a blood vessel, usually for the insertion of a catheter, is called _____. The constructed form of this term is angi/o/stomy.

angiotomy
an jee OT oh mee

8.64 The surgical incision into a blood vessel is called _____, which uses the suffix *-tomy* that means "incision, to cut." The constructed form of this term reveals three word parts, as shown in angi/o/tomy.

aortography AY or TOG rah fee	**8.65** A procedure that obtains an x-ray image, MRI, or CT scan image of the aorta is called _____. The constructed form of this term is aort/o/graphy. The image is called an **aortogram**.
arteriography ahr tee ree OG rah fee	**8.66** A procedure that obtains an image of an artery is known as _____. The constructed form of this term is arteri/o/graphy, which literally means "process of recording an artery." The image is called an **arteriogram**.
arteriotomy ahr tee ree OT oh mee	**8.67** An incision into an artery is called an _____. This constructed term is written arteri/o/tomy. It is usually performed to repair an injured artery during a procedure known as an **arterioplasty**. The conclusion of the procedure is achieved by suturing the opening, called **arteriorrhaphy**.
auscultation oss kull TAY shun *listening to ♡*	**8.68** An important part of a physical examination involves listening to internal sounds using a **stethoscope** (STETH oh skope) and is called _____. Certain sounds suggest abnormalities of heart function, especially arrhythmias and valve disorders (■ Figure 8.9).

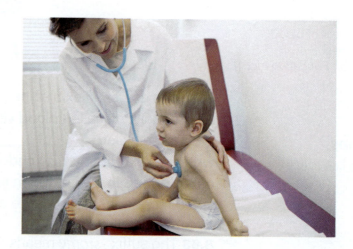

■ **Figure 8.9**
Auscultation. A pediatrician is performing auscultation on an infant to check for possible heart disorders.
Source: Image Point Fr/ Shutterstock.

? **Did You KNOW**

AUSCULTATION

Auscultation is derived from the Latin word *ausculto*, which means "to listen." During the ancient times of Aristotle, early physicians practiced this form of evaluation by pressing an ear against the patient's chest. The stethoscope, which literally means "instrument to view the chest," is a device that made this procedure much more efficient by amplifying the sounds. French physician Rene Laennec was the inventor of the first stethoscope in 1816. He rolled paper into a tube shape to listen to the chest sounds of a young female patient to avoid unwanted contact between his ear and her chest. He was excited to learn of the amplified effect of the tube and developed a wooden tube that became widely used within a few years. Today, stethoscopes include two rubber earpieces and an amplifying bell or cone.

cardiac catheterization

KAR dee ak * kath eh ter ih ZAY shun

8.69 Insertion of a narrow flexible tube, called a **catheter**, through a blood vessel leading into the heart is called _____ _____ (■ Figure 8.10). The procedure is performed to withdraw blood samples from heart chambers, measure pressures, and inject contrast medium for imaging purposes. The term *catheter* is derived from the Greek word *katheter*, which means "to send down."

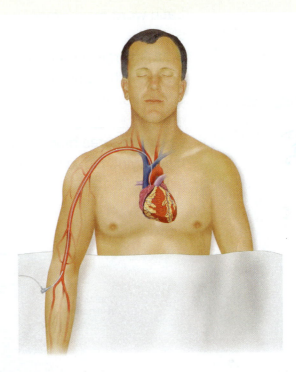

■ **Figure 8.10**
Cardiac catheterization. Insertion of a tube, called a *catheter*, through a blood vessel. In this example, the catheter is inserted into the brachial artery of the arm and is pushed through vessels until reaching the interior of the heart.

cardiac pacemaker

KAR dee ak * PAYS may ker

8.70 A **cardiac pacemaker** is a battery-powered device that is implanted under the skin and wired to the inner wall of the heart to help control abnormal heart rhythms (■ Figure 8.11). It produces timed electric pulses that replace the function of the SA node as a treatment for a heart block and certain other arrhythmias. Recently, the _____ _____ has been improved to adjust to the patient's physical activity and SA node function. This is called an *on-demand pacemaker*.

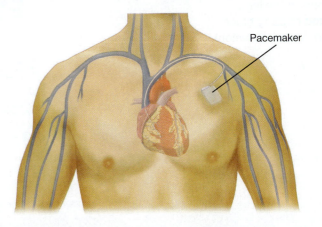

Pacemaker

■ **Figure 8.11**
Cardiac pacemaker. The pacemaker device is implanted beneath the skin near the heart.

cardiopulmonary resuscitation

KAR dee oh PULL mon air ee * ree SUSS ih TAY shun

8.71 An emergency procedure that is used to maintain some blood flow to vital organs until the heart can be restarted is commonly abbreviated **CPR**, which means _____ _____. It consists of rhythmic chest compression. If the restoration of breathing is also needed, artificial respiration may be included. The constructed form of this term is written cardi/o/pulmon/ary resuscitation. The term *resuscitation* is derived from the Latin word *resuscitatio*, which means "to revive."

coronary artery bypass graft

Most common open O surgery

8.72 A surgical procedure that involves removing a blood vessel from another part of the body and inserting it into the coronary circulation is called _____ _____ _____ _____, or **CABG**. The grafted vessel restores blood flow to an oxygen-deprived area of the heart by carrying blood around an occluded (blocked) coronary artery (■ Figure 8.12).

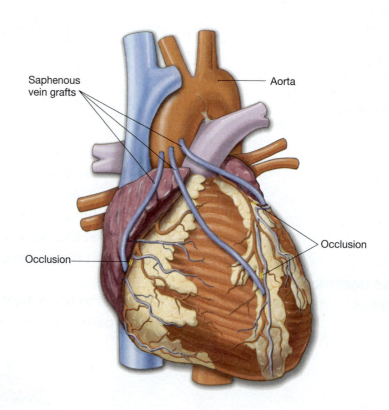

Saphenous vein grafts

Aorta

Occlusion

Occlusion

■ **Figure 8.12**
Coronary artery bypass graft (CABG). The grafts are often obtained from the patient's saphenous veins in the legs and are inserted to carry blood around the blockage (occlusion).

8.73 An artificial, metallic scaffold that is used to support an injured blood vessel, compress an atherosclerotic plaque, or anchor a surgical implant or graft is called a **stent** (■ Figure 8.13). In coronary circulation, a **coronary stent** may be implanted into a coronary artery that is occluded to restore blood flow to an oxygen-deprived part of the heart. A _____ _____ may also be used to prevent closure of a coronary artery after angioplasty (Frame 8.61).

coronary stent

■ **Figure 8.13**
Coronary stent. Insertion of a stent to open a coronary artery that is blocked by an atherosclerotic plaque is a popular surgery that improves blood flow to the heart. The top figure shows the stent, temporarily attached to a catheter, in place in the area of the occluding plaque. The middle figure shows the process of expanding the stent, which pushes the plaque to clear the occlusion. In the bottom figure, the catheter has been removed and the stent is fully expanded, and will remain in place after the surgery.
Source: Pearson Education, Inc.

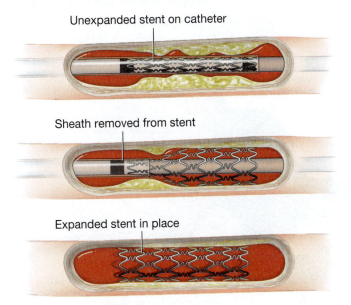

Unexpanded stent on catheter

Sheath removed from stent

Expanded stent in place

defibrillation

dee fib rih LAY shun

8.74 In cases in which an arrhythmia progresses to the state of ventricular fibrillation (Frame 8.42), an electric charge may be applied to the chest wall to stop the heart conduction system momentarily, then restart it to establish a more normal heart rhythm. This procedure is called _____. In most cases, the electric charge is applied to the skin of the chest with paddles using an **automated external defibrillator**. Abbreviated **AED**, a portable unit is illustrated in ■ Figure 8.14a. Alternatively, a smaller device may be surgically implanted under the skin with electrodes terminating directly on the heart. This device is called an **implantable cardioverter defibrillator (ICD)** and is illustrated in ■ Figure 8.14b.

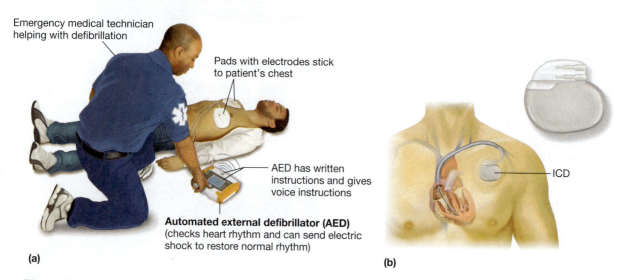

Emergency medical technician helping with defibrillation

Pads with electrodes stick to patient's chest

AED has written instructions and gives voice instructions

Automated external defibrillator (AED) (checks heart rhythm and can send electric shock to restore normal rhythm)

ICD

(a)

(b)

■ **Figure 8.14**
Defibrillator. Defibrillators are devices that supply a voltage charge to the heart in the hope of restarting the cardiac cycle (heartbeat). (a) A portable automated external defibrillator (AED). The unit includes two paddles that are pressed against the external chest wall, which deliver a brief voltage charge from a generator to the patient. AEDs are given credit for saving thousands of lives every year, mainly from sudden cardiac arrest (SCA). (b) An implantable cardioverter defibrillator (ICD), which is used during surgery and may be inserted for postsurgical maintenance.

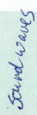 _sound waves_

Doppler sonography

DOP ler * son OG rah fee

8.75 An ultrasound procedure that evaluates blood flow through a blood vessel is called **Doppler sonography**. It is often performed on the heart or on the carotid artery of the neck to evaluate problems in blood flow in a noninvasive manner, and it may also be used to monitor pulse rate from peripheral arteries. In the term _____ _____, _sonography_ is a constructed term, written son/o/graphy, which literally means "recording process of sound."

echocardiography

ek oh kar dee OG rah fee

[handwritten: sound waves ultrasound of ♡]

8.76 An ultrasound procedure that directs sound waves through the heart to observe heart structures in an effort to evaluate heart function is called _____ (■ Figure 8.15). This is a constructed term with five word parts that is written ech/o/ cardi/o/graphy. The procedure may also be called **cardiac ultrasonography** (KAR dee ak * ul trah son OG rah fee). The record or image of the data is typically called an **echocardiogram** (ek oh KAR dee oh gram). If a heart condition is suspected, it is often performed during or immediately after exercise using a treadmill or stationary bicycle to reproduce the dysfunction for closer evaluation, in the procedure known as a **stress ECHO**.

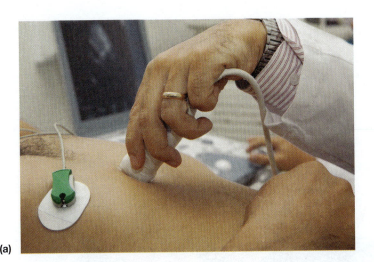

(a)

■ **Figure 8.15**
Echocardiography. (a) The procedure is performed by placing electrodes on the chest wall, which sends ultrasound pulses to the heart. A receiver, held by the physician or technician, picks up echoes from the pulses and sends them to a computer for analysis. (b) A monitor displays the flow of blood passing through the heart (red and yellow) and action of the heart valves, providing a record that may be digitally saved and printed. *Source: (a) Anamaria Mejia/ Shutterstock (b) cylonphto/123RF.com.*

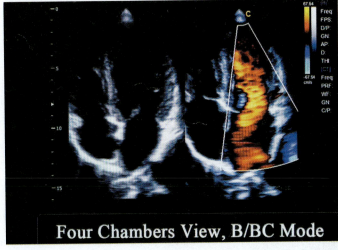

Four Chambers View, B/BC Mode

(b)

electrocardiography

ee LEK troh KAR dee AWG rah fee

8.77 In the procedure known as **electrocardiography**, electrodes are pasted to the skin of the chest to detect and record the electrical events of the heart conduction system (■ Figure 8.16). The constructed form of _____ is written electr/o/cardi/o/graphy. The record or image of the data is called an **electrocardiogram** and abbreviated **ECG** or **EKG** (the *K* is from the Greek word for heart, *kardia*) (see Figure 8.16b). Electrocardiography is used extensively to evaluate heart function and is the most common method for diagnosing a heart attack. It is particularly useful in diagnosing cardiac arrhythmias (Frame 8.10). When measured during physical activity using a treadmill or stationary bicycle, it is called a **stress ECG**.

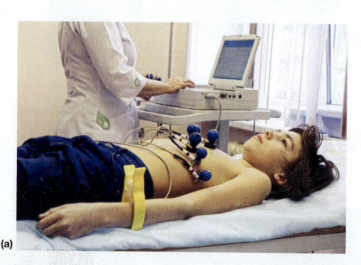

(a)

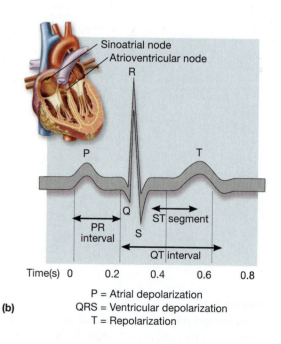

Sinoatrial node
Atrioventricular node

PR interval

ST segment

QT interval

Time(s) 0   0.2   0.4   0.6   0.8

(b)

P = Atrial depolarization
QRS = Ventricular depolarization
T = Repolarization

■ **Figure 8.16**
An electrocardiogram may be obtained while at rest (shown) or during exercise when it is called a stress ECG. (a) Electrodes are placed on the patient's chest to record the electrical events within the heart, and the results are collected by computer and displayed on a monitor. (b) Each cardiac cycle of a normal electrocardiogram includes three peaks or waves, called the *P wave*, *QRS wave*, and *T wave*.
Source (a): Lapina/Shutterstock.

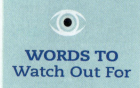

WORDS TO Watch Out For

Echocardiography and *Electrocardiography*

Echocardiography and electrocardiography are both methods of measuring heart function. The two medical terms are similar enough in construction and in meaning to be confusing. Let the word parts provide the clue. Remember that one *hears* an echo, and thus, *echocardiography* is the procedure that uses ultra*sound* technology to make measurements of heart function. Also remember a synonym for *ultrasound* is *sonography*, which means "recording process of sound."

embolectomy
EM boh LEK toh mee

8.78 The suffix *-ectomy* means "surgical excision, removal." The surgical removal of a floating blood clot, or embolus (Frame 8.40), is called _____. The constructed form of this term is embol/ectomy.

endarterectomy
END ahr teh REK toh mee

8.79 The removal of the inner lining of an artery to remove a fatty plaque is a surgical procedure called **endarterectomy**. The constructed form of _____ is end/arter/ectomy, which literally means "surgical excision or removal of within artery." The most common surgical site for this procedure is the carotid artery in the neck, which is subject to developing atherosclerotic plaques (Frame 8.26). Note that the *o* ending in the prefix *endo-* is deleted from this constructed term for ease of pronunciation.

Holter monitor

8.80 A portable electrocardiograph may be worn by the patient to monitor electrical activity of the heart over 24-hour periods. The device is called a _____ _____ and is useful in detecting periodic or transient cardiac abnormalities (■ Figure 8.17).

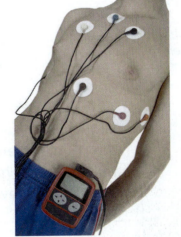

■ Figure 8.17
Holter monitor. Photograph of a portable Holter monitor on a male patient.
Source: Papa1266/Shutterstock.

nitroglycerin
NIGH troh GLIH ser ihn

under the tongue

8.81 A drug that is commonly used as an emergency vasodilator to treat severe angina pectoris (Frame 8.7) or myocardial infarction (Frame 8.49) is the compound **nitroglycerin**. The vasodilation that results from _____ temporarily improves blood flow to the heart and other vital organs.

phlebectomy
fleh BEK toh mee

8.82 Phlebectomy is constructed from the word root meaning "vein" (*phleb*) and the suffix meaning "surgical excision, removal" (*-ectomy*). From its word parts, we know that a _____ is a procedure involving the surgical removal of a vein. The constructed form of this term is phleb/ectomy.

phlebotomy
fleh BOT oh mee

8.83 A puncture into a vein to remove blood for sampling or donation is called **phlebotomy** (■ Figure 8.18). This constructed term combines the word root for vein, the combining vowel *o*, and the suffix meaning "incision or to cut" to create the term _____, which is written phleb/o/tomy. Although the word part for incision is included, a small puncture is made rather than an incision when withdrawing blood (called a **venipuncture**). A healthcare professional who performs this procedure is called a **phlebotomist** (fleh BOT oh mist).

■ **Figure 8.18**
Phlebotomy. In this common procedure, a syringe needle punctures a vein, usually in the arm, and withdraws blood for sampling or donation.
Source: Courtesy of the Public Health Image Library, Centers for Disease Control and Prevention.

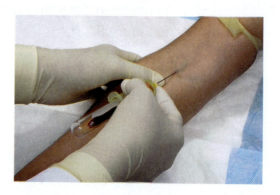

positron emission tomography scan
PAHZ ih tron * ee MISH uhn * toh MOG rah fee

8.84 A noninvasive procedure that provides blood flow images using **positron emission tomography (PET)** techniques combined with radioactive isotope labeling may be used to produce images of the heart to reveal functional defects. The procedure is called

_____ _____ _____

_____, or **PET scan**.

sphygmomanometry
SFIG moh mah NOM eh tree

taking Blood pressure

8.85 A common procedure that measures arterial blood pressure is called _____. This constructed term is written sphygm/o/man/o/metry, which literally means "the process of measuring scanty gas." It utilizes a device called a **sphygmomanometer** (sfig moh mah NOM eh ter), which consists of an arm cuff and air pressure pump with a pressure gauge (■ Figure 8.19). In recent years, the mercury pressure gauge has been replaced by aneroid dials and digital technology.

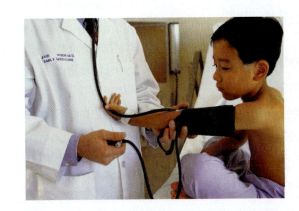

■ **Figure 8.19**
Sphygmomanometry.
Photograph of a physician taking blood pressure readings with the use of a sphygmomanometer, which includes an arm cuff and pressure gauge.
Source: Keith Brofsky/ Photodisc/Getty Images.

thrombolytic therapy
throm boh LITT ik * THAIR ah pee

8.86 Treatments to dissolve unwanted blood clots are often necessary after surgery to prevent the development of emboli (Frame 8.40). It is also performed soon after a myocardial infarction (Frame 8.49) to minimize damage to the heart and is credited with saving many lives. Known as _____ _____, it includes the use of drugs such as streptokinase and tissue plasminogen activator (TPA). The constructed term *thrombolytic* is made up of the combining form that means "clot" (*thromb/o*) and the suffix that means "pertaining to loosen or dissolve" (*-lytic*).

Stress EKG , Stress tolerance test

treadmill stress test

8.87 If a heart condition is suspected, a cardiologist will often require the patient to undergo exercise during echocardiography or electrocardiography (or both) in an effort to examine heart function under stress. The most common term for this procedure is _____ _____

_____.

valvuloplasty
VAL vyoo loh plass tee

8.88 The surgical repair of a heart valve is called _____. The constructed form of this term is written valvul/o/plasty. If repair is not possible due to the extent of the damage or defect, valve replacement may be required using an artificial valve or a porcine (pig) valve.

PRACTICE: Treatments, Procedures, and Devices of the Cardiovascular System

The Right Match

Match the term on the left with the correct definition on the right.

_____ 1. cardiac pacemaker

_____ 2. defibrillation

_____ 3. phlebotomy

_____ 4. Holter monitor

_____ 5. coronary stent

_____ 6. PET scan

_____ 7. stress ECHO

_____ 8. nitroglycerin

_____ 9. auscultation

_____ 10. Doppler sonography

a. an artificial metallic scaffold that is implanted to open a blocked coronary artery

b. a drug that is commonly used as an emergency vasodilator

c. a patient undergoes exercise before or during echocardiography to examine heart function under stress

d. a battery-powered device that is implanted under the skin and wired to the wall of the heart

e. puncture into a vein, usually to remove blood for sampling or donation

f. a portable electrocardiograph worn by the patient

g. an electric charge applied to the chest wall to stop the heart conduction system momentarily, then restart it with a more normal heart rhythm

h. a noninvasive procedure that provides blood flow images using positron emission tomography techniques combined with radioactive isotope labeling

i. an ultrasound procedure that evaluates blood flow

j. a physical examination that involves listening to internal sounds

Break the Chain

Analyze these medical terms:

a) Separate each term into its word parts; each word part is labeled for you (**p** = prefix, **r** = root, **cf** = combining form, and **s** = suffix).

b) For the Bonus Question, write the requested definition in the blank that follows.

1. a) arteriogram _____/___/_____
                    cf   s

   b) *Bonus Question*: What is the definition of the suffix? _____

2. a) echocardiography _____/___/_____/___/_____
                       cf   cf   s

   b) *Bonus Question*: What is the definition of the *first* combining form? _____

3. a) embolectomy _____/_____
                   r   s

   b) *Bonus Question*: What is the definition of the word root? _____

4. a) sphygmomanometry   _____/___/_____/___/_____
                                                 cf   cf   s

    b) *Bonus Question*: What is the definition of the suffix? _____

5. a) phlebotomist   _____/___/_____/_____
                                                 cf   r   s

    b) *Bonus Question*: What is the definition of the combining form? _____

6. a) electrocardiography   _____/___/_____/___/_____
                                                 cf   cf   s

    b) *Bonus Question*: What is the definition of the suffix? _____

7. a) cardiopulmonary   _____/___/_____/_____
                                                 cf   r   s

    b) *Bonus Question*: What is the definition of the word root in the first word? _____

8. a) endarterectomy   _____/_____/_____
                                         p   r   s

    b) *Bonus Question*: What is the definition of the prefix? _____

9. a) valvuloplasty   _____/___/_____
                                         cf   s

    b) *Bonus Question*: What is the definition of the suffix? _____

Abbreviations of the Cardiovascular System

The abbreviations that are associated with the cardiovascular system are summarized here. Study these abbreviations and review them in the exercise that follows.

Abbreviation	Definition
AED	automated external defibrillator
A-fib	atrial fibrillation
AI	aortic insufficiency
AS	aortic stenosis
ASD	atrial septal defect
ASHD	arteriosclerotic heart disease
AV	atrioventricular
CABG	coronary artery bypass graft
CAD	coronary artery disease
CHD	coronary heart disease
CHF	congestive heart failure
CP	chest pain

Abbreviation	Definition
CPR	cardiopulmonary resuscitation
ECG, EKG	electrocardiogram
ICD	implantable cardioverter defibrillator
LA	left atrium
LV	left ventricle
MI	myocardial infarction
MVP	mitral valve prolapse
PET	positron emission tomography
RA	right atrium
RV	right ventricle
SCA	sudden cardiac arrest
VSD	ventricular septal defect

PRACTICE: Abbreviations

Fill in the blanks with the abbreviation or the complete medical term.

Abbreviation

1. _____
2. ASD
3. _____
4. MI
5. _____
6. CPR
7. _____
8. AV
9. _____
10. CAD
11. _____
12. RV
13. _____
14. MVP

Medical Term

congestive heart failure

_____

coronary artery bypass graft

_____

positron emission tomography

_____

arteriosclerotic heart disease

_____

electrocardiogram

_____

automated external defibrillator

_____

ventricular septal defect

_____

CHAPTER REVIEW

Word Building

Construct medical terms from the following meanings. (Some are built from word parts, some are not.) The first question has been completed as an example.

1. generalized disease of the heart muscle — **_cardiomyo_**pathy
2. inflammation of the heart and blood vessels — angio_____
3. narrowing of a blood vessel — angio_____
4. tumor arising from a blood vessel — angi_____
5. hardening of the arteries — _____sclerosis
6. abnormally slow heart rate — _____cardia
7. a sensation of pain in the heart — cardio_____
8. incision into an artery to remove plaque — end_____ectomy
9. abnormal hypertrophy of the heart — cardio_____
10. inflammation of the inner heart membrane — endo_____
11. an abnormal heart rhythm — a_____
12. high blood pressure that is persistent — _____tension
13. death of a portion of the myocardium — _____cardial in_____
14. inflammation of the myocardium — myo_____
15. a process of recording heart electrical activity — _____cardiography

Define the Combining Form

In the space provided, write the definition of the combining form, followed by one example of the combining form used to build a medical term in Chapter 8.

		Definition	Use in a Term
1.	angi/o	_____	_____
2.	cardi/o	_____	_____
3.	hem/o	_____	_____
4.	phleb/o	_____	_____
5.	sten/o	_____	_____
6.	scler/o	_____	_____
7.	thromb/o	_____	_____
8.	ech/o	_____	_____
9.	arter/o	_____	_____
10.	coron/o	_____	_____
11.	electr/o	_____	_____
12.	valvul/o	_____	_____
13.	isch/o	_____	_____
14.	sphygm/o	_____	_____

Complete the Labels

Complete the blank labels in the illustrations by writing the labels in the spaces provided.

1. _____

2. _____

3. _____

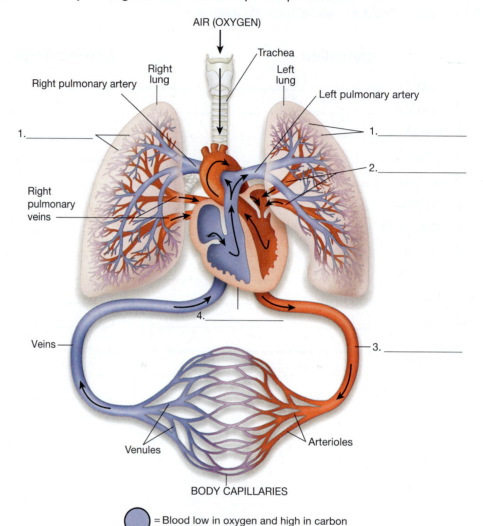

■ **Figure 8.20**
The cardiovascular system.

4. _____

5. _____

6. _____

7. _____

8. _____

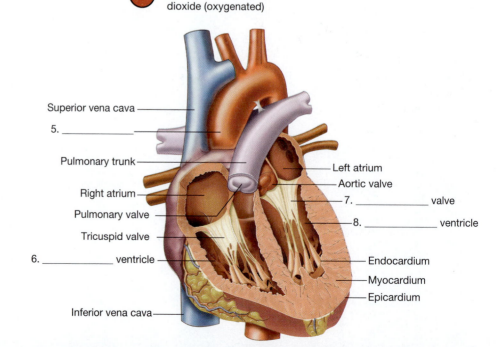

■ **Figure 8.21**
Internal anatomy of the heart.
The heart is sectioned to reveal
its internal features.

MEDICAL REPORT EXERCISES

Robert Gorman

Read the following medical report, then answer the questions that follow.

PGH

PEARSON GENERAL HOSPITAL

5500 University Avenue, Metropolis, New York
Phone: (211) 594-4000 • Fax (211) 594-4001

Medical Consultation: Cardiology

Patient: Robert Gorman

Dob: 3/14/1954   **Age**: 62   **Sex**: Male

Provider: Richard Freemann, MD

Date: 10/22/2016

Patient ID: 123456

Allergies: NKDA

Subjective:

"I have been experiencing chest pain for the past couple of weeks, unlike any I've felt before. I am also tired most of the time and have lost my appetite."

62 y/o male patient has a recent history of mild chest pain, shortness of breath, and malaise. No murmur has yet been reported. The patient says he underwent tooth extractions a month ago and had been given antibiotics by the dentist, but since he wasn't feeling ill, he did not take them. Patient reports his father died at 79 y/o due to CHF.

Objective:

Vital Signs: **T**: 98.6°F; **P**: 80; **R**: 23; **BP**: 144/102

Ht: 5'8"

Wt: 183 lb

General Appearance: Some pallor and edema present in the face and neck. Mild diaphoresis. No noticeable discolorations of the skin.

Heart: Rate at 80 bpm, with possible murmur at mitral valve.

Lungs: Clear without signs of disease.

AbD: Bowel sounds normal all four quadrants.

MS: Joints and muscles symmetric. No swelling, masses, or deformity.

CV: ECG normal. Stress ECHO shows minor vegetations of mitral valve.

Assessment:

Endocarditis with cardiovalvulitis on left side

Plan:

Long-term IV drip with nonpenicillin antibiotic. If there is no improvement in 4 weeks, consult for valvuloplasty.

Photo Source: Aletia2011/Fotolia.

Comprehension Questions

1. What complaints support the diagnosis? _____
_____
_____

2. Why is the patient history an important part of this diagnosis? _____
_____
_____

3. What is the meaning of the abbreviation CHF? _____
_____
_____

Case Study Questions

The following Case Study provides further discussion regarding the patient in the medical report. Fill in the blanks with the correct terms. Choose your answers from the following list of terms. (Note that some terms may be used more than once.)

angina pectoris	angiostenosis	atherosclerosis	block
cardiologist	cardiology	cardiovalvulitis	electrocardiography
endocarditis	myocardial infarction	stress ECHO	valvuloplasty

A patient named Robert Gorman complained of pain in the heart area of the chest, or

(a) _____, and was subsequently referred to (b) _____ for immediate

diagnosis and treatment. The specialist, a (c) _____, diagnosed the pain as having a

cause from insufficient blood supply to the heart. The patient was given medication and educated about

heart disease management. Several weeks later, the patient was readmitted due to continued complaints

of chest pain. After evaluating heart electrical events with (d) _____, the physician

performed a technique using sound waves to evaluate heart activity during physical exercise, known as a(n)

(e) _____ _____. The ECG showed a normal conduction system, thereby

ruling out damage to the conduction system, or a heart (f) _____. The stress ECHO also

showed mostly normal results, ruling out damage to the heart muscle, or a(n) (g) _____

_____, because the heart muscle was receiving sufficient levels of oxygen. Because blood

flow was normal, the narrowing of a coronary artery, generally called a(n) (h) _____, was eliminated as a cause, which also eliminated the common plaque-forming disease that causes a stenosis,

known as (i) _____. However, the stress ECHO did reveal abnormal valvular activity during

ventricular contraction, or systole, indicating a valvular disorder called (j) _____. A course

of treatment was ordered that included a long-term, nonpenicillin antibiotic therapy with an IV drip. If

the patient did not improve, consideration for a surgical operation to repair a damaged valve, called (k)

_____, would be made.

Danika Price

For a greater challenge, read the following medical report and answer the critical thinking questions that follow from the information in the chapter.

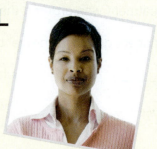

PEARSON GENERAL HOSPITAL

5500 University Avenue, Metropolis, New York
Phone: (211) 594-4000 • Fax (211) 594-4001

Medical Consultation: Cardiology

Date: 12/09/2016

Patient: Danika Price

Patient ID: 123456

Dob: 04/15/1974   **Age**: 42   **Sex**: Female   **Allergies**: NKDA

Provider: Donald H. Surley, MD

Subjective:

"I have been experiencing pain in my upper abdomen that comes and goes. It started about a week ago, and it interrupts my sleep."

42 y/o female patient describes the pain as recent, within 1 week, occurring between the median and radiating to the left upper quadrant. According to her it is a sharp, intermittent pain, which increases in intensity when she stands from a sitting or lying position.

Objective:

Vital Signs: **T**: 98.6°F; **P**: 83; **R**: 21; **BP**: 135/90

Ht: 5'7"

Wt: 135 lb

General Appearance: No pallor, edema, or diaphoresis of the skin. No noticeable discolorations of the skin. No masses.

Heart: Rate at 83 bpm. Heart sounds with auscultation appear normal.

Lungs: Clear without signs of disease.

AbD: Bowel sounds normal all four quadrants. Tenderness of the LUQ with palpation.

MS: Joints and muscles symmetric. No swelling, masses, or deformity.

CV: ECG normal. Aortogram reveals abnormal swelling of the aorta inferior to the celiac trunk.

Assessment:

Aortic aneurysm of upper abdominal aorta inferior to celiac trunk

Plan:

Angioplasty with stent insertion at aortic aneurysm.

Photo Source: Monkey Business Images/Shutterstock.

Comprehension Questions

1. What is the actual cause of the abdominal pain reported by the patient? _____

   _____

   _____

2. What procedure provided the evidence for the diagnosis? _____

   _____

   _____

3. What is an angioplasty and how might it correct an aortic aneurysm? _____

   _____

   _____

Case Study Questions

The following case study provides additional discussion of the patient's condition in the medical report. Fill in the blanks with the correct terms from your readings in this chapter.

Danika Price, a 42-year-old female patient with a history of persistently high blood pressure, or

(l) _____, complained of intermittent pain sensations in the upper abdomen. Upon evaluation

during which an x-ray was taken of the aorta, called a(n) (m) _____, it became apparent that

the source of the pain was from abdominal spasms of the aorta wall, called (n) _____, due to

an abnormal dilation of the vessel wall known as a(n) (o) _____. To prevent a possible rupture

of the wall of the aorta, a surgical repair called a(n) (p) _____ was scheduled. During the

repair, an incision was made into the wall of the vessel in a procedure called a(n) (q) _____

and the vessel wall received a stent to strengthen it. The patient made a complete recovery, and received

education on ways to control her essential hypertension.

MyLab Medical Terminology™

MyLab Medical Terminology is a premium online homework management system that includes a host of features to help you study. Registered users will find:

- A multitude of quizzes and activities built within the MyLab platform
- Powerful tools that track and analyze your results—allowing you to create a personalized learning experience
- Videos and audio pronunciations to help enrich your progress
- Streaming lesson presentations (Guided Lectures) and self-paced learning modules
- A space where you and your instructors can view and manage your assignments

Chapter 9

The Respiratory System

 Learning Objectives

After completing this chapter, you will be able to:

9.1 Define and spell the word parts used to create terms for the respiratory system.

9.2 Break down and define common medical terms used for symptoms, diseases, disorders, procedures, treatments, and devices associated with the respiratory system.

9.3 Build medical terms from the word parts associated with the respiratory system.

9.4 Pronounce and spell common medical terms associated with the respiratory system.

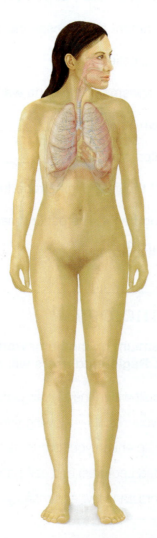

Anatomy and Physiology Terms

The following table provides the combining forms that commonly apply to the anatomy and physiology of the respiratory system. Note that the combining forms are colored red to help you identify them when you see them again later in the chapter.

Combining Form	Definition	Combining Form	Definition
alveol/o	air sac, alveolus	phragm/o, phragmat/o	partition
bronch/o, bronch/i	airway, bronchus	pleur/o	rib, pleura
hem/o, hemat/o	blood	pneum/o, pneumon/o	air, lung
laryng/o	voice box, larynx	pulmon/o	lung
lob/o	a rounded part, lobe	rhin/o	nose
muc/o	mucus	sept/o	putrefying; wall, partition
nas/o	nose	sinus/o	cavity
ox/i	oxygen	thorac/o	chest, thorax
pharyng/o	throat, pharynx	trache/o	windpipe, trachea

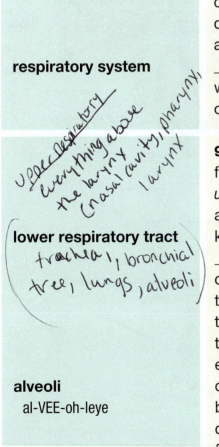

respiratory system

upper respiratory
everything above
the larynx, pharynx
(nasal cavity, pharynx,
larynx

lower respiratory tract
trachea, bronchial
tree, lungs, alveoli

alveoli
al-VEE-oh-leye

9.1 The **respiratory** (RESS pih rah tor ee) **system** brings oxygen into the bloodstream, where it is transported to all body cells. The system gets its name from its function: The process of providing cells with oxygen is commonly known as **respiration**. This term is derived from the Latin word *respiratio*, which means "to breathe again." In addition to bringing oxygen into the bloodstream, the _____ _____ also removes the waste product, carbon dioxide, from the blood and channels it outside the body.

9.2 When you inhale through the nose, air enters the body and flows through a series of chambers and tubes, known as the *upper respiratory tract*. It includes the nasal cavity, pharynx, and larynx. The lower portion of the respiratory system, known as the _____ _____ _____, consists of the trachea in the neck and chest; the bronchial tree, which branches extensively throughout the lungs; the tiny air sacs within the lungs known as alveoli; and the lungs themselves. Gas exchange occurs within the lungs across the walls of alveoli and adjacent capillaries and begins when air enters your alveoli during inhalation. The oxygen in the air then diffuses from the _____ into capillaries to enter the bloodstream. Carbon dioxide diffuses in the opposite direction (from capillaries to alveoli), enabling you to remove the carbon dioxide from your blood with exhalation.

oxygen

carbon dioxide

9.3 The functions of the respiratory system may be summarized as follows:

- Provides a stream of _____ into the blood through the process of inhalation, followed by diffusion.
- Removes _____ _____ from the blood through the process of diffusion, followed by exhalation.

9.4 Review the anatomy of the respiratory system by studying
■ Figure 9.1a and Figure 9.1b.

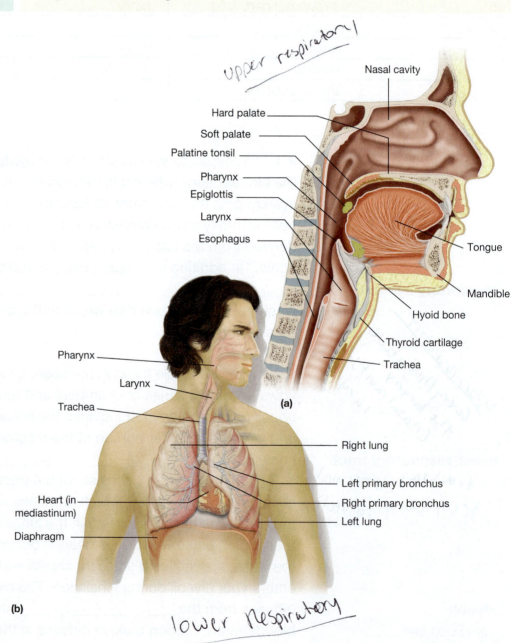

upper respiratory

Nasal cavity
Hard palate
Soft palate
Palatine tonsil
Pharynx
Epiglottis
Larynx
Esophagus
Tongue
Mandible
Hyoid bone
Thyroid cartilage
Trachea

(a)

Pharynx
Larynx
Trachea
Right lung
Left primary bronchus
Heart (in mediastinum)
Right primary bronchus
Left lung
Diaphragm

(b)

lower respiratory

■ **Figure 9.1**
The respiratory system.
(a) Sagittal section of the head and neck, revealing the organs of the upper respiratory tract: the nose, pharynx, and larynx.
(b) The organs of the lower respiratory tract, which includes the trachea, right and left primary bronchi, bronchial tree, and lungs.

Medical Terms of the Respiratory System

respiratory

9.5 Oxygen is a molecule that is required for energy production during cell metabolism. If cells are not continually supplied with oxygen, they perish because they are unable to perform their functions without energy. Many diseases of the respiratory system reduce the amount of oxygen that is normally supplied to body cells. Severe cases can lead to a failure of oxygen delivery and result in large-scale death of cells and ultimately the death of the patient. Respiratory diseases may also increase the levels of carbon dioxide, the toxic metabolic waste product. The buildup of carbon dioxide in the blood and other tissues combines with water to form acid, which becomes life-threatening quickly.

The most common symptoms of respiratory disease are breathing problems. If these problems are not identified and treated early, additional complications may arise. In general, _____ disease may be caused by congenital conditions, infections, allergies, tumors, heart disease, or injury.

pulmonologist

cancer

9.6 The clinical treatment of a respiratory disease is performed by a physician with a specialization in treating the body region, the particular disorder, or a set of similar disorders. For example, lung disease is treated by a pulmonary specialist, or _____, disease of the pharynx is treated by an **ear**, **nose**, **and throat (ENT) specialist**, or **otolaryngologist**, and lung cancer is treated by a _____ specialist, or **oncologist**. Often assisting the physician is a **respiratory therapist** who has received special training in the operation of equipment used to diagnose or treat breathing problems.

9.7 In the following sections, you will study the prefixes, combining forms, and suffixes that combine to build the medical terms of the respiratory system.

Signs and Symptoms of the Respiratory System

Here are the word parts that commonly apply to the signs and symptoms of the respiratory system that are covered in the following section. Note that the word parts are color-coded to help you identify them: prefixes are yellow, combining forms are red, and suffixes are blue.

Prefix	Definition
a-, an-	without, absence of
brady-	slow
dys-	bad, abnormal, painful, difficult
epi-	upon, over, above, on top
eu-	normal, good
hyper-	excessive, abnormally high, above
hypo-	deficient, abnormally low, below
tachy-	rapid, fast

Combining Form	Definition
bronch/o	airway, bronchus
capn/o	carbon dioxide
hem/o	blood
laryng/o	voice box, larynx
orth/o	straight
ox/i	oxygen
rhin/o	nose
thorac/o	chest, thorax

Suffix	Definition
-algia	condition of pain
-dynia	condition of pain
-emia	condition of blood
-oxia	condition of oxygen
-phonia	condition of sound or voice
-pnea	breath
-ptysis	to cough up
-rrhagia	abnormal discharge
-spasm	sudden involuntary muscle contraction
-staxis	dripping

KEY TERMS A–Z

anoxia
ah NOK see ah

9.8 The suffix meaning "condition of oxygen" is -oxia. When the prefix that means "without, absence of" is added, the term _____ is made, which is the absence of oxygen. Anoxia occurs when oxygen delivery to the body's tissues or organs is absent due to any cause. The constructed form of **anoxia** is an/oxia.

aphonia
ah FOH nee ah

9.9 The suffix -phonia means "condition of sound or voice." Adding the prefix that means "without, absence of" forms the term _____, which is the absence of voice. The constructed form of this term is a/phonia.

apnea
AP nee ah
a/pnea

sleep apnea

9.10 The suffix -pnea means "breath." Adding the prefix that means "without, absence of" forms the term _____, which is a longer-than-normal pause between breaths. This constructed term is _____/_____. A common form of apnea is known as **sleep apnea**, in which one or more pauses in breathing or shallow breaths occur while sleeping. In _____ _____, the pauses may last for a few seconds to several minutes, usually anywhere from 5 to 30 or more times per hour. When normal breathing resumes, a choking or snorting sound is often made.

bradypnea
brad ip NEE ah

9.11 Adding the prefix *brady-*, which means "slow," to the suffix that means "breath" produces the term for an abnormal slowing of the breathing rhythm, _____. The constructed form of **bradypnea** is brady/pnea.

---

part of asthma attacks & wheezing

bronchospasm
BRONG koh spazm

9.12 A narrowing of the airway caused by the contraction of smooth muscles in the walls of the tiny tubes known as bronchioles within the lungs is called **bronchospasm**. The constructed form of this term is bronch/o/spasm. A _____ is a common sign of the respiratory disease, asthma (Frame 9.31).

Occurs near time of death

Cheyne-Stokes respiration
chain stohks * ress pih RAY shun

9.13 The sign known as **Cheyne-Stokes respiration** is a repeated pattern of distressed breathing marked by a gradual increase of deep breathing, followed by shallow breathing and apnea. _____-_____ _____ is a sign of brain dysfunction or congestive heart failure.

---

dysphonia
diss FOH nee ah

9.14 The prefix *dys-* means "bad, abnormal, painful, or difficult." When used with the suffix that means "condition of sound or voice," the term _____ is formed. It is the symptom of a hoarse voice. The constructed form of **dysphonia** is dys/phonia.

---

dyspnea
DISP nee ah

difficult breathing

9.15 Adding the prefix *dys-* to the suffix that means "breath" forms the term _____. It is the symptom of difficult breathing, usually caused by a respiratory disease or cardiac disorder. In contrast, a normal breathing rhythm is called **eupnea** (yoop NEE ah). The constructed form of dyspnea is dys/pnea, and eupnea is eu/pnea.

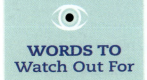

WORDS TO Watch Out For

Terms with No Word Roots

Many terms related to the respiratory system contain no word root (or combining form), such as *dysphonia*, *dyspnea*, *epistaxis*, *hyperpnea*, and *hypopnea*. Don't let those terms confuse you when you're interpreting their meanings.

SOB = shortness of breath

epistaxis
ep ih STAK siss

9.16 A nosebleed is clinically called **epistaxis**. It is a constructed term that literally means "dripping upon" and is written epi/staxis. An _____ can be a sign of high blood pressure, a nasal sinus infection, inhalation of a toxic irritant or particle, or a blow to the face. It is also called **rhinorrhagia** (rye noh RAH jee ah), another constructed term. The constructed form is rhin/o/rrhagia and literally means "abnormal discharge of nose."

hemoptysis
hee MOP tih siss

9.17 The symptom of coughing up and spitting out blood is called _____, which combines the combining form *hem/o* that means "blood" and the suffix *-ptysis* that means "to cough up." The constructed form of this term is hem/o/ptysis.

hemothorax
hee moh THOH raks

9.18 A term composed of two word parts that literally means "chest blood" is _____. It is the pooling of blood within the pleural cavity surrounding the lungs (■ Figure 9.2). The term is written hem/o/thorax. Note that this term has no prefix or suffix; it is constructed of a combining form (*hem/o*) and a noun (*thorax*).

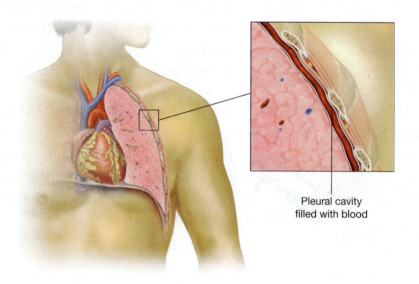

Pleural cavity
filled with blood

■ **Figure 9.2**
Hemothorax. The clinical sign of hemothorax is the presence of blood in the pleural cavity, which surrounds both lungs.

hypercapnia
HIGH per KAP nee ah

hypocapnia
HIGH per KAP nee ah

9.19 The prefixes *hyper-* and *hypo-* have opposite meanings. For example, excessive levels of carbon dioxide in the blood is a sign of respiratory failure and is called _____, since the combining form for carbon dioxide is *capn/o*. The opposite sign, in which carbon dioxide blood levels are deficient, or abnormally low, is _____.

hyperpnea
HIGH perp NEE ah

hyperventilation
HIGH per vent ih LAY shun

9.20 The sign of abnormally deep breathing or an abnormally high rate of breathing is called _____ and is common among patients suffering from the respiratory disease, emphysema (Frame 9.42). Hyperpnea is also a common symptom of heart failure. By contrast, the sign of abnormally rapid shallow breathing is more common among patients experiencing anxiety (panic) attacks and is called _____. The constructed form of **hyperpnea** is written hyper/pnea, and that of **hyperventilation** is hyper/ventilation.

common w/ Drug overdose

hypopnea
high POPP nee ah

9.21 The opposite sign of hyperpnea is abnormally shallow breathing and is called _____. This constructed term is written hypo/pnea.

hypoventilation
HIGH poh vent ih LAY shun

9.22 A reduced breathing rhythm that fails to meet the body's gas exchange demands is called _____. The constructed form of this term is hypo/ventilation. It is opposite to an accelerated shallow breathing rhythm, which you learned is called *hyperventilation* (Frame 9.20).

hypoxemia
high pahk SEE mee ah
hypoxia
high PAHK see ah

9.23 Abnormally low levels of oxygen in the blood is a sign of a respiratory deficiency called **hypoxemia**. This constructed term is written hyp/ox/emia. Notice that the letter *o* in *hypo-* is dropped because the combining form, ox/i, begins with a vowel. This rule makes _____ easier to pronounce. Similarly, this rule is also used to form the term **hypoxia**, which is written as hyp/ox/ia. _____ is the sign of abnormally low levels of oxygen throughout the body.

Serious problem – from anaphalaxis

laryngospasm
lair ING goh spazm

9.24 A **laryngospasm** is the closure of the glottis, the opening into the larynx, due to muscular contractions of the throat. _____ is a constructed term with three word parts: laryng/o/spasm.

orthopnea
or THAHP nee ah

9.25 The combining form *orth/o* means "straight." When the suffix for breath is added, the term **orthopnea** is formed. _____ is the limited ability to breathe when lying down and becomes relieved when sitting upright. The constructed form of this term is orth/o/pnea.

paroxysm pahr AHK sizm *Severe coughing (from whooping cough)*	**9.26** The term **paroxysm** refers to a sudden onset of symptomatic sharp pain or a convulsion. _____ is derived from the Greek word *paroxysmos*, which means "to sharpen or to irritate." When used with the respiratory system, *paroxysm* refers to a severe coughing spell.
sputum SPYOO tum	**9.27** Respiratory diseases often include the symptom of **sputum**, which is an expectorated (coughed out from the lungs) matter. _____ contains mucus, inhaled particulates, and sometimes pus or blood.
tachypnea tak ihp NEE ah	**9.28** The prefix *tachy-* means "rapid or fast." When combined with the suffix that means "breath," it forms the term _____. The constructed form of this term for rapid breathing is written *tachy/pnea*.
thoracalgia thor ah KAL jee ah *Chest pain (from bones or muscles)*	**9.29** The symptom of pain in the chest region is called _____. The constructed form of this term is written *thorac/algia*; notice the combining vowel (the *o*) has been dropped because the suffix begins with a vowel. An alternate term with the same meaning is **thoracodynia** (THOR ah koh DIN ee ah).

PRACTICE: Signs and Symptoms of the Respiratory System

The Right Match

Match the term on the left with the correct definition on the right.

_____ 1. thoracalgia

_____ 2. apnea

_____ 3. eupnea

_____ 4. bradypnea

_____ 5. paroxysm

_____ 6. hemoptysis

_____ 7. sputum

_____ 8. hemothorax

_____ 9. hypercapnia

_____ 10. hypoxemia

_____ 11. Cheyne-Stokes respiration

a. severe coughing spell (in respiratory system)

b. coughing up and spitting out blood

c. expectorated (spit-out) matter that contains mucus, inhaled particulates, and sometimes pus and blood

d. normal breathing

e. slow breathing

f. pause in breathing

g. excessive carbon dioxide blood levels

h. deficient levels of oxygen in the blood

i. pain in the chest region

j. blood in the pleural cavity

k. pattern of repeated distressed breathing marked by a gradual increase of deep breathing, followed by shallow breathing and apnea

Break the Chain

Analyze these medical terms:

    a) Separate each term into its word parts; each word part is labeled for you (**p** = prefix, **r** = root, **cf** = combining form, and **s** = suffix).

    b) For the Bonus Question, write the requested definition in the blank that follows.

The first set has been completed for you as an example.

---

1. a) bronchospasm   **_bronch/o/spasm_**
                                    cf   s

    b) *Bonus Question*: What is the definition of the suffix? **_sudden involuntary muscle contraction_**

---

2. a) dysphonia   _____/_____
                                 p   s

    b) *Bonus Question*: What is the definition of the suffix? _____

---

3. a) dyspnea   _____/_____
                                 p   s

    b) *Bonus Question*: What is the definition of the prefix? _____

---

4. a) epistaxis   _____/_____
                                 p   s

    b) *Bonus Question*: What is the definition of the suffix? _____

---

5. a) hyperpnea   _____/_____
                                 p   s

    b) *Bonus Question*: What is the definition of the suffix? _____

---

6. a) laryngospasm   _____/___/_____
                                 cf   s

    b) *Bonus Question*: What is the definition of the combining form? _____

Diseases and Disorders of the Respiratory System

Here are the word parts that commonly apply to the diseases and disorders of the respiratory system that are covered in the following section. Note that the word parts are color-coded to help you identify them: prefixes are yellow, combining forms are red, and suffixes are blue.

Prefix	Definition
a-	without, absence of
epi-	upon, over, above, on top

Combining Form	Definition
atel/o	incomplete
bronch/o, bronch/i	airway, bronchus
carcin/o	cancer
coccidioid/o	Coccidioides immitis (a fungus)
coni/o	dust
cyst/o	bladder, sac
embol/o	plug
fibr/o	fiber
glott/o	opening into the windpipe
laryng/o	voice box, larynx
myc/o	fungus
nas/o	nose
pharyng/o	throat, pharynx
pleur/o	rib, pleura
pneum/o, pneumon/o	air, lung
pulmon/o	lung
py/o	pus
rhin/o	nose
sinus/o	cavity
sphyx/o	pulse
sten/o	narrow
tonsill/o	almond, tonsil
trache/o	windpipe, trachea
tubercul/o	little swelling

Suffix	Definition
-al	pertaining to
-ary	pertaining to
-ectasis	expansion, dilation
-genic	pertaining to producing, forming
-ia	condition of
-ic	pertaining to
-ism	condition or disease
-itis	inflammation
-oma	tumor
-osis	condition of

KEY TERMS A–Z

asphyxia
ass FIK see ah

9.30 The word root meaning "pulse" is *sphyx*. It is included in the term **asphyxia**, which is the absence of respiratory ventilation. In other words, it is the inability to breathe. The constructed form of _____ is a/sphyx/ia and literally means "condition of without pulse."

asthma

AZ mah

inflammation of the small airways (bronchia ls) [handwritten]

9.31 A chronic condition of the lungs that is characterized by widespread narrowing of the bronchioles, bronchospasms (Frame 9.12), and formation of mucous plugs is known as **asthma**. The term is derived from the Greek word *asthma*, which means "to pant." Illustrated in ■ Figure 9.3, _____ produces the symptoms of wheezing, shortness of breath (SOB), chest pain, and frequent coughing during an episode, the frequency of which varies with every patient. It is regarded as an inflammatory response to an allergic substance by the lungs. According to the American Academy of Allergy, Asthma, and Immunology roughly 25 million Americans suffer from this chronic disease, 10 million of whom are under the age of 18 years. When asthma is complicated with bronchitis (see Frame 9.34), it is referred to as **asthmatic bronchitis** (az MAHT ik * brong KYE tiss).

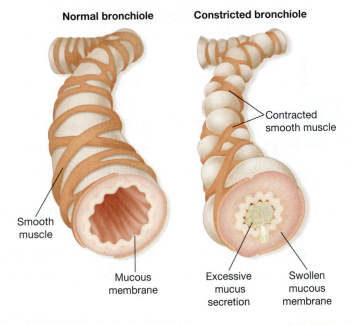

Normal bronchiole | **Constricted bronchiole**

Contracted smooth muscle

Smooth muscle

Mucous membrane

Excessive mucus secretion

Swollen mucous membrane

■ **Figure 9.3**
Asthma. A normal bronchiole (left) compared to an asthmatic bronchiole (right). During an asthma "attack," the bronchioles undergo spasms that reduce the airway diameter. In addition, the mucous membrane lining the bronchioles swells, and thickened mucous secretions form plugs that further reduce the airway.

atelectasis

at eh LEK tah siss

9.32 The alveoli in the lungs normally retain a small amount of air even during a forced expiration, which prevents them from collapsing completely. In the condition called **atelectasis**, trauma or disease disables this protective mechanism and causes the alveoli to collapse, preventing air from entering. _____ is a constructed term composed of two word parts, *atel*, which means "incomplete," and *-ectasis*, which means "expansion, dilation." Its constructed form is written *atel/ectasis*. When the alveoli in a lung collapse due to the abnormal entry of air into the pleural cavity, the condition is commonly called **collapsed lung** (Frame 9.54).

bronchiectasis

BRONG kee EK tah siss

9.33 Another term that uses the suffix *-ectasis* is _or stretched_ [handwritten], which is a chronic, abnormal dilation (widening) of the bronchi. The constructed form of this term is *bronchi/ectasis*.

results in chronic infection [handwritten]

bronchitis
brong KYE tiss

bronchiolitis
brong kee oh LEYE tiss

[handwritten margin note: acute--infections allergies; Chronic--from cigs leads to COPD]

9.34 Recall that the suffix that means "inflammation" is *-itis*. This will be used in many terms in this section. Inflammation of the bronchi is called _____. The constructed form of this term is bronch/itis. Bronchi are large tubes that branch into much smaller tubes within the lungs known as bronchioles (the suffix *-oles* means "tiny"). When these small air tubes undergo inflammation, the condition is called _____, written with its word parts as bronchiol/itis. Acute bronchitis is usually associated with a respiratory tract infection. Chronic bronchitis is usually caused by smoking, although allergies may cause this condition in some people. Bronchiolitis can be caused by either infection or allergy and can become life-threatening if the swelling closes off airflow to the alveoli.

bronchogenic carcinoma
brong koh JENN ik * kar sih NOH mah

9.35 An aggressive form of cancer arising from cells within the bronchi is known as **bronchogenic carcinoma** (■ Figure 9.4). The constructed form of this term is written bronch/o/genic carcin/oma. According to the National Cancer Institute (NCI), in 2016 there were approximately 224,000 new cases and 158,000 deaths due to _____ _____ in the United States, making it the most deadly form of any type of cancer. According to the American Lung Association, each year more people die from bronchogenic carcinoma than from the next three most common cancers combined (colon, breast, and prostate). It is commonly referred to as **lung cancer** and includes two major types: small cell lung cancer (SCLC) and non–small cell lung cancer (NSCLC). It is well established that smoking tobacco products is the cause of at least 90% of all cases of bronchogenic carcinoma.

■ **Figure 9.4**
Bronchogenic carcinoma (lung cancer). (a) An illustration of a sectioned lung with tumors that originated from the bronchial wall. (b) Photograph of part of a lung removed after death. The yellow area is a large tumor and the blackened areas suggest the patient was a heavy smoker. *Photo Source: Courtesy of National Institutes of Health, National Cancer Institute Visuals Online.*

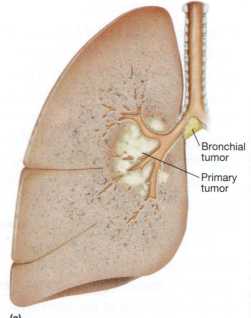

Bronchial tumor
Primary tumor

(a)

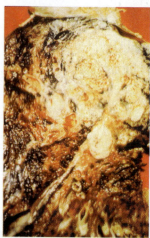

(b)

bronchopneumonia
BRONG koh noo MOH nee ah

9.36 An acute inflammatory disease involving the bronchioles and the alveoli is called **bronchopneumonia**. This constructed term contains four word parts: bronch/o/pneumon/ia. It is usually caused by a bacterial infection that involves the bronchi and the soft tissue of the lungs, causing the alveoli to fill with fluid and leading to the loss of air space. _____ often occurs in a lobe of a lung, lending it the alternate name of **lobar pneumonia**.

chronic obstructive pulmonary disease

[handwritten: COPD no cure, emphysema & chronic bronchitis]

9.37 A reduced flow of air to and from the alveoli in the lungs may be the result of chronic bronchitis (Frame 9.34) or emphysema (Frame 9.42). When both conditions appear simultaneously, the diagnosis is given as **chronic obstructive pulmonary disease**, abbreviated **COPD**. _____ _____ _____ is a progressive disease (gets worse with time) that makes breathing very difficult and is primarily caused by smoking tobacco products.

coccidioidomycosis
kok SIDD ee oy doh mye
KOH siss

[handwritten: fungal infection of lungs AKA - valley fever]

9.38 The combining form *myc/o* means "fungus." A fungal infection of the upper respiratory tract, which often spreads to the lungs and other organs, is called **coccidioidomycosis**. This constructed term is coccidioid/o/myc/osis and is based on the name of the causative fungus, *Coccidioides immitis*. Also called **valley fever** due to its place of origin in the San Joaquin Valley of California, _____ is caused by inhaling spores of the fungal pathogen.

coryza *[handwritten: URI]*
koh RYE zah

[handwritten: Common cold]

9.39 The common cold is caused by a virus that infects the upper respiratory tract, resulting in local inflammation. The condition is clinically called **coryza**, which is derived from the Greek word for runny nose, *koryza*. Because a cold is an acute illness, it is often called **acute** _____. It is also called **rhinitis** (rye NYE tiss), due to the inflammation of the nasal mucosa.

croup
kroop

[handwritten: Barking cough from virus swollen larynx]

9.40 A viral infectious disease that is relatively common among infants and young children produces a characteristic hoarse cough with a sound resembling the bark of a dog or seal. Commonly known as **croup**, the cough results from a swelling of the larynx in response to a viral infection. The clinical term for _croup_ is **laryngotracheobronchitis** (lair RING goh TRAY kee oh brong KYE tiss). The constructed form of this term reveals six word parts: laryng/o/trache/o/bronch/itis.

cystic fibrosis
SISS tik * fye BROH siss

(handwritten: Affects children / Genetic)

(handwritten: mucus too thick)

9.41 A severe hereditary disease that is characterized by excess mucus production in the respiratory tract, digestive tract, and elsewhere is called **cystic fibrosis** and is abbreviated **CF**. This constructed term is written cyst/ic fibr/osis. _____ _____ literally means "condition of fibrous cysts (bladders)" and is named after the characteristic fibrosis and cysts that form in the pancreas. CF causes difficulty breathing because of the dense mucus that obstructs the airways. It strikes roughly 1 in 3,000 children in the United States and is commonly fatal before the age of 40 years, usually from chronic infections.

(handwritten: from smoking)

emphysema
em fih SEE mah

9.42 A chronic lung disease characterized by the symptoms of dyspnea (Frame 9.15), a chronic cough, formation of a barrel chest due to labored breathing, and a gradual deterioration caused by chronic hypoxemia (Frame 9.23) and hypercapnia (Frame 9.19) is called **emphysema**. It is a Greek word that means "to inflate." The symptoms arise when the alveolar walls deteriorate, resulting in a loss of elasticity that causes an inability to exhale normally, making breathing extremely difficult. Smoking is the leading cause of _____, and when it is combined with chronic bronchitis, the patient is diagnosed with chronic obstructive pulmonary disease (COPD), described in Frame 9.37. Emphysema is illustrated in ■ Figure 9.5.

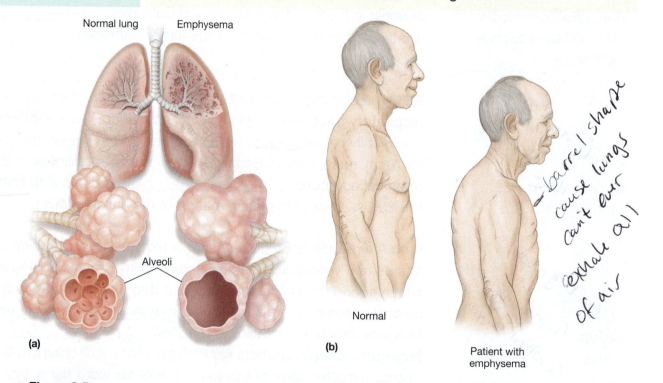

Normal lung   Emphysema

Alveoli

(a)

Normal

(b)

Patient with emphysema

(handwritten: barrel shape cause lungs can't ever exhale all of air)

■ **Figure 9.5**
Emphysema. (a) Illustration comparing normal lungs and emphysemic lungs. The insets illustrate how alveolar walls deteriorate in emphysema, reducing their surface area by convergence.
(b) Comparison of a patient with and without emphysema. Characteristic signs of emphysema include reduced weight, a barrel chest, and a drawn facial appearance, all due to the need to inhale deeply and forcibly exhale with nearly every breath.

epiglottitis
ep ih glah TYE tiss

[handwritten: acute lifethreatening bacterial infection]
[handwritten: prevent himp vaccine]

9.43 Inflammation of the epiglottis is called **epiglottitis**. This constructed term includes three word parts: epi/glott/itis. *[handwritten: cant breath]* _____ is usually caused by a bacterial infection that spreads from the throat to the epiglottis and can be very serious because of the danger of it causing airway obstruction, especially among children.

laryngitis *[handwritten: - most viral]*
LAIR in JYE tiss

9.44 An acute inflammation of the larynx is called _____. The constructed form of this term is laryng/itis. It is characterized by the symptom of dysphonia (Frame 9.14).

legionellosis
lee juh nell OH siss

9.45 A form of pneumonia (Frame 9.52) that is caused by the bacterium *Legionella pneumophila* is called **Legionnaires' disease**, or _____. *[handwritten: 1976]*

? **Did You KNOW**

LEGIONNAIRES' DISEASE

Legionellosis was first identified in 1976, when many members at an American Legion convention became afflicted with an infection that caused 21 deaths. It took intensive research to reveal the causative bacteria and why it spread so quickly: it was delivered throughout the hotel ventilation system under ideal conditions for the bacteria to proliferate.

nasopharyngitis
nay zoh FAIR in JYE tiss

9.46 Recall that the suffix *-itis* means "inflammation." Inflammation of the nose and pharynx is thereby called _____. The constructed form of this term is written nas/o/pharyng/itis. It may be caused by an allergic reaction or bacterial or viral infection.

pertussis
per TUSS siss

[handwritten: Whooping cough]
[handwritten: leads to seizures & death]

9.47 An acute infectious disease characterized by inflammation of the larynx, trachea, and bronchi that produces spasmodic coughing is called **pertussis**. The term is a Latin word that means "intense cough." _____ is commonly known as **whooping cough** because of the noise produced at the end of a cough when the larynx spasms, producing a long inspirational noise. If not treated, it can become fatal due to the exhaustive coughing and obstructed airflow. Pertussis is a preventable disease with early childhood vaccination (often called *DTaP*).

pharyngitis FAIR in JYE tiss	**9.48** Inflammation of the pharynx is called _____. The constructed form of this term is written pharyng/itis. Pharyngitis is commonly called "sore throat."
pleural effusion PLOO ral * eh FYOO zhun	**9.49** Effusion refers to the leakage of fluid. In the disease _____ _____, fluid leaks into the pleural cavity. It usually occurs as a response by the body to injury or infection of the pleural membranes surrounding the lungs. *Pleural* is a constructed term, pleur/al.
pleuritis ploo RYE tiss	**9.50** Inflammation of the pleural membranes is called _____. This constructed term is written pleur/itis. It is also called **pleurisy**. Inflammation of the pleural membranes and the lungs is a disease called **pleuropneumonia** (PLOO roh noo MOH nee ah).
pneumoconiosis noo moh KOH nee OH siss	**9.51** Inflammation of the lungs, when caused by the chronic inhalation of fine particles, is called **pneumoconiosis**. The constructed form of this term is pneum/o/coni/osis, which literally means "condition of dusty lungs." The term arose because the disease is usually caused by mining and manufacturing activities. The inflammation leads to the formation of a fibrotic (scar) tissue around alveoli, reducing their ability to stretch with incoming air, which impedes the efficiency of gas exchange. The most common forms of _____ are **asbestosis** (az bess TOH siss), caused by inhalation of asbestos fibers, and **silicosis** (sill ih KOH siss), caused by inhalation of fine silicone dust.

Industrial dust exposure (black lung-coal miners)

mesothelioma

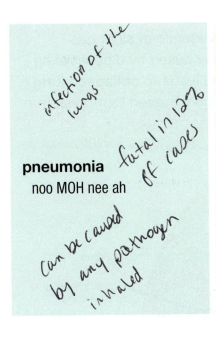

pneumonia
noo MOH nee ah

[handwritten notes: infection of the lungs; fatal in 13% of cases; Can be caused by any pathogen inhaled]

9.52 Inflammation of soft lung tissue (excluding the bronchi) that results in the formation of an exudate (fluid) within alveoli is the general condition known as **pneumonia**. The constructed form of this term is pneumon/ia. The exudate fills the alveoli, which impedes the efficiency of gas exchange (■ Figure 9.6). The filling of alveoli with exudate has the same effect as drowning, so _____ is sometimes referred to as "drowning in your own fluids." Pneumonia is usually caused by bacterial, viral, or fungal pathogens, which trigger the inflammatory response, although it can also be caused by smoke inhalation. Viral and bacterial pneumonia are leading causes of death worldwide. Fungal pneumonia is relatively rare, although infection by the fungus *Pneumocystis jiroveci* is a common sign of HIV/AIDS.

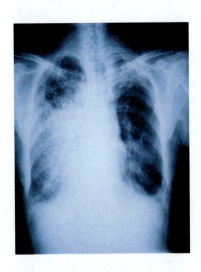

■ **Figure 9.6**
Pneumonia. This common lung inflammation may be caused by bacteria, viruses, or fungi and is often diagnosed with a chest x-ray. In this chest x-ray of infected lungs, the inflammation appears as the cotton-like whitish areas, known as *opacities*.
Source: Joloei/Shutterstock.

pneumonitis
NOO moh NYE tiss

9.53 An inflammatory condition of the lungs that is independent of a particular cause is called _____. The constructed form of this term is written pneumon/itis. Pneumonitis is often associated with pulmonary edema (Frame 9.55), which is the accumulation of fluid within the lungs.

pneumothorax
NOO moh THOH raks

air in the chest
— lungs spring a leak
(from gunshot)

9.54 A **pneumothorax** is the abnormal presence of air or gas within the pleural cavity (■ Figure 9.7). It is caused by a penetrating injury to the chest or severe coughing and leads to **collapsed lung** (Frame 9.32). _____ is a constructed term: pneum/o/thorax.

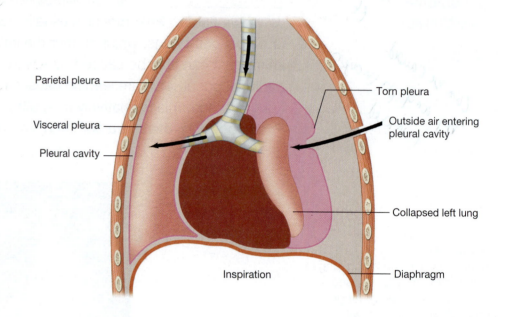

■ **Figure 9.7**
Pneumothorax. The abnormal presence of air or gas within the pleural cavity is usually caused by a penetrating chest wound. This illustration shows a movement of air into the pleural cavity, which has collapsed the left lung while pushing the heart and trachea to the right side.

Parietal pleura

Visceral pleura

Pleural cavity

Torn pleura

Outside air entering pleural cavity

Collapsed left lung

Inspiration

Diaphragm

pulmonary edema
PULL mon air ee * eh
DEE mah

fluid accumulating in lungs

9.55 The accumulation of fluid within the lungs is a response to infection or injury and is called **pulmonary edema**. The most common cause of _____ _____ is cardiovascular disease, including congestive heart failure. Pulmonary edema may also arise from adult respiratory distress syndrome (ARDS), which you learn about soon in Frame 9.58. Pulmonary edema is often associated with pneumonia (Frame 9.52) and pneumonitis (Frame 9.53). *Pulmonary* is a constructed term with two word parts, pulmon/ary, and *edema* means "swelling."

pulmonary embolism
PULL mon air ee * EM
boh lizm

Blood clot from leg

9.56 A blood clot that moves along with the bloodstream is called an **embolus** (EM boh lus). It is derived from the Greek word *embolos*, which means "a plug." An embolus can become dangerous if it lodges in a blood vessel, causing an occlusion that blocks the flow of blood to form an **embolism**. A blockage in the pulmonary circulation by a blood clot is called a _____ _____. Abbreviated **PE**, it is often a complication to an injury or surgery elsewhere in the body. *Pulmonary embolism* is a constructed term: pulmon/ary embol/ism.

pyothorax
pye oh THOH raks

(handwritten: abcess in chest (from stabwound))

9.57 The presence of pus in the pleural cavity is called **pyothorax**. This constructed term is written py/o/thorax. _____ is also known as **empyema** (em pye EE mah), which is composed of mostly Greek word parts that mean "leakage of pus within."

neonatal respiratory distress syndrome

(handwritten: babies get surfactant @ 8 mth of pregnancy)

(handwritten: Common from being on a ventilator)

9.58 A severe respiratory disease that is characterized by rapid respiratory failure is known as **respiratory distress syndrome (RDS)**. It occurs in two different forms. One form affects newborns and is called **neonatal respiratory distress syndrome (NRDS)**. It is caused by insufficient surfactant, which is an oily substance produced by alveolar cells. Surfactant prevents alveoli from sticking together following a deep exhalation, and thereby helps to prevent atelectasis (Frame 9.32). _____

_____ _____ _____ mainly strikes premature infants because they have not yet developed the ability to produce surfactant. The second form of RDS affects adults and is called **adult** (or **acute**) **respiratory distress syndrome (ARDS)**. It is caused by severe lung infections or injury that result in damage to lung capillary walls and bronchioles, causing a rapid accumulation of purulent fluid into alveoli and bronchioles that places the patient in immediate danger of "drowning in their own fluids." Thus, ARDS often involves pneumonia (Frame 9.52) and pulmonary edema (Frame 9.55). It requires swift medical intervention with blood transfusions, anti-inflammatory drugs, and antibiotics to save the patient's life.

rhinitis
rye NYE tiss

9.59 Inflammation of the mucous membrane lining the nasal cavity is called **rhinitis**. The constructed form of this term is rhin/itis. Acute _____ is one of the clinical terms for the common cold (Frame 9.39).

severe acute respiratory syndrome

(handwritten: 2003 arose in china)
(handwritten: new cold)

9.60 A severe, rapid-onset viral infection resulting in respiratory distress that includes acute lung inflammation, alveolar damage, and atelectasis (Frame 9.32) is often referred to by its abbreviation, **SARS**. The long form is _____

_____ _____ _____.

It is usually caused by a virus and can become fatal due to the aggressive immunological response that injures alveoli and bronchioles.

sinusitis
sigh nuss EYE tiss

[handwritten: 7 sinuses]

9.61 Similar to rhinitis (Frame 9.59), the condition known as _____ is an inflammation of the mucous membranes. It affects the nasal cavity and also the paranasal sinuses that are located within the frontal, sphenoid, ethmoid, and maxillary bones of the skull. The constructed form of this term is sinus/itis.

tonsillitis
TAHN sill EYE tiss

9.62 Inflammation of one or more tonsils is called _____. This constructed term is tonsill/itis.

tracheitis
tray kee EYE tiss

[handwritten: - severe chest cold - chemicals - smoke from fire]

9.63 Inflammation of the trachea is called _____. The constructed form of this term is trache/itis. It is usually caused by a bacterial infection that travels downward from the larynx. If the inflammation leads to a narrowing of the trachea, it is called _____ because the combining form that means "narrow" is sten/o. Also constructed of word parts, it includes four: trache/o/sten/osis.

tracheostenosis
TRAY kee oh steh NOH siss

[handwritten: place tube in trachea to treat]

tuberculosis
too BER kyoo LOH siss

[handwritten: - common w/ Aids pt's medication for a full year]

9.64 Infection of the lungs by the bacterium *Mycobacterium tuberculosis* causes the disease _____, abbreviated **TB** (■ Figure 9.8). This term is constructed of two word parts, tubercul/osis, and literally means "condition of a little swelling." The little swelling, or tubercle, is a colony of bacteria within the soft tissue of the lung that forms a hardened barrier, preventing white blood cells from entering and destroying the bacteria. In time, the bacterial colonies multiply throughout the lung until necrosis and inflammation overwhelm the function of gas exchange. In its active state, TB is a severely life-threatening disease, ranking as the world's second most lethal infectious disease (HIV/AIDS is first) with over 1 million deaths each year, according to the World Health Organization.

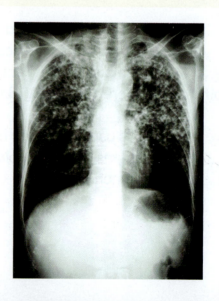

■ **Figure 9.8**
Tuberculosis. A chest x-ray is often used to diagnose TB in a patient. The white clusters in the lungs indicate the presence of TB colonies, called *tubercles*.
Source: Puwadol Jaturawutthichai/Shutterstock.

upper respiratory infection	9.65 A generalized infection of the upper respiratory tract (nasal cavity, pharynx, and larynx) is called a(n) _____ _____ _____, or **URI**.

common cold-virus

PRACTICE: Diseases and Disorders of the Respiratory System

Linkup

Link the word parts in the list to create the terms that match the definitions. You may use word parts more than once. Remember to add combining vowels when needed—and that some terms do not use any combining vowel. The first one is completed as an example.

Prefix	Combining Form	Suffix
a-	bronch/o, bronch/i	-ary
	coni/o	-ectasis
	embol/o	-ia
	legionell/o	-ism
	pleur/o	-itis
	pneum/o	-genic
	pulmon/o	-osis
	sinus/o	
	sphyx/o	
	sten/o	
	tonsill/o	
	trache/o	
	tubercul/o	

Definition

Term

1. inflammation of the pleurae; also called pleurisy — *pleuritis*
2. inflammation of the mucous membranes of the nasal cavity and also the paranasal sinuses — _____
3. dilation of the bronchi — _____
4. narrowing of the trachea — _____
5. the absence of respiratory ventilation, or suffocation — _____
6. inflammation of a tonsil — _____
7. lung cancer — _____
8. inflammation of the lungs caused by the chronic inhalation of fine particles, which leads to the formation of a fibrotic tissue around the alveoli — _____
9. infection of the lungs by the bacterium *Mycobacterium tuberculosis* — _____
10. pneumonia caused by the bacterium *Legionella pneumophila* — _____
11. blockage in the pulmonary circulation by a mobile blood clot — _____

The Right Match

Match the term on the left with the correct definition on the right.

_____ 1. emphysema

_____ 2. pertussis

_____ 3. asthma

_____ 4. severe acute respiratory syndrome

_____ 5. croup

_____ 6. atelectasis

_____ 7. tracheitis

_____ 8. tuberculosis

_____ 9. coryza

_____ 10. pyothorax

a. severe viral infection resulting in respiratory distress that includes lung inflammation, alveolar damage, and atelectasis

b. condition of pus in the pleural cavity

c. inflammation of the trachea

d. collapse of alveoli in the lungs

e. also known as whooping cough

f. clinical term for the common cold

g. condition of the lungs that is characterized by widespread narrowing of the bronchioles and formation of mucous plugs

h. chronic lung disease named by a Greek word that means "to inflate"

i. a barking cough caused by an acute obstruction in the larynx among children

j. a highly contagious bacterial disease

Treatments, Procedures, and Devices of the Respiratory System

Here are the word parts that commonly apply to the treatments, procedures, and devices of the respiratory system that are covered in the following section. Note that the word parts are color-coded to help you identify them: prefixes are yellow, combining forms are red, and suffixes are blue.

Prefix	Definition
anti-	against, opposite of
endo-	within

Combining Form	Definition
aden/o	gland
angi/o	blood vessel
bronch/o	airway, bronchus
dilat/o	to widen
laryng/o	voice box, larynx
lob/o	a rounded part, lobe
ot/o	ear
ox/i	oxygen
pleur/o	pleura, rib
pneum/o, pneumon/o	lung, air
pulmon/o	lung
rhin/o	nose
sept/o	putrefying; wall, partition
spir/o	breathe
thorac/o	chest, thorax
trache/o	windpipe, trachea

Suffix	Definition
-al	pertaining to
-ary	pertaining to
-centesis	surgical puncture
-ectomy	surgical excision, removal
-gram	a record or image
-graphy	recording process
-ion	process
-logist	one who studies
-meter	measure, measuring instrument
-metry	measurement, process of measuring
-oid	resembling
-plasty	surgical repair
-scope	instrument used for viewing
-scopy	process of viewing
-stomy	surgical creation of an opening
-tomy	incision, to cut

KEY TERMS A–Z

acid-fast bacilli smear

stained w/ red dye [handwritten]

9.66 A clinical test performed on sputum to identify the presence of bacteria that react to acid is called **acid-fast bacilli smear**, abbreviated **AFB**. An _____-_____ _____ _____ is frequently used with chest x-rays to confirm a diagnosis of tuberculosis (Frame 9.64). An AFB smear is shown in ■ Figure 9.9.

■ **Figure 9.9**
Acid-fast bacilli smear. Photograph through a microscope of a sample taken during an AFB procedure. The red structures are *Mycobacterium tuberculosis*, the cause of TB.
Source: Courtesy of Public Health Image Library, Centers for Disease Control and Prevention.

rod shaped [handwritten]

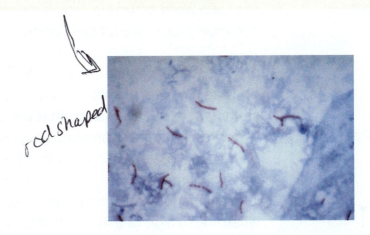

Common → Snoring & sleep apnea enlarged adenoids are most cause [handwritten]

adenoidectomy
ADD eh noyd EK toh mee

9.67 A pharyngeal tonsil is called an **adenoid** (ADD eh noyd). This constructed term, written aden/oid, means "resembling a gland." In some cases, a chronically inflamed adenoid is surgically removed to avoid complications, including obstruction of the nasopharynx. Remember that the suffix *-ectomy* means "surgical excision, removal." So, combine that with the term *adenoid*, and it creates the name for this procedure, _____. The constructed form of this term reveals three word parts: aden/oid/ectomy. Because the adenoid is one of several types of tonsils, its removal may also be called **tonsillectomy** (TAHN sil EK toh mee).

antihistamine
an tih HISS tah meen

9.68 A histamine is a compound released by certain cells in response to allergens. Histamines cause bronchial constriction and blood vessel dilation. A therapeutic drug that inhibits the effects of histamines is called an _____, which uses the prefix that means "against, opposite of." Because antihistamines cause bronchial dilation, they are useful as a treatment against swollen airways.

arterial blood gases	**9.69** A clinical test on arterial blood to identify the levels of oxygen and carbon dioxide is called _____ _____ _____. It is abbreviated **ABGs**.
aspiration ass pih RAY shun	**9.70** The removal of fluid, air, or foreign bodies with suction is a procedure called **aspiration**. _____ is derived from the Latin word *aspiratus*, which means "to breathe on," and is a common procedure for clearing the airway of obstructions.
auscultation aw skull TAY shun	**9.71** A procedure that involves listening to sounds within the body as part of a physical examination, often with the aid of a stethoscope, is called **auscultation**. The term _____ is derived from the Latin word *ausculto*, which means "to listen to." As part of a physical examination that addresses the respiratory system, auscultation involves listening to breathing sounds during inhalation and exhalation (■ Figure 9.10). Abnormal sounds include wheezing, a sign of asthma (Frame 9.31); rales, a sign of pulmonary edema (Frame 9.55) or atelectasis (Frame 9.32); and gurgles, a sign of pneumonia (Frame 9.52).

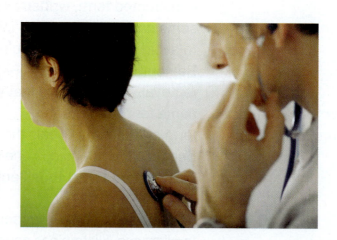

■ **Figure 9.10**
Auscultation. A stethoscope is pressed against the body wall to listen for sound waves associated with breathing.
Source: Image Point Fr/ Shutterstock.

bronchodilation BRONG koh dye LAY shun	**9.72** A procedure that uses a bronchodilating agent to relax the smooth muscles of the airways in an effort to stop bronchial constriction, thereby allowing the patient to breathe easier, is called _____. The constructed form of this term is bronch/o/dilat/ion, which means "process of widening the airway."

bronchography
brong KOG rah fee

9.73 The suffix *-graphy* means "recording process." The x-ray imaging of the bronchi is called _____. This procedure produces an x-ray image of the bronchi called a **bronchogram** (BRONG koh gram) and uses a contrast medium to highlight the bronchial tree. In many respiratory clinics, bronchography is being replaced by bronchoscopy (Frame 9.74) and CT scans to provide improved observation of the bronchi.

bronchoscopy
brong KOSS koh pee

9.74 Remember that the suffix *-scopy* means "process of viewing." The evaluation of the bronchi using a flexible fiber-optic tube mounted with a small lens at one end and attached to an eyepiece and computer monitor at the other end is called _____. This constructed term is bronch/o/scopy. The instrument is a modified endoscope, known as a **bronchoscope** (BRONG koh skope), which is inserted through the nose to observe the trachea and bronchi (■ Figure 9.11).

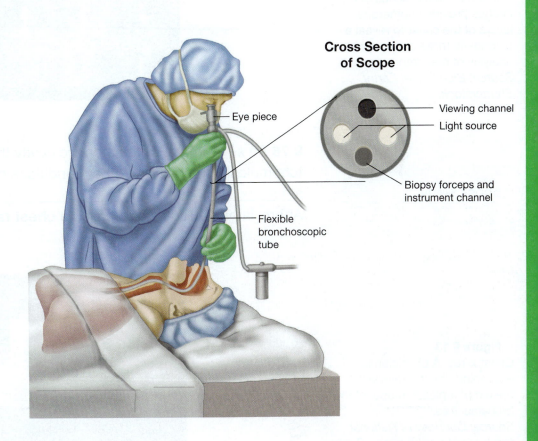

Cross Section of Scope

Eye piece

Viewing channel

Light source

Biopsy forceps and instrument channel

Flexible bronchoscopic tube

■ **Figure 9.11**
Bronchoscopy.

"pictures of cuts"

chest CT scan

high radiation exposure

Cut scan

9.75 Diagnostic imaging of the chest by a computed tomography (CT) instrument is called _____ _____ _____ (■ Figure 9.12). The procedure is used to diagnose respiratory tumors, pleural effusion, pleuritis, and other diseases by providing three-dimensional images of the thoracic cavity.

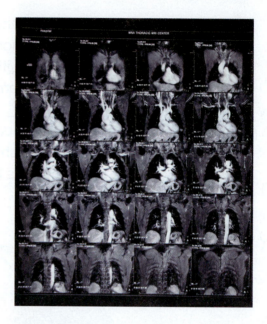

■ **Figure 9.12**
Chest CT scan. A series of CT images provides numerous layers of the chest to reveal a diagnostic three-dimensional analysis of respiratory disease. *Source: Blue Planet Earth/ Shutterstock.*

chest x-ray

9.76 An x-ray image of the thoracic cavity that is used to diagnose tuberculosis, tumors, and other conditions of the lungs is called a _____ _____ (■ Figure 9.13). Abbreviated **CXR**, it is also called a **chest radiograph**.

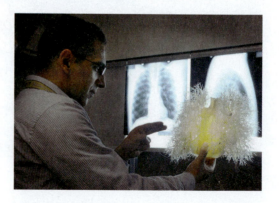

■ **Figure 9.13**
Chest x-ray. A physician is examining chest x-rays with the aid of a plastic model of the bronchial tree. *Source: Courtesy of National Institutes of Health Image Bank.*

CPAP

machine for sleep apnea

9.77 A device that is commonly used to regulate breathing during sleep as a treatment for sleep apnea (Frame 9.10) is called **continuous positive airway pressure**, abbreviated _____. The CPAP machine includes a mask that fits over the mouth and nose, or just the nose, and gently blows air to encourage rhythmic breathing (■ Figure 9.14).

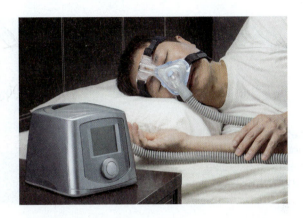

■ **Figure 9.14**
Continuous positive airway pressure (CPAP) device. The sleeping subject is receiving the benefits of the flow of air generated by the CPAP device. *Source: Chalermpon Poungpeth/ Shutterstock.*

ear, nose, and throat specialist

9.78 A physician specializing in the treatment of upper respiratory tract disease is called an **ENT**, which is the abbreviation of _____ _____ _____ _____ _____.

Alternate terms include **otolaryngologist** (OH toh LAIR in GAHL oh jist), **otonasolaryngologist** (OH toh NAY so LAIR in GAHL oh jist), and **otorhinolaryngologist** (oh toh RYE no LAIR in GAHL oh jist). The constructed form of otorhinolaryngologist is ot/o/rhin/o/ laryng/o/logist.

endotracheal

9.79 Insertion of a noncollapsible breathing tube into the trachea through the nose or mouth is called **endotracheal intubation** (EHN doh TRAY kee al * in too BAY shun). It is performed to open the airway or, if the patient is comatose, to keep the airway open. _____ is a constructed term, endo/trache/al, which means "pertaining to within the trachea."

expectorant
ek SPEK toh rant

9.80 A drug that breaks up mucus and promotes the coughing reflex to expel the mucus is called an **expectorant**. The term _____ is derived from the Latin word *expectoro*, which means "spit out of the chest."

incentive spirometry

in SEHN tiv * spy RAH meh tree

Patient measured breathing

9.81 A valuable postoperative breathing therapy is called **incentive spirometry** (■ Figure 9.15). It involves the use of a portable **spirometer** (Frame 9.93) to promote deeper breathing to improve lung expansion after an operation. Usually self-administered, _____ _____ reduces pulmonary complications and helps to correct atelectasis (Frame 9.32).

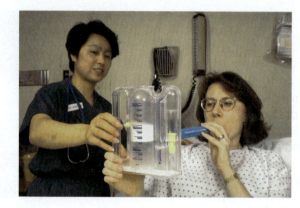

■ **Figure 9.15**
Incentive spirometry. A portable incentive spirometer is useful for encouraging patients to exercise their breathing function following an operation.

inhaler

Controller prevention rescue

9.82 An inhaler is a small handheld device containing a prescription medication, such as albuterol, that delivers a specific dosage of aerosolized medicine for inhalation to open (dilate) the bronchiolar airways. An _____ is commonly used as a primary self-administered response to asthma (Frame 9.31) and may be prescribed for other breathing disorders as well. Two types are in general use: a "controller inhaler" is used regularly to help prevent asthma symptoms by controlling lung inflammation, and a "rescue inhaler" is used to stop asthma symptoms once they have begun.

laryngectomy

lair in JEK toh mee

cig smoking = laryngeal cancer = remove voicebox

9.83 Surgical removal of the larynx is performed during a _____. The constructed form of this term is written laryng/ectomy. It is often required as a treatment for laryngeal cancer and is usually followed by training or insertion of a device to enable the patient to communicate orally. Laryngectomy patients have a permanent tracheostomy (Frame 9.102).

laryngoscopy
lair ring GOSS koh pee

9.84 A diagnostic procedure that uses a modified endoscope, called a **laryngoscope** (lair RING goh skope), to visually examine the larynx is called _____.

laryngotracheotomy
lair ring goh TRAY kee
OTT oh mee

9.85 A surgical incision into the larynx and trachea is usually performed to provide a secondary opening for inspiration and expiration, allowing air to bypass the upper respiratory tract. Remember that the suffix -*tomy* means "incision, to cut." Combine that with the combining forms for larynx and trachea, and you form the term for this procedure, _____. The constructed form of this term reveals five word parts: laryng/o/trache/o/tomy.

lobectomy
loh BEK toh mee

9.86 Surgical removal of a single lobe of a lung is sometimes required as a treatment for lung cancer, if the tumor is isolated in one lobe (the right lung has three lobes, and the left lung has two). The procedure is called _____. It may involve the removal of more than one lobe if required. Lobectomy is a constructed term: lob/ectomy.

mechanical ventilation

9.87 A medical treatment to provide supplemental oxygen to patients in respiratory distress is called **mechanical ventilation**. It provides assisted breathing using a **ventilator**, which pushes air into the patient's airway (■ Figure 9.16). _____ _____ is often used by a respiratory therapist in a clinical setting or by an emergency medical technician at the site of injury and in transit to a hospital.

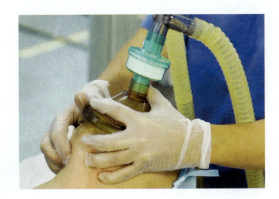

■ **Figure 9.16**
Mechanical ventilation. The photograph shows a patient receiving breathing assistance by the use of a portable mechanical ventilator.
Source: Beerkoff/Shutterstock.

nebulizer
NEBB yoo lye zer

for asthma

9.88 A device used to convert a liquid medication to a mist and deliver it to the lungs with the aid of deep inhalation is called a **nebulizer** (■ Figure 9.17). The term _____ is derived from the Latin word *nebula*, which means "fog."

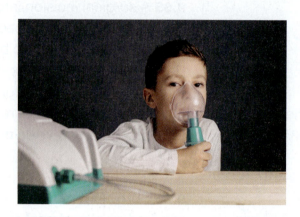

■ **Figure 9.17**
Nebulizer. The nebulizer converts a liquid medication to a mist that is easily inhaled. A face mask, such as the one shown here, is often included to direct the mist.
Source: Kleber Cordeiro/ Shutterstock.

oximetry
ok SIM eh tree

9.89 The suffix *-metry* means "measurement, process of measuring," and the combining form that means "oxygen" is *ox/i*. Therefore, the procedure that measures oxygen levels in the blood using an instrument called an **oximeter** (ok SIM eh ter) is called _____. The constructed form of this term is *ox/i/metry*. A small, widely used oximeter that provides a digital readout of oxygen levels is called a **pulse oximeter** (■ Figure 9.18) because it also monitors pulse rate. The pulse oximeter is usually attached to a finger and includes sensors with a computer chip that determines oxygen levels carried by hemoglobin in the red blood cells moving through capillaries in the dermis of the skin.

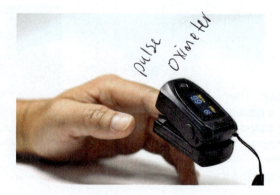

pulse oximeter

■ **Figure 9.18**
Pulse oximetry. The small device provides a digital readout of oxygen levels in the blood.
Source: toysf400/Shutterstock.

pleurocentesis
ploor oh sehn TEE siss

9.90 The suffix *-centesis* means "surgical puncture." The surgical puncture and aspiration of fluid from the pleural cavity is a diagnostic procedure called _____. After aspiration, the fluid is analyzed for the presence of bacteria and white blood cells, the presence of which indicates pleuritis (Frame 9.50). *Pleurocentesis* is a constructed term, pleur/o/centesis. It is also called **thoracentesis** (Frame 9.98) or **thoracocentesis**.

pneumonectomy
NOO moh NEK toh mee

9.91 Many terms in this section have used the suffix that means "surgical excision, removal," *-ectomy*. A word root that means "lung" is *pneumon*. Therefore, surgical removal of a lung is called _____, or **pneumectomy** (noo MEK toh mee). It is performed as a radical treatment for lung cancer, in which tumors have progressed throughout one lung. The constructed form of **pneumonectomy** is pneumon/ectomy. If the surgery is limited to the removal of a single lobe, recall that the procedure is called a *lobectomy* (Frame 9.86).

pulmonary angiography
PULL mon air ee * AN jee
OG rah fee

9.92 A diagnostic procedure that evaluates the blood circulation of the lungs is called **pulmonary angiography**. In this procedure, x-ray images are taken of the lungs following the injection of a contrast medium into the pulmonary circulation. _____ _____ is a constructed term represented as pulmon/ary angi/o/graphy, which literally means "recording of blood vessel pertaining to lung."

pulmonary function tests

Done to evaluate Breathing

9.93 A series of diagnostic tests performed to determine the cause of lung disease by evaluating lung capacity through the use of spirometry (Frame 9.81) is called _____ _____ _____ (abbreviated **PFTs**). Spirometry involves breathing into a tube connected to an instrument, called a **spirometer**. Both are terms that use the combining form that means "breathe," *spir/o*. Spirometry measures the amount of air inhaled and exhaled during a normal breathing cycle, called *tidal volume (TV)*, the amount of air forcefully exhaled, called *expiratory reserve volume (ERV)*, the volume of air forcefully inhaled, called *inspiratory reserve volume (IRV)*, and other values shown in ■ Figure 9.19.

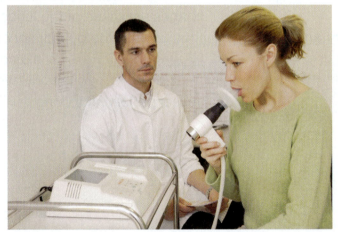

Inspiratory reserve volume - 3100 mL —

Tidal volume - 500 mL —
Expiratory reserve volume - 1200 mL —

Residual volume - 1200 mL —

(a)

■ **Figure 9.19**
Pulmonary function test (PFT): spirometry. (a) Normal respiratory volumes, as measured during spirometry. A patient's spirometry data are compared to this chart to identify breathing deficiencies. (b) Photograph of a patient exhaling into a spirometer during a pulmonary function test, with the assistance of a respiratory therapist.
Source: Phanie/ScienceSource.

(b)

pulmonologist
PUL moh NAHL oh jist

9.94 A physician specializing in the treatment of diseases affecting the lower respiratory tract, particularly the lungs, is called a **pulmonary specialist** or _____.

resuscitation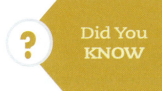
ree SUSS ih TAY shun

9.95 An emergency procedure that is used to restore breathing is known as **pulmonary resuscitation**. The most common form is **cardiopulmonary** _____, or **CPR**, which uses chest compressions with the patient lying supine (on the back).

?   Did You KNOW

RESUSCITATION

The term _resuscitation_ is derived from the Latin word _resuscito_, which means "to rise up again" or "revive." Its present meaning refers to any procedure that involves a restoration of body functions such as breathing and blood flow to vital organs and includes the popular technique of compressing the chest and heart called _cardiopulmonary resuscitation (CPR)_. It also includes mouth-to-mouth resuscitation, in which air is blown into the patient's mouth while holding the nose, and the Heimlich maneuver, during which an obstruction (usually food) may be dislodged by reaching around a standing patient and pushing upward on the diaphragm to force an expulsion of air.

---

rhinoplasty
RYE noh plass tee

9.96 Add the combining form that means "nose" (_rhin/o_) to the suffix that means "surgical repair" to form the term _____, which is the surgical repair of the nose. This constructed term is rhin/o/plasty. Although this procedure is commonly used to modify the external appearance of the nose during cosmetic surgery, it may include **septoplasty** (SEP toh plass tee), during which deviation of the nasal septum is corrected to improve breathing. The combining form in this term, _sept/o_, means "wall, partition."

TB skin test

9.97 A simple skin test to determine the presence of a tuberculosis infection is called a **TB skin test**. During a _____ _____ _____, a purified protein derivative (PPD) sample of the TB bacillus is injected beneath the epidermis of the skin (called an *intradermal injection*). A reddened, swollen skin lesion at the injection site a few days later indicates a previous exposure (■ Figure 9.20) and requires follow-up confirmation with a chest x-ray (Frame 9.76), a sputum AFB smear (Frame 9.66), or both. The TB skin test is also called **PPD skin test** and **Mantoux skin test** (after French physician Charles Mantoux).

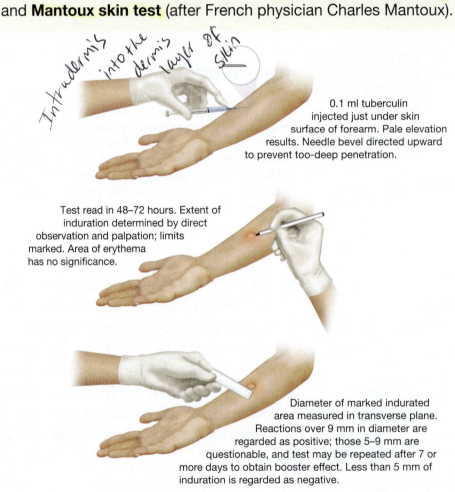

Intradermis into the dermis layer of skin

0.1 ml tuberculin injected just under skin surface of forearm. Pale elevation results. Needle bevel directed upward to prevent too-deep penetration.

Test read in 48–72 hours. Extent of induration determined by direct observation and palpation; limits marked. Area of erythema has no significance.

Diameter of marked indurated area measured in transverse plane. Reactions over 9 mm in diameter are regarded as positive; those 5–9 mm are questionable, and test may be repeated after 7 or more days to obtain booster effect. Less than 5 mm of induration is regarded as negative.

■ **Figure 9.20**
The TB (PPD) skin test. It is in common use as an initial screening for tuberculosis.

thoracentesis
THOR ah sehn TEE siss

9.98 The suffix that means "surgical puncture" is *-centesis*. Surgical puncture using a needle and syringe into the thoracic cavity to aspirate pleural fluid for diagnosis or treatment is called a _____. It is also called **thoracocentesis** (THOR ah koh sehn TEE siss) or **pleurocentesis** (Frame 9.90). Thoracentesis is a constructed term, thora/centesis; note that, in this term, the syllable *co* is removed from the combining form *thorac/o*. The procedure is often used to treat pleural effusion (Frame 9.49) by draining the excess fluid from the pleural cavity.

thoracostomy
THOR ah KOSS toh mee

9.99 The suffix *-stomy* means "surgical creation of an opening." Surgical puncture into the chest cavity, usually for the insertion of a drainage or air tube, is called a _____. The constructed form of this term is written thorac/o/stomy. The procedure is often termed "placing a chest tube."

thoracotomy
THOR ah KOTT oh mee

9.100 Recall the suffix that means "incision, to cut." Add this to the combining form that means "chest, thorax," and you form the term _____, which is a surgical incision into the chest wall. The constructed form of this term is thorac/o/tomy.

tracheoplasty
TRAY kee oh PLASS tee

9.101 The suffix *-plasty* means "surgical repair." Surgical repair of the trachea is called _____. The constructed form of this term reveals three word parts: trache/o/plasty.

tracheostomy
TRAY kee OSS toh mee

9.102 Recall the suffix that means "surgical creation of an opening." Surgical creation of an opening into the trachea, usually for the insertion of a breathing tube, is called _____. This constructed term is trache/o/stomy. The procedure is shown in ■ Figure 9.21.

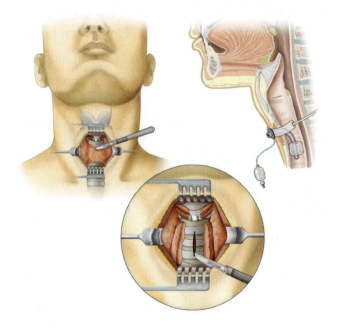

■ **Figure 9.21**
Tracheostomy. A tracheotomy, or incision into the trachea, is performed to create an opening into the trachea as shown in this series of illustrations.

tracheotomy
TRAY kee OTT oh mee

9.103 Surgical incision into the trachea is a required part of a tracheostomy (Frame 9.102). The incision is called a _____. The constructed form of this term is trache/o/tomy.

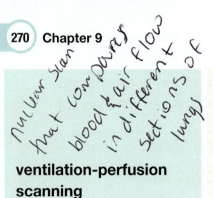

nuclear scan that compares blood & air flow in different sections of lungs

ventilation-perfusion scanning

9.104 A diagnostic tool that uses nuclear medicine, or the use of radioactive material, to evaluate pulmonary function is called **ventilation-perfusion scanning**. It can identify pulmonary embolism (Frame 9.56) and pulmonary edema (Frame 9.55).

_____-_____ _____

math

is also called **lung scan** and **V/Q scan** (the Q stands for "quotient").

flow

PRACTICE: Treatments, Procedures, and Devices of the Respiratory System

The Right Match

Match the term on the left with the correct definition on the right.

_____ 1. pulmonary function tests

_____ 2. pulse oximeter

_____ 3. bronchodilation

_____ 4. arterial blood gases

_____ 5. TB skin test

_____ 6. auscultation

_____ 7. ventilation-perfusion scanning

_____ 8. nebulizer

_____ 9. pulmonary angiography

_____ 10. expectorant

a. breaks up mucus and promotes coughing

b. also called PPD skin test and Mantoux skin test

c. measurement of oxygen and carbon dioxide blood levels

d. device used to convert a liquid medication to a mist and deliver it to the lungs

e. physical examination that includes listening to sounds within the body

f. a blood oxygen measuring device that reads oxygen levels by noninvasive physical contact with a finger

g. procedure that uses a bronchodilating agent in an inhaler to reduce bronchial constriction

h. x-ray of lung blood vessels

i. diagnostic tool that uses nuclear medicine, or the use of radioactive material, to evaluate pulmonary function

j. use of spirometry to evaluate lung function

Break the Chain

Analyze these medical terms:

a) Separate each term into its word parts; each word part is labeled for you (**p** = prefix, **r** = root, **cf** = combining form, and **s** = suffix).

b) For the Bonus Question, write the requested definition in the blank that follows.

1. a) tracheotomy   _____/___/_____
                                      cf   s

   b) *Bonus Question*: What is the definition of the suffix? _____

2. a) thoracentesis   _____/_____
                                   r   s

   b) *Bonus Question*: What is the definition of the word root? _____

3. a) pneumonectomy   _____/_____
                                   r   s

   b) *Bonus Question*: What is the definition of the word root? _____

4. a) bronchoscopy   _____/___/_____
                                      cf   s

   b) *Bonus Question*: What is the definition of the suffix? _____

5. a) adenoidectomy   _____/_____/_____
                                   r   s   s

   b) *Bonus Question*: What is the definition of the first suffix? _____

6. a) bronchodilation   _____/___/_____/_____
                                      cf   r   s

   b) *Bonus Question*: What is the definition of the suffix? _____

7. a) lobectomy   _____/_____
                                   r   s

   b) *Bonus Question*: What is the definition of the word root? _____

8. a) rhinoplasty   _____/___/_____
                                      cf   s

   b) *Bonus Question*: What is the definition of the combining form? _____

9. a) septoplasty   _____/___/_____
                                      cf   s

   b) *Bonus Question*: What is the definition of the suffix? _____

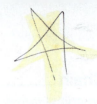

Abbreviations of the Respiratory System

The abbreviations that are associated with the respiratory system are summarized here. Study these abbreviations and review them in the exercise that follows.

Abbreviation	Definition
ABGs	arterial blood gases
AFB	acid-fast bacilli smear
ARDS	adult (acute) respiratory distress syndrome
CF	cystic fibrosis
COPD	chronic obstructive pulmonary disease
CPAP	continuous positive airway pressure device
CPR	cardiopulmonary resuscitation
CXR	chest x-ray
ENT	ear, nose, and throat specialist
NRDS	neonatal respiratory distress syndrome

Abbreviation	Definition
NSCLC	non–small cell lung cancer
PE	pulmonary embolism
PPD	purified protein derivative
PFTs	pulmonary function tests
RDS	respiratory distress syndrome
SARS	severe acute respiratory syndrome
SCLC	small cell lung cancer
SOB	shortness of breath
TB	tuberculosis
URI	upper respiratory infection
V/Q scan	ventilation-perfusion scanning

PRACTICE: Abbreviations

Fill in the blanks with the abbreviation or the complete medical term.

Abbreviation

1. _____
2. _____
3. ARDS
4. _____
5. CPR
6. _____
7. URI
8. _____
9. COPD
10. _____
11. AFB
12. _____
13. SOB
14. _____
15. PPD

Medical Term

continuous positive airway pressure device

tuberculosis

_____

chest x-ray

_____

cystic fibrosis

_____

small cell lung cancer

_____

pulmonary embolism

_____

neonatal respiratory distress syndrome

_____

pulmonary function tests

_____

CHAPTER REVIEW

Word Building

Construct medical terms from the following meanings. (Some are built from word parts, some are not.)
The first question has been completed as an example.

1. inflammation of the larynx   _____*laryng*itis

2. absence of oxygen   _____oxia

3. inflammation of the bronchi   bronch_____

4. respiratory failure characterized by atelectasis   respiratory _____

5. physical exam that includes listening to body sounds   _____ (do this one on your own!)

6. deficient oxygen levels in the blood   hyp_____

7. difficulty breathing   _____pnea

8. excessive carbon dioxide levels in the blood   hyper_____

9. abnormal dilation of the bronchi   bronchi _____

10. lung inflammation due to dust inhalation   _____coniosis

11. cancer arising from cells within the bronchi   bronchogenic _____

12. an inherited disease of excessive mucus production   cystic _____

13. inflammation of the trachea   trache_____

14. the absence of respiratory ventilation   _____sphyxia

15. x-ray image of the bronchi   broncho_____

16. surgical puncture and aspiration of fluid from the pleural cavity   thora_____

17. measurement of oxygen levels in the blood   oxi_____

Define the Combining Form

In the space provided, write the definition of the combining form, followed by one example of the combining form used to build a medical term in Chapter 9.

	Definition	**Use in a Term**
1. bronch/o	_____	_____
2. laryng/o	_____	_____
3. ox/i	_____	_____
4. rhin/o	_____	_____
5. atel/o	_____	_____
6. pleur/o	_____	_____
7. pneum/o, pneumon/o	_____	_____
8. pulmon/o	_____	_____

Complete the Labels

Complete the blank labels in ■ Figure 9.22 by writing the labels in the spaces provided.

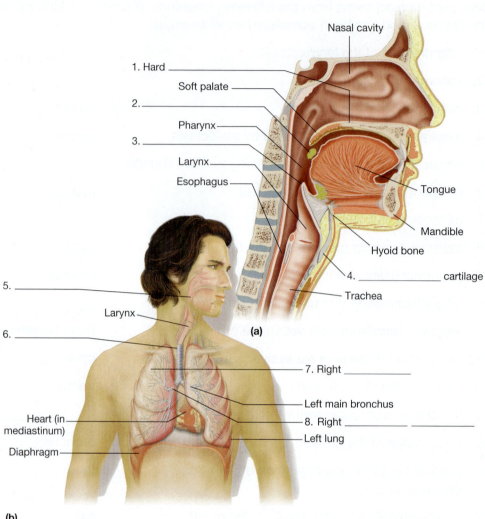

Nasal cavity

1. Hard

Soft palate

2.

Pharynx

3.

Larynx

Esophagus

Tongue

Mandible

Hyoid bone

4. _____ cartilage

Trachea

(a)

5.

Larynx

6.

7. Right _____

Left main bronchus

Heart (in mediastinum)

8. Right _____ _____

Left lung

Diaphragm

(b)

■ **Figure 9.22**
The respiratory system.

1. _____

2. _____

3. _____

4. _____

5. _____

6. _____

7. _____

8. _____

MEDICAL REPORT EXERCISES

Geoffrey Piscotti

Read the following medical report, then answer the questions that follow.

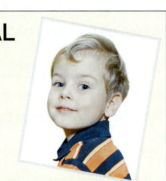

PEARSON GENERAL HOSPITAL

5500 University Avenue, Metropolis, New York
Phone: (211) 594-4000 • Fax (211) 594-4001

Medical Consultation: Pediatrics **Date**: 11/04/2014

Patient: Geoffrey Piscotti **Patient ID**: 123456

Dob: 04/22/2008 **Age**: 6 **Sex**: Male **Allergies**: NKDA

Provider: Maria S. Zargas, MD

Subjective:

Described with help from Mom: "My chest hurts when I breathe, so I cough a lot. I'm tired a lot, and I have a stuffy nose that sometimes bleeds."

6 y/o male has difficulty breathing. His mother indicates it is interrupting his sleep, leaving him tired during the day. He coughs frequently and expressed sputum tinged with blood while in the examination room. Mother is a respiratory therapist in downtown clinic with known TB exposures. Father is a schoolteacher.

Objective:

Vital Signs: **T**: 99.5°F; **P**: 88; **R**: 25; **BP**: 135/90

Ht: 3'5"

Wt: 55 lb

General Appearance: Skin with pallor, mild diaphoresis. Mild edema of the face around the eyes. Eyes unclear with mild conjunctivitis.

Heart: Rate at 88 bpm. Heart sounds with auscultation appear normal.

Lungs: Bronchial, tracheal congestion present; congestion in left lung during auscultation with minor rales and gurgles.

HEENT: Swelling of nasal cavity with evidence of recent epistaxis; erythema and swelling of throat.

AbD: Bowel sounds normal all four quadrants.

MS: Joints and muscles symmetric. No swelling, masses, or deformity.

Lab: Skin test positive for TB. AFB positive for TB. TB in left lung confirmed by chest x-ray.

Assessment:

Active TB

Plan:

Admit and provide oxygen assist with TB antibiotic cocktail by IV drip. After release and return home, follow with long-term antibiotic cocktail supervised by adult with weekly clinic visits. Report infection to County Health and CDC.

Photo Source: Pavel L Photo and Video/Shutterstock.

Comprehension Questions

1. What complaints support the diagnosis? _____

_____

_____

2. Based on the family history, how do you think the TB infection originated? _____

_____

_____

3. What is the meaning of the abbreviation TB? _____

_____

_____

Case Study Questions

The following Case Study provides further discussion regarding the patient in the medical report. Fill in the blanks with the correct terms. Choose your answers from the following list of terms. (Note that some terms may be used more than once.)

acid-fast	bronchitis	coryza (or acute rhinitis)
chest x-rays	bronchodilating	tuberculosis (TB)

Geoffrey Piscotti, a 6-year-old boy with a previous healthy history, was admitted into an emergency clinic

when his mother became concerned about his respiratory function. She explained that he had come home

from school 3 weeks ago with a common cold, or (a) _____. He began coughing violently

shortly afterward, preventing him from sleeping. Physical exams showed an acute inflammation of the larynx,

trachea, and bronchi, indicating the acute condition known as (b) _____, which was bacterial

in origin. Following the prescribed use of antibiotic therapy and the use of inhaled (c) _____

agents to reduce bronchial constriction, the patient recovered initially. Several months passed and then the

coughing returned and the boy complained of low energy. Following a (d) _____ skin test

and a sputum test that included (e) _____-_____ bacilli, positive results indicated

an active lung infection known as (f) _____. TB was confirmed with the use of radiographic

images of the thorax, or (g) _____ _____. The course of treatment included

a cocktail of antibiotics administered over a 6-month period.

Shareena Mushreen

For a greater challenge, read the following medical report, then answer the critical thinking questions that follow.

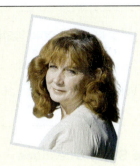

PEARSON GENERAL HOSPITAL

PGH

5500 University Avenue, Metropolis, New York
Phone: (211) 594-4000 • Fax (211) 594-4001

Medical Consultation: EENT

Patient: Shareena Mushreen

Dob: 3/08/1949   **Age**: 68   **Sex**: Female

Provider: George T. Cohn, MD

Date: 12/09/2017

Patient ID: 123456

Allergies: NKDA

Subjective:

"For the past week I have found it hard to breathe. When I take a big breath, my chest hurts badly. I cough frequently, and I'm tired a lot."

65 y/o female complains of chest pain when breathing deeply, coughing, headache, and malaise. She is a recent immigrant from Eastern Europe and works in a textile factory.

Objective:

Vital Signs: **T**: 100.8°F; **P**: 79; **R**: 20; **BP**: 139/97

Ht: 5'2"

Wt: 155 lb

General Appearance: Skin with pallor, mild diaphoresis. Mild edema of the face around the eyes and neck.

Heart: Rate at 79 bpm. Heart sounds with auscultation appear normal.

Lungs: Congestion during auscultation with prominent gurgles of both lungs.

HEENT: Swelling of nasal cavity and throat; mild erythema of throat and larynx. Oxygen 63%. PFT shows reduced IRV and VC 25%.

AbD: Bowel sounds normal all four quadrants.

MS: Joints and muscles symmetric. No swelling, masses, or deformity.

Lab: Chest x-ray positive for pneumonia. AFB negative for TB. Blood culture positive for *P. jiroveci*, but no HIV antibodies present.

Assessment:

Pneumonia with *P. jiroveci*

Plan:

Admit stat and isolate in oxygen tent with IV drip antibiotics specific against *P. jiroveci*. Monitor continuously. Once stable, release with oral antibiotics and weekly visits until cleared. Report infection to County Health and CDC.

Photo Source: David Jenks/Shutterstock.

Comprehension Questions

1. Why would the diagnosed condition of pneumonia cause the patient complaint? _____

_____

2. Why is additional testing recommended to explore the source of the infection? _____

_____

3. What is the source of the infection causing the pneumonia? _____

_____

Case Study Questions

The following case study provides additional consideration of the patient in the medical report. Recall the terms from this chapter to fill in the blanks with the correct terms.

A 65-year-old female, Shareen Mushareen, complained of difficulty breathing and chest pain, two symptoms

called (h) _____ and (i) _____. Her personal physician began with a chest

(j) _____ using a stethoscope, followed by fingertip assessment of oxygen levels in the blood using

a (k) _____ and a measurement of breathing volumes, using a (l) _____. The tests

indicated reduced oxygen levels in the blood, called (m) _____, in combination with reduced lung

capacity. Breathing sounds suggested labored breathing with some gurgling sounds. The physician diagnosed

the condition as a lung inflammation with alveolar fluids, called (n) _____, caused by an unknown

infectious agent. To identify the source of the infectious agent, sputum and blood tests were performed that

included (o) _____ _____ bacilli, HIV testing, and histological blood tests. The tests

showed the infectious agent as a fungus that is an opportunistic pathogen in immune-suppressed patients, known

as (p) _____ _____. This disease, called (q) _____, is a common

diagnostic indicator of patients suffering from HIV infection. An antibody test for HIV was administered, with negative

results. The patient was admitted for continual monitoring during antibiotic therapy and was kept within an oxygen

tent to improve oxygen blood levels. After the treatment, blood tests confirmed the pathogen had been defeated.

MyLab Medical Terminology™

MyLab Medical Terminology is a premium online homework management system that includes a host of features to help you study. Registered users will find:

- A multitude of quizzes and activities built within the MyLab platform
- Powerful tools that track and analyze your results—allowing you to create a personalized learning experience
- Videos and audio pronunciations to help enrich your progress
- Streaming lesson presentations (Guided Lectures) and self-paced learning modules
- A space where you and your instructors can view and manage your assignments

Chapter 10

The Digestive System

Learning Objectives

After completing this chapter, you will be able to:

10.1 Define and spell the word parts used to create terms for the digestive system.

10.2 Break down and define common medical terms used for symptoms, diseases, disorders, procedures, treatments, and devices associated with the digestive system.

10.3 Build medical terms from the word parts associated with the digestive system.

10.4 Pronounce and spell common medical terms associated with the digestive system.

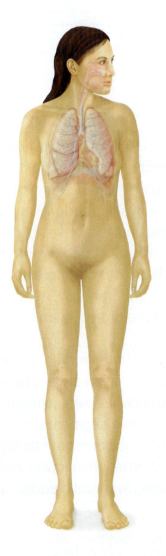

Anatomy and Physiology Terms

The following table provides the combining forms that commonly apply to the anatomy and physiology of the digestive system. Note that the combining forms are colored red to help you identify them when you see them again later in the chapter.

Combining Form	Definition	Combining Form	Definition
abdomin/o	abdomen	hepat/o	liver
an/o	anus	ile/o	to roll, ileum
append/o, appendic/o	appendix	jejun/o	empty, jejunum
bil/i	bile	lingu/o	tongue
cec/o	blind intestine, cecum	or/o	mouth
chol/e	bile, gall	pancreat/o	sweetbread, pancreas
choledoch/o	common bile duct	peps/o, pept/o	digestion
col/o, colon/o	colon	peritone/o	to stretch over, peritoneum
cyst/o	bladder, sac		
dent/o	teeth	proct/o	rectum or anus
duoden/o	twelve, duodenum	pylor/o	pylorus
enter/o	small intestine	rect/o	rectum
esophag/e, esophag/o	gullet, esophagus	sial/o	saliva
gastr/o	stomach	sigm/o	the letter s, sigmoid colon
gingiv/o	gums	stomat/o	mouth
gloss/o	tongue		

digestive

dye JEST iv

GI

10.1 The _____ system converts food into a form the body can use for energy, growth, and repair. It derives its name from its primary function, **digestion**. The term is from the Latin word *digestus*, which means "to divide, dissolve, or set in order." The digestive system performs all three: When the body digests food, it divides and dissolves it into simpler parts, called *nutrients*, which may then be absorbed into the bloodstream. From the blood, nutrients diffuse into cells to serve as fuel to power body functions. Digestion occurs gradually, as food is passed from one organ to the next through the digestive tract, or gastrointestinal (**GI**) tract. The organs of the _____ tract form a long continuous tube that includes the mouth, pharynx, esophagus, stomach, small intestine, and large intestine. The small intestine includes three segments: the duodenum, jejunum, and ileum. The large intestine also includes three segments, called the cecum, colon, and rectum. Accessory organs contribute to digestion, mainly by secreting enzymes and other chemicals into the GI tract. They include the salivary glands, liver, gallbladder, and pancreas.

digestion

10.2 You have just learned that _____, which is the breakdown of food particles into their small subunits, is the primary function of the digestive system. Chemical digestion is performed by enzymes, and mechanical digestion is achieved by chewing in the mouth and mixing and churning actions produced by muscles in the walls of the stomach. Other important functions of the digestive system include:

- Absorption of nutrients, which occurs across the wall of the small intestine

- Formation of solid waste, in the form of feces, and its elimination from the body

- Conservation of water, which occurs as water is absorbed across the walls of the small and large intestines

10.3 Review the anatomy of the digestive system by studying ■ Figure 10.1 and ■ Figure 10.2.

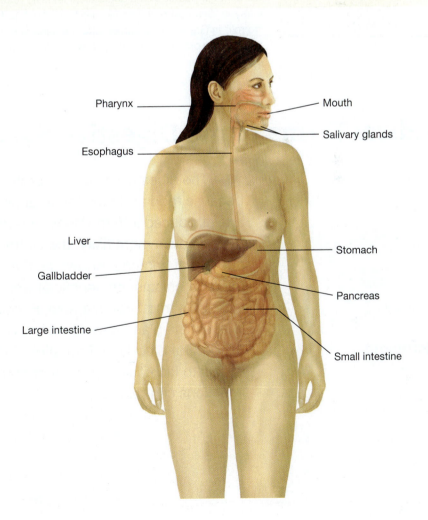

Pharynx

Mouth

Salivary glands

Esophagus

Liver

Stomach

Gallbladder

Pancreas

Large intestine

Small intestine

■ **Figure 10.1**
Organs of the digestive system.

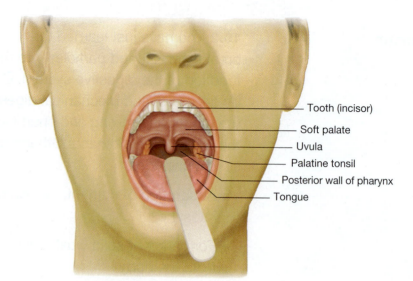

- Tooth (incisor)
- Soft palate
- Uvula
- Palatine tonsil
- Posterior wall of pharynx
- Tongue

■ **Figure 10.2**
The oral cavity. Anterior view of the open mouth.

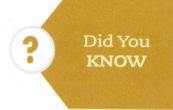

Did You KNOW

DUODENUM, JEJUNUM, AND ILEUM

The three segments of the small intestine are the duodenum, jejunum, and ileum. The term *duodenum* is derived from the Medieval Latin word *duodeni*, which means "twelve." This word first appeared in the anatomical texts in 1050 AD, taken from a monk's description of it as the "first part of the small intestine, about 12 fingerbreadths in length." *Ileum* means "to roll" in Greek and is named after its peristaltic waves of muscle contraction that roll through the organ like ocean waves. The term *jejunum* is named from the Latin word *jejunus*, meaning "empty."

Medical Terms of the Digestive System

microbiota

10.4 The digestive system is under a constant risk of infection because food and other substances that often contain pathogens are introduced into the body through the mouth every day. To make matters even more risky, the GI tract normally contains an enormous number of bacteria. Known as the *microbiota*, most of these microorganisms are beneficial when their populations are contained within the tract. For example, *E. coli* assists in the breakdown of indigestible plant materials and synthesizes vitamin K, which is needed for blood clot formation. But if the _____ is able to increase in density or spread to other body areas, severe infections can result.

infections

10.5 In addition to _____, the GI tract organs are also susceptible to inherited defects and the development of tumors. In each case, the result of the disease may be a reduction of the body's ability to digest food, eliminate wastes, absorb and conserve water, or perform other specific functions. Most digestive disorders affect overall health rather than remain localized, due to the abundance of blood vessels and lymphatics associated with GI tract organs and the functional importance of accessory organs like the liver and pancreas.

disease

10.6 The clinical treatment of a digestive disorder is performed by a physician with a specialization in treating the body region or organ, the particular disorder, or a set of disorders. For example, a _____ of the mouth or throat is treated by a **head and neck specialist**, stomach or intestinal disease is treated by a **gastroenterologist** (GAS troh EN ter AHL oh jist), a disease of the rectum is treated by a **proctologist** (prok TAHL oh jist), and a disease of the liver is treated by a **hepatobiliary** (heh PAT oh BIL ee air ee) **specialist**. Cancer is treated by an **oncologist**, often in association with a regional specialist. The area within a hospital that treats digestive disorders is often called **internal medicine**.

digestive

10.7 Because most digestive organs are located deep within the body, the diagnosis of _____ disorders can benefit from noninvasive imaging procedures. Consequently, magnetic resonance imaging (MRI), computed tomography (CT) scans, and specialized x-ray techniques are often used. Once diagnosed, most disorders may be treated with therapeutic agents or by surgery.

10.8 In the following sections, you will study the prefixes, combining forms, and suffixes that combine to build the medical terms of the digestive system.

Signs and Symptoms of the Digestive System

Here are the word parts that commonly apply to the signs and symptoms of the digestive system and are covered in the following section. Note that the word parts are color-coded to help you identify them: prefixes are yellow, combining forms are red, and suffixes are blue.

Prefix	Definition
a-	without, absence of
dia-	through
dys-	bad, abnormal, painful, difficult
re-	back

Combining Form	Definition
flux/o	flow
gastr/o	stomach
halit/o	breath
hemat/o	blood
hepat/o	liver
peps/o, pept/o	digestion
phag/o	eat, swallow
steat/o	fat

Suffix	Definition
-algia	condition of pain
-dynia	condition of pain
-emesis	vomiting
-emia	condition of blood
-ia	condition of
-megaly	abnormally large
-osis	condition of
-rrhea	discharge

KEY TERMS A–Z

aphagia
ah FAY jee ah

10.9 The prefix *a-* means "without, absence of" and the combining form *phag/o* means "eat, swallow." Combining these word parts forms the term _____, which is the inability to swallow. This constructed term contains three word parts, as shown when it is written *a/phag/ia*. Although the literal meaning is "without eating or swallowing," clinical use of the term has changed its meaning to "inability to swallow."

ascites
ah SIGH teez

10.10 The Greek word that means "bag" is *askos*. It is used to create the term **ascites**, which is an accumulation of fluid within the peritoneal cavity that produces an enlarged abdomen. _____ is a sign of liver disease, congestive heart failure, malnutrition, or irritation to the peritoneum.

constipation
kon stih PAY shun

10.11 Infrequent or incomplete bowel movements are characteristic of **constipation**. It is a sign of an intestinal disorder that causes feces lacking in water, making their passage through the rectum and anus difficult and often painful. The term _____ is derived from the Latin word *constipatus*, which means "to press together."

diarrhea
dye ah REE ah

10.12 An opposite condition to constipation is **diarrhea**, in which a frequent discharge of watery fecal material occurs. It is a constructed term with two word parts: *dia/rrhea*. _____ literally means "discharge through" and may be caused by an improper diet, but it is more commonly a sign of infection by virus, bacteria, or protozoa. It is particularly dangerous to infants, who are in danger of severe dehydration. According to the World Health Organization, more than 500,000 children die across the world each year from dehydration resulting from diarrhea.

dyspepsia diss PEPP see ah	**10.13** A common symptom of digestive difficulty that literally translates to "condition of difficult digestion" is _____. This constructed term contains three word parts, as shown in dys/peps/ia. Commonly called **indigestion**, it is accompanied by stomach or esophageal pain or discomfort.
dysphagia diss FAY jee ah	**10.14** Difficulty in swallowing is called **dysphagia**. It often accompanies a sore throat, although its chronic form can be a sign of oral or pharyngeal cancer. _____ is a constructed term: dys/phag/ia.
flatus FLAY tuss	**10.15** The term *flatus* is a Latin word that means "a blowing." It is used to describe the presence of gas, or air, in the GI tract, which is simply called _____. Gas is expelled through the anus as **flatulence** (FLAT yoo lens).
gastrodynia GAS troh DINN ee ah	**10.16** The combining form for stomach is *gastr/o*, and a suffix that means "condition of pain" is *-dynia*. Therefore, the symptom of stomach pain is known as _____. This constructed term includes three word parts and is written gastr/o/dynia. It is also known as **gastralgia** (gast RAL jee ah). Despite the availability of these terms, the primary term in present clinical use to identify the symptom of stomach pain is, simply, **abdominal pain**.
halitosis hal ih TOH siss	**10.17** The word root *halit* means "breath." It is derived from the Latin word for breath, *halitus*. Adding the suffix *-osis* forms the term **halitosis**. Although there is no word part included to give the term a negative meaning, nonetheless _____ means "bad breath." The constructed form is halit/osis.
hematemesis HEE mah TEM eh siss	**10.18** Vomiting blood is a sign of a severe digestive disorder, such as a bleeding peptic ulcer (Frame 10.62) or stomach cancer (Frame 10.43). It is called **hematemesis**, which is a constructed term with two word parts: hemat/emesis. The literal meaning of _____ is "vomiting blood."
hepatomegaly HEPP ah toh MEG ah lee	**10.19** A sign of liver disease is abnormal enlargement of the liver, called _____. This constructed term is hepat/o/megaly, which literally means "abnormally large liver."

jaundice
JAWN diss

10.20 A yellowish-orange coloration of the skin, sclera of the eyes, and deeper tissues is a collective sign of liver disease called **jaundice** (■ Figure 10.3). The condition of _____ results from the accumulation of bile pigments in the bloodstream that is normally removed by the liver.

■ **Figure 10.3**
Jaundice. Photograph of an individual with liver disease, evidenced by the yellowing of the sclera of the eyes and the skin. *Source: Courtesy of Dr. Thomas F. Sellers and Emory University, Public Health Image Library, Centers for Disease Control and Prevention, Atlanta, GA.*

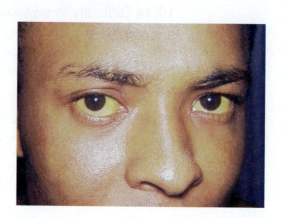

? Did You KNOW

JAUNDICE
The term *jaundice* is derived from the French word for yellow, *jaune*, to describe the yellowing appearance of the skin and sclera. An alternate term for this symptom is *icterus*, which is the Greek word meaning "yellow bird."

nausea
NAW see ah

10.21 A symptom of dizziness that includes an urge to vomit is called **nausea**. When _____ is accompanied by vomiting, it is abbreviated **N&V**. Nausea is derived from the Latin and Greek words for seasickness, *nausia*.

reflux
REE fluks

10.22 A backward flow of material in the GI tract, or regurgitation, is called **reflux**. This constructed term is re/flux. The literal meaning of _____ is "back flow."

steatorrhea
STEE at oh REE ah

10.23 Abnormal levels of fat in the feces is a sign of digestive malfunction. It is called **steatorrhea**, which is a constructed term, steat/o/rrhea. Because *steat/o* is a combining form for fat, _____ literally means "discharge of fat."

PRACTICE: Signs and Symptoms of the Digestive System

The Right Match

Match the term on the left with the correct definition on the right.

_____ 1. dysphagia

_____ 2. reflux

_____ 3. flatus

_____ 4. halitosis

_____ 5. ascites

_____ 6. diarrhea

_____ 7. nausea

_____ 8. constipation

_____ 9. jaundice

a. backward flow of material in the GI tract

b. gas trapped in the GI tract

c. difficulty in swallowing

d. infrequent or incomplete bowel movements

e. frequent discharge of watery fecal material

f. bad breath

g. from the French word for yellow

h. a symptomatic urge to vomit

i. accumulation of fluid in the peritoneal cavity

Break the Chain

Analyze these medical terms:

a) Separate each term into its word parts; each word part is labeled for you (**p** = prefix, **r** = root, **cf** = combining form, and **s** = suffix).

b) For the Bonus Question, write the requested definition in the blank that follows.

The first set has been completed for you as an example.

1. a) aphagia   ***a/phag/ia***

                               p   r   s

   b) *Bonus Question:* What is the definition of the suffix? ***condition of*** _____

2. a) dyspepsia   _____/_____/_____

                              p   r   s

   b) *Bonus Question:* What is the definition of the word root? _____

3. a) gastrodynia   _____/___/_____

                              cf   s

   b) *Bonus Question:* What is the definition of the combining form? _____

4. a) hematemesis   _____/_____

                              r   s

   b) *Bonus Question:* What is the definition of the suffix? _____

5. a) steatorrhea   _____/___/_____

                              cf   s

   b) *Bonus Question:* What is the definition of the combining form? _____

6. a) hepatomegaly   _____/___/_____

                              cf   s

   b) *Bonus Question:* What is the definition of the combining form? _____

Diseases and Disorders of the Digestive System

Here are the word parts that commonly apply to the diseases and disorders of the digestive system and are covered in the following section. Note that the word parts are color-coded to help you identify them: prefixes are yellow, combining forms are red, and suffixes are blue.

Prefix	Definition
an-	without, absence of
dys-	bad, abnormal, painful, difficult
mal-	bad

Combining Form	Definition
aden/o	gland
appendic/o	appendix
cheil/o	lip
chol/e	bile, gall
cholecyst/o	gallbladder
choledoch/o	common bile duct
cirrh/o	orange
col/o	colon
diverticul/o	diverticulum
duoden/o	twelve, duodenum
enter/o	small intestine
esophag/e, esophag/o	gullet, esophagus
gastr/o	stomach
gingiv/o	gums
gloss/o	tongue
hepat/o	liver
lith/o	stone
orex/o	appetite
pancreat/o	sweetbread, pancreas
parot/o	parotid gland
pept/o	digestion
peritone/o	to stretch over, peritoneum
polyp/o	small growth
proct/o	rectum or anus
rect/o	rectum
sial/o	saliva
volv/o	to roll

Suffix	Definition
-al	pertaining to
-ectasis	expansion, dilation
-ia	condition of
-iasis	condition of
-ic	pertaining to
-itis	inflammation
-malacia	softening
-megaly	abnormally large
-oid	resembling
-oma	tumor
-osis	condition of
-pathy	disease
-ptosis	drooping
-sis	state of
-y	process of

KEY TERMS A–Z

anorexia nervosa
AN or EKS ee ah * nerv
OH sah

appendicitis
ah pen dih SIGH tiss

10.24 An emotional eating disorder in which the patient avoids food because of a compulsion to become thin in appearance is known as **anorexia nervosa**. The medical term _____ _____ is a constructed term, an/orex/ia nervosa and literally means "nervous condition of absence of appetite." It results in extreme weight loss and nutritional deficiencies and can become fatal if left untreated.

10.25 Inflammation of the appendix is called _____. It is a constructed term, appendic/itis and is illustrated in ■ Figure 10.4. Appendicitis is considered a medical emergency because the appendix is in immediate risk of rupture, which can spread life-threatening infectious material throughout the abdominal cavity.

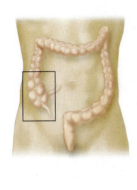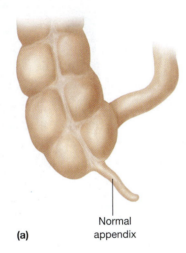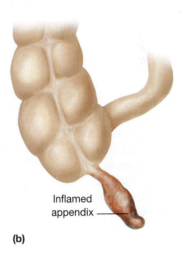

Normal appendix

Inflamed appendix

(a) (b)

■ Figure 10.4
Appendicitis. (a) A normal appendix. (b) An inflamed appendix in appendicitis.

bulimia
boo LEEM ee ah

10.26 A common eating disorder involving repeated gorging with food followed by induced vomiting or laxative abuse is known as **bulimia**. Commonly known as "bingeing and purging," the term _____ is derived from the Greek word that means "ravenous hunger," *boulimia*.

cheilitis
kye LYE tiss

10.27 Because the combining form for lip is *cheil/o*, inflammation of the lip is called _____, a constructed term written cheil/itis. Another term using this combining form is **cheilosis** (kye LOH siss). It is a general condition of the lip, which often includes splitting of the lips and corners of the mouth, usually resulting from vitamin B deficiency.

cholecystitis
koh lee siss TYE tiss

10.28 The combining form for gallbladder is *cholecyst/o*, which literally means "bladder of gall." Inflammation of the gallbladder is therefore called _____, which includes two word parts: cholecyst/itis. It is usually caused by stones lodged within the gallbladder, which are commonly called *gallstones* (shown in ■ Figure 10.5).

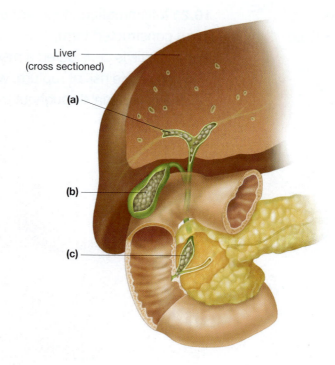

Liver
(cross sectioned)

(a)

(b)

(c)

■ **Figure 10.5**
Cholelithiasis. Common sites of gallstones in the generalized condition. (a) Stones in the hepatic duct. (b) Stones in the gallbladder. (c) Stones in the common bile duct (called *choledocholithiasis*).

choledochitis
KOH leh dok EYE tiss

choledoch/o/lith/iasis

10.29 The combining form for common bile duct, which is a tube that carries bile from the liver to the small intestine, is *choledoch/o*. Thus, inflammation of the common bile duct is called _____. Adding the combining form *lith/o* and the suffix *-iasis* to the word root to describe the presence of stones within the common bile duct forms the term **choledocholithiasis** (KOH leh doh koh lith EYE ah siss) (shown in Figure 10.5). This constructed term includes four word parts: _____/__/_____/___.

cholelithiasis
KOH lee lith EYE ah siss

10.30 A generalized condition of stones lodged within the gallbladder or bile ducts is called _____. It is illustrated in Figure 10.5. This constructed term includes four word parts, as shown when it is written chol/e/lith/iasis.

cirrhosis

ser ROH siss

10.31 A chronic, progressive liver disease characterized by the gradual loss of liver cells and their replacement by fat and other forms of connective tissue is known as **cirrhosis**. It is shown in ■ Figure 10.6. The constructed form of _____ is cirrh/osis. It literally means "condition of orange," referring to the common symptom of a yellowish-orange coloration of the skin (jaundice; Frame 10.20). Hepatitis B and C (Frame 10.52) are responsible for about 65% of cirrhosis cases. The remainder is mainly caused by chronic alcoholism, drug abuse, and obesity.

■ **Figure 10.6**
Cirrhosis. Cirrhosis is characterized by a chronic deterioration of the liver, in which healthy cells are replaced with connective tissue and fat that causes a mottled appearance. In this photograph, the liver was removed from a deceased patient in an advanced state of cirrhosis.

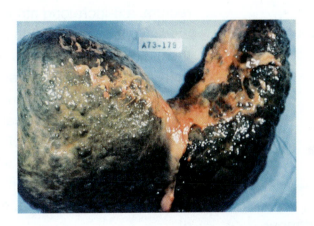

cleft palate

10.32 A **cleft palate** is a congenital defect in which the bones supporting the roof of the mouth, or hard palate, fail to fuse during fetal development, leaving a space between the oral cavity and nasal cavity (■ Figure 10.7). A _____ _____ is often accompanied by an opening in the upper lip, called a **cleft lip**.

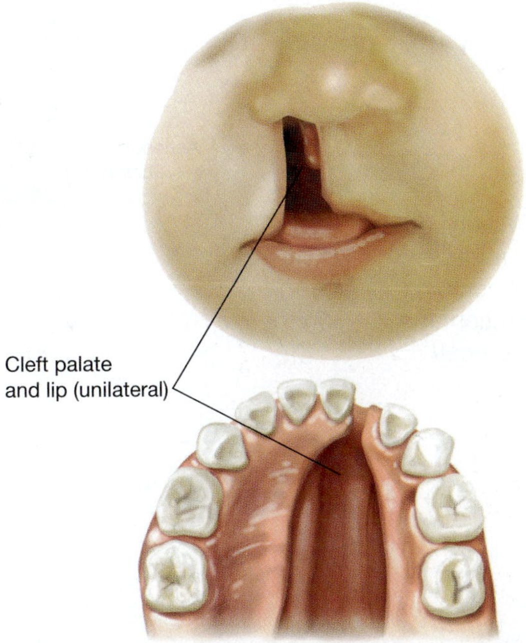

Cleft palate
and lip (unilateral)

■ **Figure 10.7**
Cleft palate. A congenital defect in which the bones of the palate (roof of the mouth) fail to fuse, leaving a space between the mouth and nasal cavity.

colitis koh LYE tiss	**10.33** Inflammation of the segment of the large intestine known as the colon is called _____. Colitis often includes excessive peristaltic contractions, mucus production, and cramping pain. If chronic bleeding of the colon wall occurs to form bloody diarrhea, the condition is called **ulcerative colitis** (UHL ser ah tiv * koh LYE tiss). Ulcerative colitis is a form of chronic inflammatory bowel disease, or IBD (Frame 10.55). *Colitis* is a constructed term, col/itis.
colon cancer KOH lun*KAN ser **colorectal cancer** kohl oh REK tal * KAN ser	**10.34** Most of the large intestine is made up of the colon, a muscular tube about 5 feet long. At its distal end, the colon becomes the rectum, a 6-inch-long straight tube that opens to the exterior at the anus. Cancer of the colon is simply called _____ _____. If the cancer occupies parts of the colon and rectum, it is known as **colorectal cancer**. *Colorectal* is a constructed term: col/o/rect/al. According to the American Cancer Society, colorectal cancer is the third most lethal form of cancer among men and women, with more than 50,000 deaths expected in 2017. Primary tumors often arise as a polyp (Frame 10.64), which is an abnormal mass of tissue that projects from the wall of the organ into the interior like a mushroom, to become an aggressive, malignant tumor. The most common sites of _____ _____ are illustrated in ■ Figure 10.8.

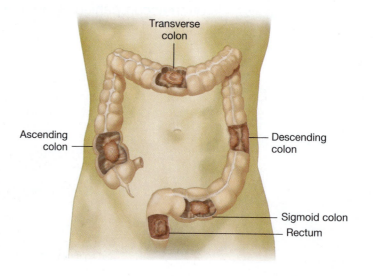

Transverse colon

Ascending colon

Descending colon

Sigmoid colon

Rectum

■ **Figure 10.8**
Cancer of the colon. When tumors are present in multiple areas of the colon and rectum, as shown in this illustration, the condition is called *colorectal cancer*.

10.35 A chronic inflammation of any part of the GI tract, most commonly the ileum of the small intestine, that involves ulcerations, scar tissue formation, and thickening adhesions of the organ wall, is called **Crohn's disease**. Also known as **regional ileitis** or **regional enteritis**, its cause is unknown and a cure is not yet available. _____ _____ is a form of chronic inflammatory bowel disease, or IBD (Frame 10.55).

Crohn's disease
KRONZ * dih ZEEZ

?　**Did You KNOW**

CROHN'S DISEASE

Dr. B. B. Crohn first described the disease that bears his name in 1932. At the time, he believed this chronic form of IBD was caused by a pathogen. Recent evidence suggests that he may have been partly correct, although the causative organism has not yet been identified. This new evidence suggests that genetic factors may play a role in its cause by reducing the body's immune response to certain bacteria or viruses, resulting in the chronic inflammation.

---

diverticulosis
DYE ver tik yoo LOH siss

diverticul/itis

10.36 In some individuals, small pouches called **diverticula** form on the wall of the colon (■ Figure 10.9). The presence of diverticula is often without symptoms or with mild bowel discomfort and is called _____. This constructed term is diverticul/osis. If the pouches become inflamed, it produces a more painful condition known as **diverticulitis** (DYE ver tik yoo LYE tiss), which increases the risk of developing colorectal cancer (Frame 10.34). The constructed form of this term is _____/_____.

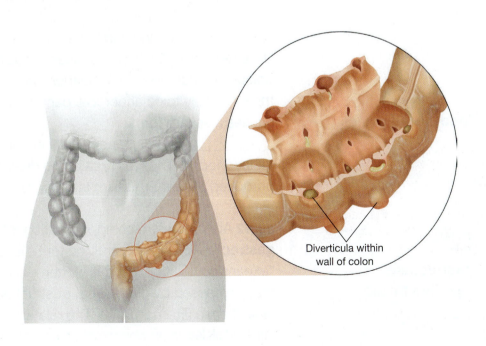

Diverticula within wall of colon

■ **Figure 10.9**
Diverticulosis. The presence of abnormal pouches in the wall of the large intestine (diverticula). If the pouches become inflamed to produce diverticulitis, the risk of developing colorectal cancer is elevated.

duodenal ulcer doo ODD eh nal * UL ser	**10.37** An ulcer, or erosion, in the wall of the duodenum of the small intestine is called a _____ _____. The constructed form of *duodenal* is duoden/al. Duodenal ulcer is further described in Frame 10.62.
[handwritten: developing country – diarrhea – bacteria] **dysentery** DIS en tair ee	**10.38** An acute inflammation of the GI tract that is caused by bacteria, protozoa, or chemical irritants is called **dysentery**. This constructed term includes three word parts, dys/enter/y and literally means "difficult intestine." _____ is characterized by severe diarrhea, often with a bloody discharge, and can become a life-threatening disease by causing dehydration.
[handwritten: or enthro • leading cause of death of infants in 3rd world countries] **enteritis** EHN ter EYE tiss	**10.39** The combining form for "intestine" is enter/o. Thus, inflammation of the small or large intestine is called _____, which can be written enter/itis to show the word parts.
esophagitis eh soff ah JYE tiss esophag/o/malacia	**10.40** Inflammation of the esophagus is called **esophagitis**. This constructed term is esophag/itis. It is often caused by acid reflux (Frame 10.22) from the stomach, which burns the esophageal lining to produce the inflammation. Chronic _____ may lead to either a morbid softening of the esophageal wall, called **esophagomalacia** (eh soff ah go mah LAY shee ah), or the development of **esophageal cancer**. The constructed form of *esophagomalacia* is written _____/__/_____.
food-borne illness	**10.41** Ingestion of food contaminated with harmful bacteria can cause symptoms of diarrhea and vomiting, even in otherwise healthy people, but in the very young, elderly, and immunosuppressed it can become life-threatening. Common causes of **food-borne illness**, or food poisoning, include *E. coli*, *Salmonella*, and *Staphylococci*. In addition, the extremely toxic anaerobic bacterium *Clostridium botulinum* causes a severe form of _____-_____ _____, especially in improperly prepared home-canned foods. The life-threatening disease caused by toxins produced by this organism is called **botulism** (BOTT choo lizm).
gastrectasis gas TREK tah siss	**10.42** Abnormal stretching, or dilation, of the stomach is called **gastrectasis**. This constructed term uses the suffix -ectasis (meaning "expansion, dilation") and is written gastr/ectasis. _____ may be caused by overeating, obstruction of the pyloric opening, or hiatal hernia (Frame 10.54). The related condition of **gastromegaly** (GAS troh MEG ah lee) is an abnormal enlargement of the stomach.

gastric cancer
GAS trik * KAN ser

10.43 Commonly known as **stomach cancer**, _____
_____ is an aggressive form of cancer arising from
cells lining the stomach (■ Figure 10.10). Risk of developing gastric
cancer increases with chronic infection of the stomach by the
bacterium *Helicobacter pylori*.

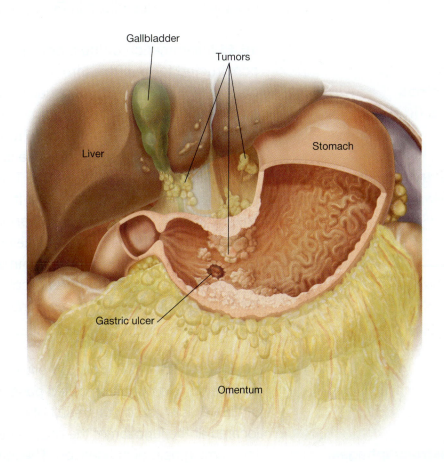

Gallbladder

Tumors

Liver

Stomach

Gastric ulcer

Omentum

■ **Figure 10.10**
Gastric cancer. In advanced
stages of gastric cancer,
malignant cells spread from their
origin in the stomach wall to
form tumors in the lymph nodes,
liver, omentum, pancreas, bile
ducts, and elsewhere.

gastric ulcer
GAS trik * UL ser

10.44 An ulcer, or erosion, in the wall of the stomach is commonly called a _____ _____. It is caused by an imbalance between the secretion of the protective mucous layer and the secretion of hydrochloric acid in the stomach, which is often the result of infection by the bacterium *Helicobacter pylori* (*H. pylori*) and elevates the risk of developing gastric cancer. Gastric ulcer is further described in Frame 10.62.

gastritis
gas TRY tiss

gastroenteritis
GAS troh en ter EYE tiss

gastr/o/enter/o/col/itis

10.45 Inflammation of the stomach is called **gastritis**. The constructed form of this term is written gastr/itis. The acute form of _____ is usually caused by an improper diet or an infection, and the chronic form may be caused by a chronic bacterial infection, peptic ulcers (Frame 10.62), or gastric cancer (Frame 10.43). If the small intestine is involved in the inflammation, it is called _____. This constructed term includes four word parts: gastr/o/enter/itis. If the first segment of the small intestine, the duodenum, is specifically involved, it is called **gastroduodenitis** (GAS troh doo oh den EYE tiss), shown with its word parts as gastr/o/duoden/itis. Inflammation of the stomach, small intestine, and colon all at once is called **gastroenterocolitis** (GAS troh EN ter oh koh LYE tiss). The constructed form of this term reveals six word parts: _____/__/_____/__/_____/_____.

gastroesophageal
GAS troh eh SOFF ah JEE al

10.46 A recurring backflow, or reflux, of stomach contents into the esophagus is a condition called **gastroesophageal reflux disease**, or **GERD**. It is usually the result of a weakened esophageal sphincter located at the junction of the esophagus and stomach and produces the burning pain of indigestion. The term _____ is constructed of word parts: gastr/o/esophag/e/al. In some cases, untreated GERD leads to **Barrett's esophagus**, in which the cells lining the esophagus undergo a change. This cellular change increases the risk of developing a rare form of cancer, known as **esophageal adenocarcinoma** (eh SOFF ah JEE al*AD eh noh kar sih NOH mah).

gastromalacia
GAS troh mah LAY shee ah

10.47 The suffix *-malacia* means "softening." The softening of the stomach wall may occur during advanced stages of stomach cancer and other chronic diseases of the stomach. It is called _____. The constructed form of this term is gastr/o/malacia.

giardiasis
jee ahr DYE ah siss

day care centers – contaminated H₂0

10.48 Infection by the intestinal protozoa *Giardia intestinalis* or *Giardia lamblia* produces symptoms of diarrhea, cramps, nausea, and vomiting (■ Figure 10.11). The disease is usually contracted by drinking contaminated water and is known as _____. The constructed form of this term is giardia/sis.

■ **Figure 10.11**
Giardiasis. Colorized electron micrograph of a *Giardia* protozoan on the surface of an epithelial cell lining the small intestine. The tiny red circles are microvilli, which number roughly 3,000 on a single intestinal cell. *Source: Courtesy of Dr. Stan Erlandsen, Public Health Image Library, Centers for Disease Control and Prevention, Atlanta, GA.*

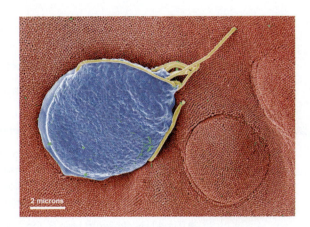

gingivitis
jin jih VYE tiss

10.49 Inflammation of the gums, or gingivae, is called _____. It is usually caused by chronic bacterial activity at the junction of the teeth and gums and normally follows the formation of dental plaque. The constructed form of this term is gingiv/itis.

glossitis
gloss EYE tiss

gloss/itis

10.50 A combining form for tongue, *gloss/o*, is derived from the Greek word *glossa*. Any disease of the tongue is called a **glossopathy** (gloss AH path ee). The constructed form is gloss/o/pathy. An example of a glossopathy is _____, which is an inflammation of the tongue often caused by exposure to allergens, toxic substances, or extreme heat or cold. The constructed form of glossitis is _____/_____.

hemorrhoids
HEM oh roydz

10.51 A varicose, or swollen, condition of the veins in the anus produces painful swellings that may break open and bleed, known as **hemorrhoids**. This term literally means "resembling leakage of blood." _____ are commonly called "piles."

hepatitis

10.52 A viral-induced inflammation of the liver is called _____. The constructed form of this term is hepat/itis. There are five known forms of hepatitis, which are categorized with the letters *A* through *E* and described in the Did You Know? box.

? Did You KNOW

HEPATITIS TYPES

There are five main categories of hepatitis, all caused by viruses:

- Type A (infectious hepatitis) is transmitted by the ingestion of contaminated food or water.

- Type B (serum hepatitis) is transmitted via body fluids, such as blood or semen. Because it can be transmitted during sexual exchange, it is considered to be an STI.

- Type C is mainly transmitted through the blood and often causes permanent liver damage. It is the most deadly of the five types; according to the Centers for Disease Control and Prevention (CDC), close to 20,000 deaths were caused by type C hepatitis in 2015, more than double all other types combined.

- Type D is similar to type B and may combine with it to severely damage the liver.

- Type E is similar to type A and is the most common form in countries that have contaminated water supplies.

In the United States, periodic testing for types B and C is recommended for healthcare professionals, and vaccination is available for type B and, hopefully soon, for type C.

malignant hepatoma

10.53 The suffix that means "tumor" is *-oma*. A tumor arising from cells within the liver is called a **malignant hepatoma** (hepp ah TOH mah). The constructed form of this term is hepat/oma. _____ _____ is also called **hepatocellular carcinoma**, or **HCC**. This form of liver cancer accounts for about 85% of the cases and is often associated with alcoholic cirrhosis or hepatitis B.

hiatal hernia

HER nee ah

10.54 A hernia is an abnormal protrusion through a body wall. Protrusion of the cardiac portion of the stomach through the hiatus of the diaphragm to enter the thoracic cavity is called a **hiatal hernia**. _____ _____ causes the symptom of heartburn that results from the movement of stomach acids into the esophagus and is illustrated in ■ Figure 10.12. Another type of digestive system hernia, called **inguinal hernia**, is a protrusion of a small intestinal segment through the abdominal wall in the inguinal region. A **direct inguinal hernia** occurs in males and is a protrusion into the scrotal cavity. Also, an **umbilical hernia** occurs when a small intestinal segment enters through a tear in the membrane covering the abdominal wall at the umbilical (navel) region. In each of these cases, the hernia may become strangulated, which restricts blood flow to the protruding organ. A **strangulated hernia** requires medical intervention to avoid loss of the affected organ.

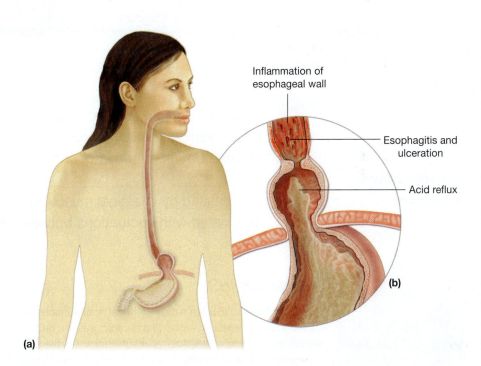

■ **Figure 10.12**
Hiatal hernia. (a) The hernia occurs when the stomach protrudes through the diaphragm and into the thoracic cavity, often leading to the movement of stomach fluids into the esophagus that creates esophageal reflux and esophagitis. (b) A close-up of a hiatal hernia.

Inflammation of esophageal wall

Esophagitis and ulceration

Acid reflux

(a)

(b)

inflammatory bowel disease

10.55 You have learned from Frames 10.33 and 10.35 that _____ _____ _____, or **IBD**, is a general term that includes the conditions ulcerative colitis and Crohn's disease. IBD is a syndrome affecting different patients in different ways. It includes a wide spectrum of conditions and symptoms that range from chronic diarrhea and enteritis to ulcerative colitis and Crohn's disease.

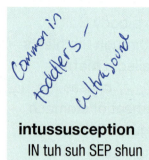

(handwritten: Common in toddlers / ultrasound)

intussusception

IN tuh suh SEP shun

10.56 Although the small intestine is anchored to the abdominal wall by the peritoneal membranes, it is subject to infolding. Infolding of a segment of the small intestine within another segment is a condition called **intussusception** and results in a reduction of intestinal motility. It is illustrated in ■ Figure 10.13. The term _____ is a combination of Latin words that collectively mean "to take within."

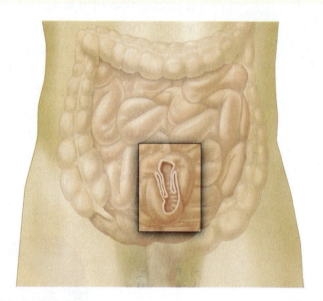

■ **Figure 10.13**
Intussusception. The condition is caused by an infolding of the small intestine, which often causes a reduction of intestinal motility.

irritable bowel syndrome

10.57 A chronic disease characterized by periodic disturbances of large intestinal (bowel) function without clear physical damage is called **irritable bowel syndrome**, or **IBS**. Episodes of _____ _____ _____ include abdominal pain caused by intestinal muscle spasms and flatus and are often associated with fluctuations between diarrhea and constipation.

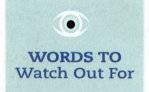

WORDS TO Watch Out For

IBD versus *IBS*

Because IBD and IBS are nearly identical abbreviations, they are often confused. IBD, which means "inflammatory bowel disease," is a chronic, severe, debilitating condition that injures the large intestine with ulcers, bleeding, and adhesions. On the softer side, IBS, which means "irritable bowel syndrome," is an uncomfortable chronic condition of irregular bowel movements that does not cause lasting tissue damage. It is marked with bouts of diarrhea, constipation, or an alternation of the two.

(handwritten: Can't absorb milk sugar — lack enzyme genetic)

lactose intolerance

LAHK tos * in TOHL er ans

10.58 All infants and many adults produce an enzyme in the small intestine that breaks down lactose, the primary sugar in milk and milk products. A lack of this enzyme results in the uncomfortable symptoms of flatus and diarrhea when dairy foods are consumed. This condition is called _____ and is abbreviated **LI**.

(handwritten: Allergy to milk is different)

malabsorption syndrome
MAL ab sorp shun * SIN drom

celiac disease
SEE lee ak

pertaining to the abdomen

10.59 The prefix *mal-* means "bad." A disorder that is characterized by difficulty absorbing one or more nutrients is called **malabsorption syndrome**. It can have severe consequences, depending on the nutrients that cannot be absorbed. An example of _____ _____ is found in people who react to ingested gluten, a plant protein found in wheat, barley, and rye. Known as **celiac disease** and, more recently, **gluten sensitivity enteropathy**, the arrival of gluten into the body triggers an immune response resulting in damage to the villi lining the small intestine, causing a failure to absorb nutrients (malabsorption) (■ Figure 10.14). Although its symptoms vary, a person suffering from _____ _____ often suffers weight loss, anemia, frequent bouts of bloody diarrhea and vomiting, cramping pain, osteoporosis, and bone and joint pain. When it strikes young children, the malabsorption may also delay growth rate and the onset of puberty. The term *celiac* means "pertaining to the abdomen" and *enteropathy* means "disease of the intestine."

■ **Figure 10.14**
Celiac disease is a form of malabsorption syndrome. The condition results from an immune reaction to glutens, which are proteins present in wheat, barley, and rye. The injury caused by the immune reaction is the destruction of villi lining the small intestine, thereby reducing the ability of the small intestine to absorb nutrients. *Source: Roberto Biasini/123RF .com.*

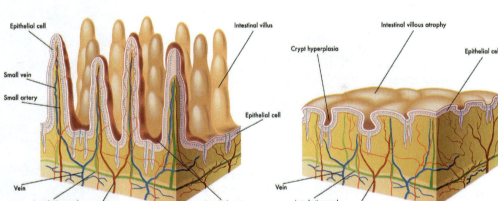

NORMAL — Epithelial cell, Small vein, Small artery, Vein, Lymphatic vessel, Arteria, Intestinal villus, Epithelial cell, Intestinal crypt

CELIAC DISEASE — Crypt hyperplasia, Intestinal villous atrophy, Epithelial cell, Vein, Lymphatic vessel, Arteria

pancreatitis
PAN kree ah TYE tiss

—alcoholism
—common bile duct obstruction

10.60 Inflammation of the pancreas is called _____. The constructed form of this term is pancreat/itis. Possible causes include tumor development and bacterial infection. If pancreatic functions are affected, the complications of **acute pancreatitis** can become life-threatening.

parotitis
pahr oh TYE tiss

parotid gland is salivary gland

10.61 The largest salivary glands are called *parotid glands* and are located around the angle of the jaw. Inflammation of one or both parotid glands is called _____. If caused by a virus, it is usually referred to as **mumps**. The term *parotitis* is a constructed term: parot/itis. It may also be referred to as **sialadenitis** (sigh AL add eh NYE tiss). The constructed form of this term reveals three word parts, sial/aden/itis, and literally means "inflammation of saliva gland."

peptic ulcer
PEPP tik * UL ser

10.62 The term **peptic** is a constructed term, pept/ic, which means "pertaining to digestion." An erosion into the inner wall of an organ along the GI tract is generally called a _____ _____. Usually, a peptic ulcer occurs in the wall of the stomach as a gastric ulcer (Frame 10.44) or in the wall of the duodenum as a duodenal ulcer (Frame 10.37). Both forms of peptic ulcer are shown in ■ Figure 10.15. The ulcer is formed when the protective mucus layer becomes eroded, exposing the inner lining to the caustic effects of hydrochloric acid. Roughly 80% of peptic ulcers are associated with an infection of *Helicobacter pylori (H. pylori)*, which triggers an immune response that reduces mucus production and increases the risk of developing gastric cancer. In severe cases, the erosion may penetrate through the wall of the organ to form a **perforated ulcer**, which is a life-threatening crisis due to hemorrhage and infection.

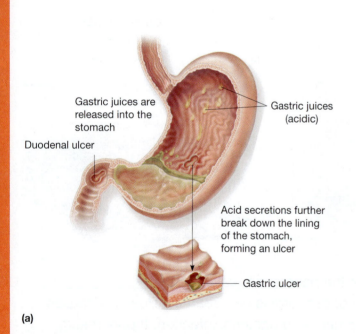

Gastric juices are released into the stomach

Gastric juices (acidic)

Duodenal ulcer

Acid secretions further break down the lining of the stomach, forming an ulcer

Gastric ulcer

(a)

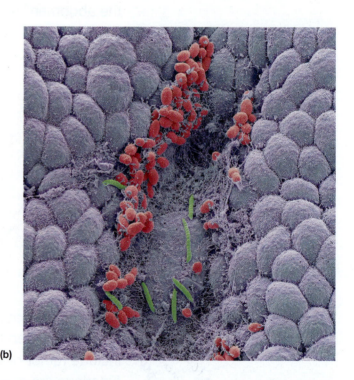

(b)

■ **Figure 10.15**
Peptic ulcer. (a) A peptic ulcer may occur in the stomach (gastric ulcer) or in the duodenum (duodenal ulcer). The most common cause is associated with infection by *H. pylori*. (b) The photograph of a gastric ulcer has been taken through the lens of a scanning electron microscope at 40,000 magnification and given color by a computer. The blue polygons are cells of the stomach lining. In the center is a cavity, which is an early gastric ulcer beginning to form. The ulcer has been caused by a reduction of protective mucus as a result of infection by the bacteria, *H. pylori*, which are the green rods. Also present are yeast cells, colored red, which sometimes accompany the *H. pylori*.
Photo Source: Steve Gschmeissner/Science Source.

peritonitis
  pair ih toh NYE tiss

10.63 The peritoneum is the extensive membrane that lines the inner wall of the abdominopelvic cavity and covers most of its organs. Inflammation of this membrane is called _____. This constructed term includes two word parts: periton/itis (the *e* on the end of the word root is dropped in this case). The inflammation is the body's response to an infection of the peritoneum, usually bacterial, that can become life-threatening without medical intervention.

polyposis
  pall ee POH siss

10.64 Any abnormal mass of tissue that projects inward from the wall of a hollow organ is called a **polyp** (PALL ip). The term means "small growth." It is usually a benign growth that may occur in the nose, throat, or large intestine. The presence of many polyps is called _____ and is illustrated in ■ Figure 10.16. The constructed form of this term is polyp/osis, which literally means "condition of small growths." Polyposis usually occurs in the colon or rectum of the large intestine, where it increases the risk for colorectal cancer (Frame 10.34).

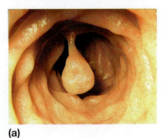

(a)

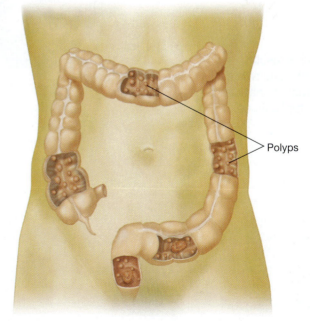

Polyps

(b)

■ **Figure 10.16**
Polyps and polyposis. A polyp is a protruding growth from a mucous membrane lining a hollow organ. (a) Photograph during a colonoscopy of a polyp in the wall of the colon. (b) In the disease polyposis, multiple polyps develop, usually along the inner wall of the large intestine.
Photo Source: Juan Gaertner/ Shutterstock.

proctitis
prok TYE tiss

10.65 A combining form meaning "rectum" or "anus" is *proct/o*. Inflammation of the anus, and usually the rectum as well, is called _____. The constructed form of this term is proct/itis.

proctoptosis
PROK top TOH siss

10.66 Recall that the suffix *-ptosis* means "drooping." A drooping, or prolapse, of the rectum is a condition called _____. The constructed form of this term is proct/o/ptosis.

volvulus
VOLL vyoo lus

10.67 A severe twisting of the intestine that leads to obstruction is called **volvulus**. The term is derived from the Latin word that means "to roll." A _____ that has caused a severe obstruction is illustrated in ■ Figure 10.17.

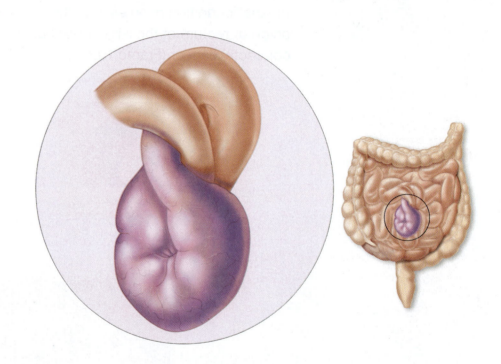

■ **Figure 10.17**
Volvulus. A volvulus results when the small intestine twists, causing an obstruction that can lead to severe complications.

PRACTICE: Diseases and Disorders of the Digestive System

The Right Match

Match the term on the left with the correct definition on the right.

_____ 1. gastrectasis

_____ 2. polyp

_____ 3. gingivitis

_____ 4. giardiasis

_____ 5. bulimia

_____ 6. duodenal ulcer

_____ 7. volvulus

_____ 8. intussusception

_____ 9. cirrhosis

_____ 10. Crohn's disease

_____ 11. irritable bowel syndrome

_____ 12. hernia

_____ 13. gastroenterocolitis

_____ 14. cheilitis

_____ 15. choledocholithiasis

_____ 16. colitis

_____ 17. diverticulitis

_____ 18. gastroesophageal reflux disease

a. infolding of a segment of the small intestine within another segment

b. a chronic inflammation of any part of the GI tract, usually of the ileum

c. intestinal infection by the protozoa *Giardia intestinalis* or *Giardia lamblia*

d. inflammation of abnormal pouches in the colon

e. twisting of the intestine causing an obstruction

f. an abnormal protrusion through a body wall

g. characterized by periodic bowel disturbances

h. a chronic liver disease

i. abnormal stretching of the stomach

j. an abnormal mass projecting inward

k. an eating disorder of bingeing and purging

l. an erosion in the wall of the duodenum of the small intestine

m. inflammation of the colon

n. inflammation of the gums

o. inflammation of the stomach and intestines

p. presence of stones in the common bile duct

q. recurring backflow of stomach contents into the esophagus

r. inflammation of the lips

Linkup

Link the word parts in the list to create the terms that match the definitions. You may use word parts more than once. Remember to add combining vowels when needed and that some terms do not use any combining vowel. The first one is completed as an example.

Prefix	Combining Form	Suffix
an-	appendic/o	-ia
dys-	chol/e	-iasis
	enter/o	-itis
	esophag/e, esophag/o	-malacia
	gastr/o	-oma
	gloss/o	-osis
	hepat/o	-ptosis
	lith/o	-y
	orex/o	
	pancreat/o	
	polyp/o	
	proct/o	

Definition

1. inflammation of the appendix
2. inflammation of the tongue
3. condition of stones lodged within the gallbladder or bile ducts
4. condition of prolapse of the rectum
5. tumor within the liver
6. softening of the stomach wall
7. inflammation of the esophagus
8. inflammation of the stomach and small intestine
9. inflammation of the pancreas
10. acute inflammation of the GI tract caused by bacteria, protozoa, or chemical irritants
11. eating disorder in which the patient restricts food intake because of a compulsion to become thin
12. condition of many polyps

Term

appendicitis
_____
_____
_____
_____
_____
_____
_____
_____
_____

_____

_____

Treatments, Procedures, and Devices of the Digestive System

Here are the word parts that commonly apply to the treatments, procedures, and devices of the digestive system and are covered in the following section. Note that the word parts are color-coded to help you identify them: prefixes are yellow, combining forms are red, and suffixes are blue.

Prefix	Definition
anti-	against, opposite of
dia-	through
endo-	within

N&V = Nausea Evomiting

Combining Form	Definition
abdomin/o	abdomen
acid/o	a solution or substance with a pH less than 7
append/o	appendix
cheil/o	lip
cholecyst/o	gallbladder
choledoch/o	common bile duct
col/o	colon
colon/o	colon
duoden/o	twelve, duodenum
esophag/e, esophag/o	gullet, esophagus
fec/o	feces
gastr/o	stomach
gingiv/o	gums
gloss/o	tongue
ile/o	to roll, ileum
lapar/o	abdomen
lith/o	stone
nas/o	nose
polyp/o	small growth
pylor/o	pylorus
vag/o	vagus nerve

Suffix	Definition
-al	pertaining to
-centesis	surgical puncture
-ectomy	surgical excision, removal
-emetic	pertaining to vomiting
gram	a record or image
-graphy	recording process
-ic	pertaining to
-plasty	surgical repair
-rrhaphy	suturing
-rrhea	discharge
-scopy	process of viewing
-spasmodic	pertaining to a sudden, involuntary muscle contraction
-stomy	surgical creation of an opening
-tomy	incision, to cut

KEY TERMS A–Z

also called
paracentisis

abdominocentesis
ab DOM ih noh sehn TEE siss

10.68 Because the suffix *-centesis* means "surgical puncture," a surgical puncture through the abdominal wall to remove fluid is a procedure called _____. The constructed form of this term is abdomin/o/centesis. An alternate term for this procedure is **paracentesis** (pair ah sehn TEE siss).

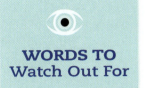

WORDS TO Watch Out For

abdomen and *abdomin/o*

The combining form meaning "abdomen" is *abdomin/o*, which is found in terms such as abdominocentesis. Notice that the combining form uses a letter *i* and not an *e*, as in *abdomen*.

---

antacid
ant ASS id

10.69 An agent that reduces the acidity of the stomach cavity is called an **antacid**. Note that the letter *i* is deleted from the prefix *anti-* because the combining form begins with a vowel, which makes _____ easier to pronounce. Most mild medications neutralize the acid pH of the stomach, whereas stronger medications inhibit the amount of acid produced and are called **proton pump inhibitors**. *Antacid* is a constructed term, ant/acid.

antiemetic
an tye ee MEH tik

10.70 An **antiemetic** is a drug that prevents or stops the vomiting reflex. The constructed form of this term is anti/emetic. _____ literally means "pertaining to against vomiting."

antispasmodic
an tye spaz MOH dik

10.71 A drug that reduces peristalsis activity in the GI tract, which arrests the muscular spasms involved in diarrhea, is called an **antispasmodic**. The constructed form of _____ is anti/spasmodic. An **antidiarrheal** (an tye dye ah REE al) may also be used to treat the symptoms of diarrhea (Frame 10.12), but usually by increasing water absorption in the colon while decreasing spasms.

appendectomy
app ehn DEK toh mee

10.72 The surgical removal of the appendix is called _____ because the suffix *-ectomy* means "surgical excision, removal." An **appendectomy** is performed to treat the acute condition of appendicitis (Frame 10.25).

bariatric surgery
behr ee AT rik

10.73 One of the most common surgeries of the GI tract is known as **bariatric surgery**. It is a procedure for treating obesity, in which the body contains an abnormally high amount of fat that threatens the health of the patient. The term *bariatric* means "treatment of weight." Some forms of _____ _____ reduce the volume of the stomach, whereas others bypass the stomach completely (■ Figure 10.18).

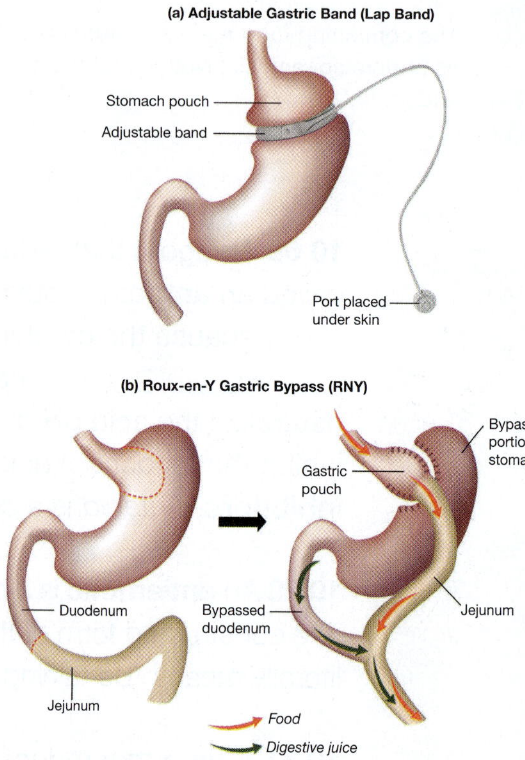

(a) Adjustable Gastric Band (Lap Band)

Stomach pouch
Adjustable band
Port placed under skin

(b) Roux-en-Y Gastric Bypass (RNY)

Bypassed portion of stomach
Gastric pouch
Duodenum
Bypassed duodenum
Jejunum
Jejunum
Food
Digestive juice

■ **Figure 10.18**
Bariatric surgery. The two most popular forms are shown, both of which are treatments for obesity. (a) Adjustable gastric band, which is reversible, and (b) Roux-en-Y gastric bypass, which is not reversible.
Source: Alila Medical Media/ Shutterstock.

cathartic
kah THAHR tik

strong medicine for constipation

10.74 An agent that stimulates strong waves of peristalsis of the colon is called a **cathartic**. Derived from the Greek word *kathartikos*, which means "purging, cleansing," a _____ is used to treat the symptom of constipation. An agent that causes mild waves of peristalsis is called a **laxative**.

cheilorrhaphy
kye LOR ah fee

suture lip(s)

10.75 Because the combining form of lip is *cheil/o* and the suffix *-rrhaphy* means "suturing," the procedure of suturing a lip is called _____. The constructed form of this term is *cheil/o/rrhaphy*.

cholecystectomy
KOH lee siss TEK toh mee

remove gallbladder

10.76 The word root for gallbladder is *cholecyst*, which literally means "bladder of gall." The surgical removal of the gallbladder is called _____. The constructed form of this term is *cholecyst/ectomy*.

?

Did You KNOW

CHOLECYSTECTOMY

Because of the prevalence of cholecystitis, cholecystectomy is the most common surgery of the abdomen performed in the United States, numbering about 500,000 each year. To reduce the invasiveness of the procedure, laparoscopic surgery using a specialized endoscope is increasing in popularity, replacing the more traditional form of "open" cholecystectomy.

---

cholecystogram
KOH lee SISS toh gram

die that shows on xray

10.77 The process of producing an x-ray image of the gallbladder is known as **cholecystography** (KOH lee siss TOG rah fee). The constructed form of this term is cholecyst/o/graphy. The x-ray image of the gallbladder is called a _____.

---

choledocholithotomy
koh lee doh koh lih THOTT oh mee

removal of stones from common bile duct

10.78 The combining form for the common bile duct is *choledoch/o*, and the combining form for stone is *lith/o*. The surgery that involves the removal of one or more obstructive gallstones from the common bile duct is called _____. This constructed term has five word parts: choledoch/o/lith/o/tomy.

---

colonoscopy
kohl on OSS koh pee

10.79 A **colonoscopy** is the visual inspection of the colon's interior (■ Figure 10.19). Because a specialized endoscope is used and the flexible end is inserted into the GI tract, a colonoscopy is a type of GI endoscopy (Frame 10.86). A _____ is routinely used as a preventative procedure in an effort to detect early signs of colorectal cancer (Frame 10.34) or to diagnose the presence of polyps (Frame 10.64), diverticulosis (Frame 10.36), or other forms of disease of the large intestine. The constructed form of this term is colon/o/scopy, which means "process of viewing the colon."

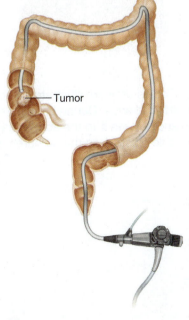

Tumor

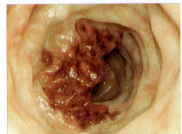

■ **Figure 10.19**
Colonoscopy. (a) Illustration of the colonoscopy procedure using a flexible colonoscope. (b) Photograph taken during a colonoscopy, during which a tumor is observable in the wall of the colon.
Photo Source: Juan Gaertner/ Shutterstock.

(a)   (b)

total colectomy

10.80 Surgical removal of the entire length of the colon is called a **total colectomy** (koh LEK toh mee). _____ _____ is commonly referred to as a **bowel resection**. If a part of the colon is removed, it is known as a **partial colectomy**, and if only the right or left segment is removed, it is called a **hemicolectomy** (*hemi-* means "half"). The constructed form of this term is hemi/col/ectomy.

colostomy

koh LAH stom ee

10.81 The suffix *-stomy* means "surgical creation of an opening." When this procedure is performed on the colon, it is called a _____. The artificial opening that is created serves as an artificial anus, usually following the excision of the distal part of the colon. The new opening is referred to as a **stoma** (STOE mah). A patient with a colostomy is taught how to manage the new opening through their GI tract, which involves the attachment of a disposable plastic bag that is secured to the skin around the stoma by a ring of adhesive wax. Once the bag fills about half way, the ring and bag are removed and discarded and the skin cleaned before a fresh bag and ring are attached. Variations of colostomy are illustrated in ■ Figure 10.20. **Colostomy** is a constructed term: col/o/stomy.

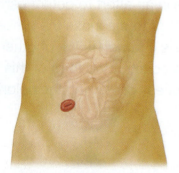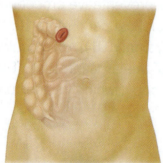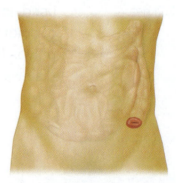

■ **Figure 10.20**
Colostomy. Alternate versions of colostomy are illustrated, each of which creates one or more new openings that serve as an artificial anus. During creation of the opening, or stoma, the surgeon rolls back the mucosa and sutures it to the abdominal wall. Waste material exiting the stoma is collected into a disposable plastic bag that adheres to the skin, and the filled bag is discarded and replaced.

fecal occult blood test
FEE kal * uh KULT

checks for blood in color - cancer

10.82 A clinical lab test performed to detect blood in the feces is called a **fecal occult blood test**, abbreviated **FOBT**. The word *occult* means "hidden, concealed," indicating that the presence of blood is often hidden in the feces and requires a lab procedure to identify it. A positive _____ _____ _____ _____ may indicate Crohn's disease (Frame 10.35), polyposis (Frame 10.64), or colorectal cancer (Frame 10.34) if hemorrhoids have been ruled out. **Fecal** is a constructed term: fec/al.

gastrectomy
gas TREK toh mee

10.83 Surgical removal of part of the stomach or, in extreme cases, the entire organ, is called _____. The constructed form of this term is gastr/ectomy. A part of the stomach may be removed to treat peptic ulcers (Frame 10.62) or severe obesity. The entire organ may be removed as a method to treat gastric cancer (Frame 10.43).

gastric lavage
GAS trik * lah VAHZH

washing of stomach (for bleeding) - used tube for poison

10.84 A cleansing procedure in which the stomach is irrigated with a prescribed solution is known as **gastric lavage**. A _____ _____ is performed after ingestion of a toxic substance or drug overdose or to remove irritants before or after surgery. A similar irrigation procedure may be performed on the colon to remove unwanted substances and is called **colonic irrigation**. If the unwanted material is a fecal blockage in the colon or rectum, an **enema** (EN eh mah) is used instead.

gavage
gah VAHZH

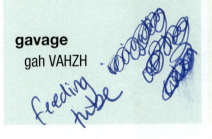

feeding tube

10.85 The process of feeding a patient through a tube inserted into the nose that extends through the esophagus to enter the stomach is called **gavage**. The term _____ is derived from the French word *gaver*, which means "to force-feed." The tube used in this procedure is called a **nasogastric tube**. The term *nasogastric* is constructed of four word parts and is written nas/o/gastr/ic.

GI endoscopy
en DAH sko pee

colonoscopy
kohl on OSS koh pee

10.86 Visual examination of the interior of the GI tract organs is made possible by the use of endoscopes in the procedure known as _____ _____, an example of which is shown in ■ Figure 10.21. The endoscope is a long, flexible tube with fiber optics, a camera, and surgical tools at one end and an eyepiece tube that can be connected to a viewing monitor at the other end. The endoscope may undergo modifications for insertion into each organ of the GI tract. Procedures using modified endoscopes to examine upper GI tract organs enter through the mouth and include **esophagoscopy** (eh SOFF ah GOSS koh pee), which examines the esophagus, **gastroscopy** (gas TROSS koh pee), which views the stomach, and **esophagogastroduodenoscopy** (eh SOFF ah goh GAS troh DOO oh dehn OSS koh pee) (**EGD**), which examines the esophagus, stomach, and duodenum. Endoscopic procedures using an endoscope that enters through the anus to examine the lower GI tract include _____, which views the colon, **sigmoidoscopy** (SIG moyd OSS koh pee), which examines the sigmoid colon, and **proctoscopy** (prok TOSS koh pee), which observes the rectum. Notice that all of these are constructed terms that are formed by adding the combining form of the organ (or organs) to the suffix *-scopy*, which means "process of viewing." For example, the constructed form of esophagogastroduodenoscopy is esophag/o/gastr/o/duoden/o/scopy.

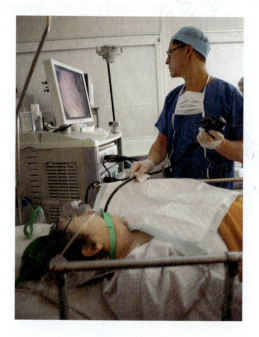

■ **Figure 10.21**
GI endoscopy. The visual examination of the interior of the GI tract. Shown here is a photograph of a gastroscopy procedure, in which the surgeon is viewing a monitor while adjusting the gastroscope with his left hand and moving the flexible tube with his right hand through the patient's mouth until it reaches the stomach cavity.
Source: A. Benoist/BSIP SA/ Alamy Stock Photo.

GI series

10.87 A **GI series** is a common term applied to several diagnostic techniques that provide radiographic examination of the GI tract. In most cases, the radiographic substance barium sulfate is administered to highlight the GI tract organ or organs within a series of x-ray photographs. The x-rays expose abnormalities in the organs, such as ulcers or tumors. In an **upper _____ _____ (UGI)**, a **barium swallow**, **barium shake**, or **barium meal** is ingested to enhance x-ray images of the esophagus, stomach, and duodenum (■ Figure 10.22a). An enema is the introduction of a substance into the rectum and colon to prepare for an evaluation, to evacuate the bowel, to administer drugs, or to introduce nutrients. A **barium enema (BE)** is the administration of barium sulfate into the rectum and colon for a **lower GI series (LGI)** of x-rays (■ Figure 10.22b).

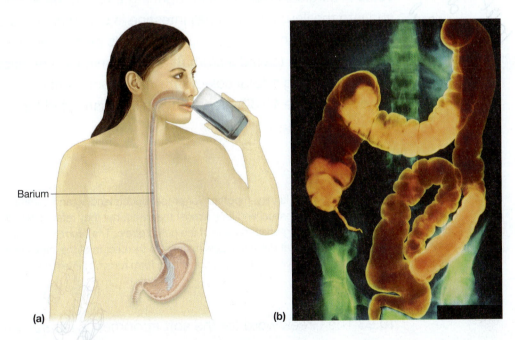

Barium

(a)   (b)

■ **Figure 10.22**
GI series. (a) Upper GI series begins with a barium swallow, barium shake, or barium meal. (b) Lower GI series begins with administration of a barium enema to provide the x-ray of the large intestine shown here.
Photo Source: CNRI/Science Source.

gingivectomy
JIN jih VEK toh mee

10.88 Surgical removal of diseased tissue in the gums, or gingivae, is called _____. The constructed form of this term is gingiv/ectomy.

glossorrhaphy
gloss OR ah fee

10.89 An injury that involves a severe bite through the tongue often requires surgery to close the wound with sutures. This surgery is called _____, which is a constructed term with three word parts: gloss/o/rrhaphy.

hemorrhoidectomy
HEM oh royd EK toh mee

10.90 Surgical removal of hemorrhoids is performed during a _____. The constructed form of this term is hemorrhoid/ectomy.

herniorrhaphy
her nee OR ah fee

10.91 Recall that the suffix -rrhaphy means "suturing." The term **herniorrhaphy** therefore means "suturing a hernia" and is a corrective response to any one of the various types of hernias described in Frame 10.54. Thus, a _____ is a common surgical procedure to repair an abnormal protrusion through a body wall.

ileostomy
ILL ee OSS toh mee

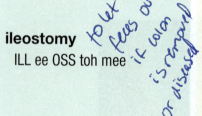
to let feces out if colon is removed or diseased

10.92 A surgical creation of an opening through the abdominal wall and into the ileum of the small intestine is called an **ileostomy** (see Figure 10.20). An _____ is performed to establish an alternative anus (called a *stoma*) for the elimination of waste material, usually following a total colectomy in which the entire colon is removed (Frame 10.80). **Ileostomy** is a constructed term: ile/o/stomy.

WORDS TO Watch Out For

Ilium and *Ileum*

Spelling medical terms correctly is very important for proper understanding and communication. Two terms, *ilium* and *ileum*, sound identical and look almost the same, but they refer to two different body parts. The *ilium* is the upper, wing-shaped bone of the pelvic girdle. The *ileum* is the third and final segment of the small intestine that delivers waste material to the cecum of the large intestine. You might remember that *ileum* has an *e* if you think of the combining form for small intestine: *enter/o*, with an *e*.

laparotomy
lap ah ROTT oh mee

laparoscopy
lap ah ROSS koh pee

10.93 The Greek word for the soft abdomen is *lapara*, which serves as the origin for a combining form for abdomen, *lapar/o*. The surgical procedure that involves an incision through the abdominal wall, often from the base of the sternum to the pubic bone, is called a _____. The constructed form of this term is lapar/o/tomy. In some cases, a **laparoscopy** may be performed instead, during which a modified endoscope equipped with a camera and surgical instruments, called a **laparoscope**, is inserted through the abdominal wall via one or more small incisions (■ Figure 10.23). The _____ has an advantage over a laparotomy because it is minimally invasive, thereby posing less risk of infection to the patient.

■ **Figure 10.23**
Laparoscopy. (a) Laparoscopy is an abdominal surgery using a specialized endoscope, called a *laparoscope*, inserted through the wall of the abdomen via a small incision. (b) In this photograph of laparoscopic surgery, several laparoscopes are used simultaneously: one with a camera and two with surgical instruments attached.
Photo Source: Samrith Na Lumpoon/Shutterstock.

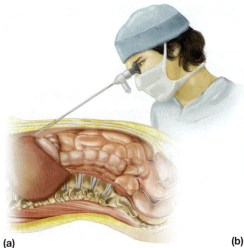

(a)

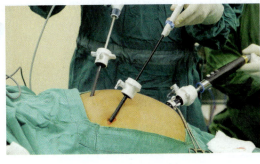

(b)

polypectomy
pall ih PEK toh mee

10.94 Because polyps (Frame 10.64) represent benign tumors that can become inflamed and change form to become malignant, surgical removal is sometimes necessary. The surgical removal of polyps is known as _____ and is usually performed during a colonoscopy (Frame 10.86). The constructed form of this term is polyp/ectomy.

pyloroplasty
pye LOR oh plass tee

babies vomiting milk at 2 weeks

10.95 Surgical repair of the pylorus region of the stomach, which may include repair of the pyloric valve, is known as a _____. The constructed form of this term is pylor/o/plasty.

stool culture and sensitivity

10.96 If a pathogen is a suspected cause of a disease that affects the GI tract, a test may be performed called a **stool culture and sensitivity**. Abbreviated **C&S**, a _____ _____ _____ _____ includes obtaining stool (fecal) samples, using the samples to grow microorganisms in culture, and identifying the microorganisms to determine which antibiotics will effectively kill the pathogens.

vagotomy
vay GOTT oh mee

10.97 The vagus nerve is a cranial nerve that innervates much of the GI tract, providing sensory information to the brain relating to digestion and stimulating peristalsis of GI tract organs. The surgical dissection of branches of the vagus nerve may be performed in an effort to reduce gastric juice secretion as a treatment for chronic gastric ulcers (Frame 10.44). This procedure is called _____. The constructed form of this term is vag/o/tomy.

PRACTICE: Treatments, Procedures, and Devices of the Digestive System

The Right Match

Match the term on the left with the correct definition on the right.

_____ 1. colonoscopy

_____ 2. abdominocentesis

_____ 3. antacid

_____ 4. gastric lavage

_____ 5. cholecystography

_____ 6. cheilorrhaphy

_____ 7. ileostomy

_____ 8. stool culture and sensitivity

_____ 9. upper GI series

_____ 10. gavage

a. test that uses a stool sample to grow and identify microorganisms in a culture

b. process of feeding a patient through a tube inserted into the nose that descends into the stomach

c. also known as paracentesis

d. procedure of suturing a lip

e. procedure of producing an x-ray image of the gallbladder

f. endoscopy of the colon

g. cleansing procedure in which the stomach is irrigated with a prescribed solution

h. an agent that neutralizes stomach acid

i. surgical creation of an opening through the abdominal wall and into the ileum of the small intestine

j. a barium substance ingested to enhance x-ray images of the esophagus, stomach, and duodenum

Break the Chain

Analyze these medical terms:

    a) Separate each term into its word parts; each word part is labeled for you (**p** = prefix, **r** = root, **cf** = combining form, and **s** = suffix).

    b) For the Bonus Question, write the requested definition in the blank that follows.

1. a) antiemetic   _____ / _____
                                        p   s

    b) *Bonus Question:* What is the definition of the suffix? _____

2. a) glossorrhaphy   _____ / __ / _____
                                           cf   s

    b) *Bonus Question:* What is the definition of the combining form? _____

3. a) sigmoidoscopy   _____ / __ / _____
                                           cf   s

    b) *Bonus Question:* What is the definition of the combining form? _____

4. a) hemorrhoidectomy   _____ / _____
                                       (noun)   s

    b) *Bonus Question:* What is the definition of the suffix? _____

5. a) laparotomy   _____ / __ / _____
                                           cf   s

    b) *Bonus Question:* What is the definition of the combining form? _____

6. a) pyloroplasty   _____ / __ / _____
                                           cf   s

    b) *Bonus Question:* What is the definition of the suffix? _____

7. a) antispasmodic   _____ / _____
                                        p   s

    b) *Bonus Question:* What is the definition of the prefix? _____

8. a) gingivectomy   _____ / _____
                                       r   s

    b) *Bonus Question:* What is the definition of the word root? _____

9. a) vagotomy   _____ / __ / _____
                                           cf   s

    b) *Bonus Question:* What is the definition of the suffix? _____

Abbreviations of the Digestive System

The abbreviations that are associated with the digestive system are summarized here. Study these abbreviations and review them in the exercise that follows.

Abbreviation	Definition
BE	barium enema
C&S	stool culture and sensitivity
EGD	esophagogastroduodenoscopy
FOBT	fecal occult blood test
GERD	gastroesophageal reflux disease
GI	gastrointestinal
HCC	hepatocellular carcinoma

Abbreviation	Definition
IBD	inflammatory bowel disease
IBS	irritable bowel syndrome
LGI	lower GI series
LI	lactose intolerance
N&V	nausea and vomiting
UGI	upper GI series

PRACTICE: Abbreviations

Fill in the blanks with the abbreviation or the complete medical term.

Abbreviation	Medical Term
1. BE	_____
2. _____	inflammatory bowel disease
3. UGI	_____
4. _____	gastroesophageal reflux disease
5. N&V	_____
6. _____	upper GI series
7. IBS	_____
8. _____	lower GI series
9. C&S	_____
10. _____	gastrointestinal
11. FOBT	_____
12. _____	esophagogastroduodenoscopy
13. LI	_____

CHAPTER REVIEW

Word Building

Construct medical terms from the following meanings. (Some are built from word parts, some are not.) The first question has been completed as an example.

1. indigestion _____***dys***pepsia

2. enlargement of the liver _____y

3. difficulty swallowing _____phag_____

4. inflammation of the lip _____itis

5. inflammation of the gallbladder cholecyst_____

6. condition of gallstones chole_____

7. inflammation of the colon _____itis

8. cancer of the colon and rectum _____al cancer

9. inflammation of the small intestine enter_____

10. softening of the stomach wall gastro_____

11. condition of diverticula diverticul_____

12. tumor of the liver _____oma

13. inflammation of a salivary gland _____itis

14. surgical removal of hemorrhoids _____ectomy

15. surgical creation of an opening into the colon _____ostomy

16. endoscopic evaluation of the rectum proct_____

17. endoscopic evaluation of the abdominal cavity _____oscopy

18. surgical repair of the tongue with sutures gloss_____

19. surgical removal of a polyp polyp_____

Define the Combining Form

In the space provided, write the definition of the combining form, followed by one example of the combining form used to build a medical term in Chapter 10.

	Definition	**Use in a Term**
1. gastr/o	_____	_____
2. cholecyst/o	_____	_____
3. choledoch/o	_____	_____
4. enter/o	_____	_____
5. duoden/o	_____	_____
6. gingiv/o	_____	_____
7. col/o	_____	_____
8. pept/o	_____	_____

Complete the Labels

Complete the blank labels in ■ Figures 10.24 and 10.25 by writing the labels in the spaces provided.

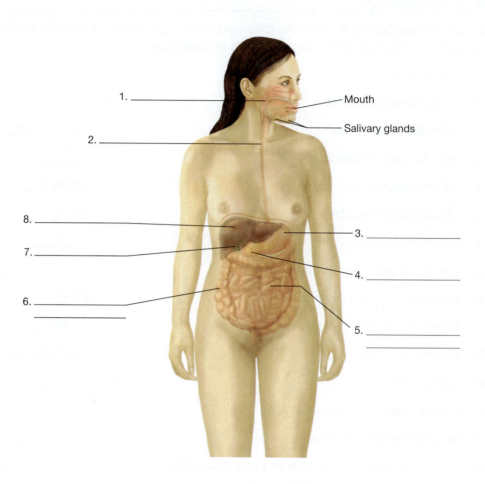

1. ———————————————— Mouth

2. ————————————————

8. ————————————————

7. ————————————————

3. ————————————

4. ————————————

6. ————————————————

5. ————————————

— Salivary glands

■ **Figure 10.24**
Organs of the digestive system.

1. _____

2. _____

3. _____

4. _____

5. _____

6. _____

7. _____

8. _____

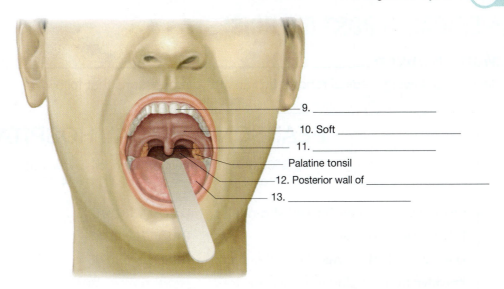

9. _____

10. Soft _____

11. _____

Palatine tonsil

12. Posterior wall of _____

13. _____

■ **Figure 10.25**
The oral cavity. Anterior view
of the open mouth.

9. _____

10. _____

11. _____

12. _____

13. _____

MEDICAL REPORT EXERCISES

Maria Nguyen

Read the following medical report, then answer the questions that follow.

PEARSON GENERAL HOSPITAL

PGH

5500 University Avenue, Metropolis, New York
Phone: (211) 594-4000 • Fax (211) 594-4001

Medical Consultation: Internal Medicine

Date: 09/18/2017

Patient: Maria Nguygen

Patient ID: 123456

Dob: 02/10/1994   **Age:** 23   **Sex:** Female   **Allergies:** NKDA

Provider: Joanne M. Morgenthaler, MD

Subjective:

"I have severely painful irregular bowel habits. I am not able to compete at school, date, or even keep friends."

23 y/o female is in tremendous discomfort with intermittent bouts of diahrrea, constipation, and abdominal cramping. It appears to be affecting her quality of life, causing anxiety and depression.

Objective:

Vital Signs: T: 98.7°F; **P:** 82; **R:** 20; **BP:** 122/75

Ht: 5'3"

Wt: 105 lb

General Appearance: Patient is underweight; skin with pallor, mild diaphoresis. Edema around the eyes.

Heart: Rate at 82 bpm. Heart sounds with auscultation appear normal.

Lungs: Clear without signs of disease.

AbD: Active peristalsis with gurgles and possible spasms in RLQ and LLQ: ileocecal junction, transverse colon. Severe tenderness at these locations during palpation.

MS: Joints and muscles symmetric. No swelling, masses, or deformity.

Lab: Lactase positive. UGI negative. BE test positive for swelling, spasms of transverse colon.

Colonoscopy: Performed on 09/14/2017, shows positive for erythema and mild ulceration at distal ileum

Laparoscopy: Performed on 09/17/2017, positive for ileitis, spastic colon.

Assessment:

Crohn's disease

Plan:

Treat with oral antispasmodics and anti-inflammatory. Educate about dietary and behavioral management of Crohn's disease. Review status in 2 weeks.

Comprehension Questions

1. What is the diagnosis? _____

   _____

   _____

2. Which findings support the diagnosis? _____

   _____

   _____

3. What is a laparoscopy? _____

   _____

   _____

Case Study Questions

The following Case Study provides further discussion regarding the patient in the medical report. Fill in the blanks with the correct terms. Choose your answers from the following list of terms. (Note that some terms may be used more than once.)

barium enema	diarrhea	inflammatory bowel
constipation	flatus	lactose intolerance
Crohn's disease	irritable bowel syndrome	laparoscopy

A 23-year-old female named Maria Nguyen was admitted following a history of 4 weeks of intermittent

watery stools, or (a) _____, accompanied with trapped gas, or (b) _____,

occasional reduced peristalsis of the large intestine, or (c) _____, abdominal pain,

and vomiting. Initial diagnosis by her personal GP was the lack of the digestive enzyme lactase,

known as (d) _____ _____, although IBS, or (e) _____

_____ _____, was ruled as another possibility. With time, symptoms

of pain and bowel irregularity increased, raising the concern that the woman might be suffering from a

chronic inflammation of the ileum, or (f) _____ _____, a type of IBD, or

(g) _____ _____ disease. Once admitted, thorough testing, including a

lactase enzyme test, BE (also known as (h) _____ _____), a UGI series, and

an endoscopy into the abdomen, called a (i) _____, ensued. The laparoscopy confirmed the

initial diagnosis of Crohn's disease.

Mark Swanson

For a greater challenge, read the following medical report, then answer the critical thinking questions that follow.

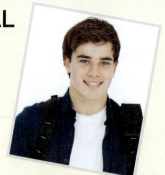

PGH PEARSON GENERAL HOSPITAL

5500 University Avenue, Metropolis, New York
Phone: (211) 594-4000 • Fax (211) 594-4001

Medical Consultation: Internal Medicine   **Date:** 08/04/2017

Patient: Mark Swanson   **Patient ID:** 123456

Dob: 11/11/1993   **Age:** 24   **Sex:** Male   **Allergies:** NKDA

Provider: Arthur Broward, MD

Subjective:

"I have abdominal cramps after eating nearly anything. At times, at least once a week, I have either diarrhea or constipation, which is often painful."

24 y/o male struggles with abdominal discomfort, with alternating bouts of diarrhea and constipation that he says limits his enjoyment of eating and makes sports, studying, and hanging out with friends very difficult and uncomfortable. Patient history reveals abdominal complaints of bloating, cramping, and excessive flatulence since age 8. Father is LI with chronic colitis and hemorrhoid complaints. Mother w/out digestive complaints.

Objective:

Vital Signs: T: 98.7°F; **P:** 78; **R:** 20; **BP:** 124/88

Ht: 5'10"

Wt: 142 lb

General Appearance: Skin with mild pallor. Lean build, timid behavior.

Heart: Rate at 78 bpm. Heart sounds with auscultation appear normal.

Lungs: Clear without signs of disease.

AbD: RLQ and LLQ with active audible peristalsis. RUQ and LUQ relatively quiet.

MS: Joints and muscles symmetric. No swelling, masses, or deformity.

Lab: C&S negative.

Colonoscopy: On 07/28/2017, with no polyps or ulcerations. Two minor internal hemorrhoids present. Mild erythema in cecal and sigmoidal walls.

Assessment:

LI and IBS

Plan:

Educate improved dietary regimen to include daily use of probiotics, fiber supplements, and lactase supplements to improve bowel functions. Reschedule visit in 3 months.

Comprehension Questions

1. Which parent's genes had more likely contributed to the diagnosed diseases? _____

   _____

   _____

2. What complaints suggest IBS as a diagnosis? _____

   _____

   _____

3. What does the abbreviation IBS mean? _____

   _____

   _____

Case Study Questions

The following case study provides additional discussion regarding the patient in the medical report. Fill in the blanks from information provided in the chapter.

Mark Swanson, a 24-year-old male patient with a pediatric history of abdominal discomfort, had

experienced weight loss, leading to an initial diagnosis of the mental disorder (m) _____

_____. However, a gastroenterologist examined him further to look for evidence of physical

disease. Tests were ordered that included endoscopy of the colon, or (n) _____, and a test for

bacterial infection known as a (o) _____ test (abbreviation). He was found to have no known

infection, and his large intestine wall was mildly irritated but without major disease. Also found was the presence

of two internal (p) _____. Due to this evidence of mild disease and his family history of

(q) _____ _____, his physician instructed Mark to undergo diet education

in order to manage his LI and (r) _____ _____ _____. It

is hoped that the education will improve his dietary habits and will serve to reduce his discomfort.

MyLab Medical Terminology™

MyLab Medical Terminology is a premium online homework management system that includes a host of features to help you study. Registered users will find:

- A multitude of quizzes and activities built within the MyLab platform
- Powerful tools that track and analyze your results—allowing you to create a personalized learning experience
- Videos and audio pronunciations to help enrich your progress
- Streaming lesson presentations (Guided Lectures) and self-paced learning modules
- A space where you and your instructors can view and manage your assignments

Chapter 11

The Urinary System

Learning Objectives

After completing this chapter, you will be able to:

11.1 Define and spell the word parts used to create terms for the urinary system.

11.2 Break down and define common medical terms used for symptoms, diseases, disorders, procedures, treatments, and devices associated with the urinary system.

11.3 Build medical terms from the word parts associated with the urinary system.

11.4 Pronounce and spell common medical terms associated with the urinary system.

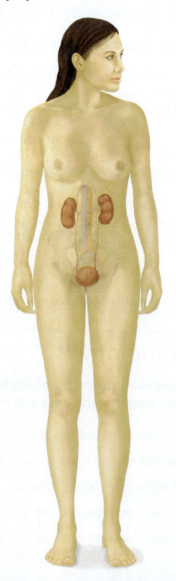

Anatomy and Physiology Terms

The following table provides the combining forms that commonly apply to the anatomy and physiology of the urinary system. Note that the combining forms are colored red to help you identify them when you see them again later in the chapter.

Combining Form	Definition	Combining Form	Definition
albumin/o	albumin (a protein)	nephr/o	kidney
blast/o	germ, bud, developing cell	pyel/o	renal pelvis
glomerul/o	little ball, glomerulus	ren/o	kidney
gluc/o	sweet, sugar	ureter/o	ureter
glyc/o, glycos/o	sweet, sugar	urethr/o	urethra
meat/o	opening, passage	ur/o, urin/o	urine

urinary

YOO rih nair ee

kidneys

11.1 The _____ system functions as the sanitation engineer of the body, maintaining the purity and health of the body's fluids by removing unwanted waste materials and recycling other materials. The kidneys are its most important organs. They filter gallons of fluids from the bloodstream every day, removing metabolic wastes, toxins, excess ions, and water that leave the body as urine, while returning needed materials back into the blood. Because waste removal is essential for your survival, the kidneys are vital organs; a loss of both _____ requires medical intervention to sustain life. Other organs of the urinary system transport urine or store it before it can be released to the exterior of the body. They are the paired ureters, the urinary bladder, and the urethra.

urine

11.2 You have just learned that the primary function of the kidneys is the removal of metabolic wastes, toxins, excess ions, and water from the bloodstream. This function is performed by the formation of urine as a watery waste. _____ is formed by three processes occurring in the kidneys: filtration of the blood to produce a filtrate; reabsorption of excess water, ions, and nutrients in the filtrate to return them to the bloodstream; and secretion of excess ions as waste into the filtrate. In addition to forming urine, the kidneys also perform other vital functions:

- Regulation of blood pressure
- Regulation of pH within body fluids
- Regulation of water and salt concentrations
- Regulation of red blood cell production

11.3 Review the anatomy of the urinary system by studying ■ Figure 11.1, ■ Figure 11.2, and ■ Figure 11.3.

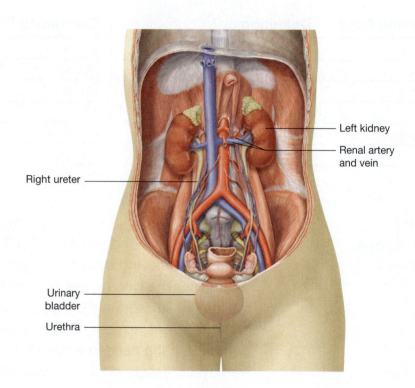

Left kidney

Renal artery and vein

Right ureter

Urinary bladder

Urethra

■ **Figure 11.1**
Organs of the urinary system. This illustration is an anterior view of a female with the abdominal wall and digestive organs removed.

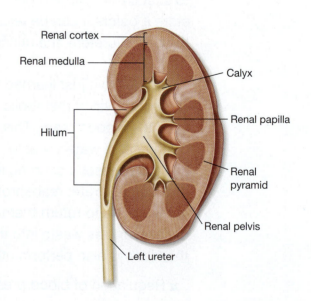

Renal cortex

Renal medulla

Calyx

Hilum

Renal papilla

Renal pyramid

Renal pelvis

Left ureter

■ **Figure 11.2**
The kidney. This illustration of a sectioned kidney reveals its internal features.

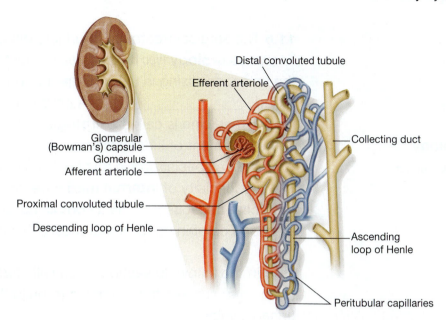

Figure 11.3
The nephron. The microscopic nephron is the basic subunit of each kidney.

Medical Terms for the Urinary System

mucous membrane

11.4 For many people, the major pathological challenge to the health of the urinary system is infection, due to communication to the exterior by way of the urinary meatus. Although the urethra, urinary bladder, and ureters are each protected by a _____ _____, bacteria and viruses are sometimes able to gain entry into the internal organs through the meatus. Once established, they are capable of spreading through the urinary tract, bringing disease to the kidneys and beyond. Also, the close location of the urinary meatus to the anus in females enables some bacterial populations that normally form the intestinal microbiota to infect the urinary tract. In addition to _____, other sources of disease afflicting the urinary system include diabetes, hypertension, tumors, stones, inherited disorders, and heart disease.

infections

urine

11.5 Because _____ originates from the bloodstream and the urinary system releases urine on a regular basis, urine testing provides a convenient means for testing general health. Many diseases can be diagnosed from a urine sample that contains abnormal contents, such as blood cells, bacteria, albumin (a protein normally found in blood), glucose, and high levels of creatinine (a protein product of metabolism).

urology

nephrology
neh FROL oh jee

11.6 The surgical treatment of urinary disease is a medical discipline known as **urology** (yoo RAHL oh jee). In most hospitals and clinics, the unit specializing in the treatment of urinary diseases is also called _____. A physician specializing in this field of medicine is called a **urologist**. The field that specializes in the treatment of kidney disease is _____. A physician specializing in this field is a **nephrologist**. Nephrology is a subspecialty of **internal medicine**, and is often called **renal medicine** because *ren/o* is a combining form for kidney (*nephr/o* is a second combining form that means "kidney").

11.7 In the following sections, you will study the prefixes, combining forms, and suffixes that combine to build the medical terms of the urinary system.

Signs and Symptoms of the Urinary System

Here are the word parts that commonly apply to the signs and symptoms of the urinary system and are covered in the following section. Note that the word parts are color-coded to help you identify them: prefixes are yellow, combining forms are red, and suffixes are blue.

Prefix	Definition
an-	without, absence of
dia-	through
dys-	bad, abnormal, painful, difficult
poly-	excessive, over, many

Combining Form	Definition
albumin/o	albumin (a protein)
azot/o	urea, nitrogen
bacteri/o	bacteria
glycos/o	sweet, sugar
hem/o, hemat/o	blood
ket/o, keton/o	ketone
noct/o	night
olig/o	few in number
protein/o	protein
py/o	pus

Suffix	Definition
-emia	condition of blood
-uresis	urination
-uria	pertaining to urine, urination

KEY TERMS A–Z

albuminuria
AL byoo men YOO ree ah

11.8 A **urinalysis** (Frame 11.84) is a clinical procedure that examines the composition of urine. The most common type of urinalysis involves dipping an indicator stick into a urine specimen and reading the results that compare with a known standard. Diseases of the urinary system and other parts of the body may be diagnosed with this valuable clinical tool. For example, albumin is a protein normally present in the bloodstream. If it appears in the urine, it is a physical sign of abnormal renal filtration. The sign is called _____. This constructed term contains two word parts, as you can see in albumin/uria.

anuria
an YOO ree ah

11.9 The inability to pass urine is the clinical sign known as **anuria**. In this term, the prefix *an-*, which means "without," is added to the suffix *-uria*, which means "pertaining to urine, urination," to create the medical term _____. It is a sign of kidney disease and is defined as the production of less than 100 mL of urine per day (the normal urine output per day varies between 800 and 2,000 mL). Its constructed form is an/uria.

azotemia
az oh TEE mee ah

11.10 The sign of abnormally high levels of urea and other nitrogen-containing compounds in the blood is called **azotemia**. _____ is a constructed term: azot/emia. The combining form *azot/o* means "urea, nitrogen," although it originates from a Greek word, *azo*, which means "without life."

bacteriuria
bak teer ee YOO ree ah
bacteri/uria

11.11 The abnormal presence of bacteria in the urine is a sign of a urinary tract infection and is called _____. This constructed term includes two word parts, which are revealed when the term is written as _____/_____.

diuresis
DYE yoo REE siss

11.12 The temporary, excessive discharge of urine is a symptom known as **diuresis**. It literally means "urination through." The constructed form of this word is di/uresis. Note the *a* in the prefix *dia-* is not used in order to make the term easier to pronounce. _____ may be induced with drugs, called *diuretics*, to reduce high blood pressure by increasing urine volume.

dysuria
diss YOO ree ah

11.13 Recall that the prefix *dys-* means "bad, abnormal, painful, or difficult." When *dys-* is combined with the suffix for "pertaining to urine, urination," the resulting term refers to difficulty or pain experienced during urination. It is a symptom of a urinary tract disease often caused by a bacterial infection. The symptom is called _____. It is a constructed term with two word parts: dys/uria.

glycosuria
glye kohs YOO ree ah

11.14 The combining form *glycos/o* means "sweet, sugar." The abnormal presence of glucose (sugar) in the urine is a sign of an endocrine disease, such as diabetes mellitus. The sign is called _____, which is a constructed term: glycos/uria.

hematuria
HEE mah TOO ree ah

11.15 The abnormal presence of blood in the urine is a sign of a urinary system disorder. It is called _____, which means "pertaining to bloody urine or urination" (■ Figure 11.4). The constructed form of this term is hemat/uria.

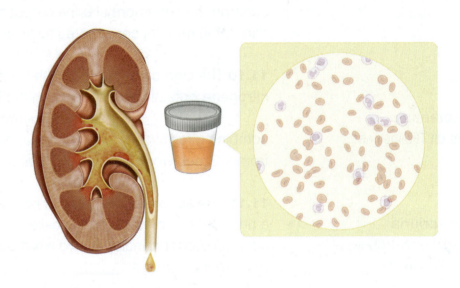

■ **Figure 11.4**
Hematuria. An analysis of urine is performed to evaluate kidney function. In this illustration, the beaker contains urine that is red, indicating the sign of blood within the urine, which is confirmed by microscopic analysis.

ketonuria
kee tohn YOO ree ah

11.16 The abnormal presence of ketone bodies in the urine is called **ketonuria**. The constructed form of _____ uses the combining form for ketone bodies (*keton/o*) and is keton/uria. It is a common sign of a metabolic disorder, a high-protein/low-carbohydrate diet, starvation, or diabetes mellitus.

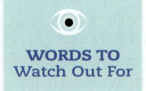

WORDS TO
Watch Out For

Terms with No Combining Vowels

Most of the terms related to the signs and symptoms of the urinary system contain no combining vowel. For example, terms such as *ketonuria* and *hematuria* contain only a word root and suffix. This is because the suffixes in this section (*-emia*, *-uresis*, *-uria*) all begin with a vowel, so no combining vowel is needed to make the terms easier to pronounce.

nocturia
nok TOO ree ah

11.17 The need to urinate frequently at night is a possible symptom of diabetes mellitus or benign prostatic hyperplasia (BPH). It is called **nocturia**. As a constructed term, _____ includes two word parts, noct/uria.

oliguria all ig YOO ree ah	**11.18** Reduced urination becomes a clinical problem when the volume of urine declines to less than 500 mL within a 24-hour period. It is known as **oliguria** and is a possible sign of a kidney disorder. _____ may also be a sign of congestive heart failure, dehydration, or a blockage in the urinary tract. The constructed form of this term is olig/uria.
polyuria pall ee YOO ree ah	**11.19** The chronic, abnormal production of large volumes of urine requires frequent urination and is a common sign of an endocrine disease, usually diabetes insipidus or diabetes mellitus. The sign is called _____, which is a constructed term with two word parts: poly/uria.
proteinuria proh tee NYOO ree ah	**11.20** In Frame 11.8 you learned that albuminuria is the presence of the protein albumin in the urine. The presence of any protein in the urine is called _____, so albuminuria is a form of proteinuria. The constructed form of this term is protein/uria.
pyuria pye YOO ree ah	**11.21** Pus is a mixture of white blood cells, bacteria, and cell debris that forms during an infection. Its appearance in the urine indicates a urinary tract infection. The presence of pus in urine is called _____, with the constructed form py/uria. The combining form that means "pus" is py/o.

PRACTICE: Signs and Symptoms of the Urinary System

The Right Match

Match the term on the left with the correct definition on the right.

_____ 1. albuminuria   a. urination at night

_____ 2. bacteriuria   b. presence of blood in the urine

_____ 3. diuresis   c. presence of bacteria in the urine

_____ 4. glycosuria   d. chronic excessive urination

_____ 5. hematuria   e. ketone bodies in the urine

_____ 6. ketonuria   f. presence of sugar in the urine

_____ 7. nocturia   g. presence of albumin in the urine

_____ 8. oliguria   h. reduced urination

_____ 9. polyuria   i. literally "urination through"

Break the Chain

Analyze these medical terms:

    a) Separate each term into its word parts; each word part is labeled for you (**p** = prefix, **r** = root, **cf** = combining form, and **s** = suffix).

    b) For the Bonus Question, write the requested definition in the blank that follows.

The first set has been completed as an example.

1. a) proteinuria   ***protein/uria***
                                        r   s

    b) *Bonus Question:* What is the definition of the suffix? ***pertaining to urine or urination***

2. a) azotemia   _____/_____
                                      r   s

    b) *Bonus Question:* What is the definition of the word root? _____

3. a) dysuria   _____/_____
                                      p   s

    b) *Bonus Question:* What is the definition of the suffix? _____

4. a) anuria   _____/_____
                                      p   s

    b) *Bonus Question:* What is the definition of the prefix? _____

5. a) pyuria   _____/_____
                                      r   s

    b) *Bonus Question:* What is the definition of the word root? _____

6. a) glycosuria   _____/_____
                                      r   s

    b) *Bonus Question:* What is the definition of the word root? _____

7. a) bacteriuria   _____/_____
                                      r   s

    b) *Bonus Question:* What is the definition of the word suffix? _____

8. a) ketonuria   _____/_____
                                      r   s

    b) *Bonus Question:* What is the definition of the word root? _____

Diseases and Disorders of the Urinary System

Review some of the word parts that commonly apply to the diseases and disorders of the urinary system and are covered in the following section. Note that the word parts are color-coded to help you identify them: prefixes are yellow, combining forms are red, and suffixes are blue.

Prefix	Definition
dys-	bad, abnormal, painful, difficult
en-	within, upon, on, over
epi-	upon, over, above, on top
hypo-	deficient, abnormally low, below
poly-	excessive, over, many

Combining Form	Definition
azot/o	urea, nitrogen
bacteri/o	bacteria
blast/o	germ, bud, developing cell
cyst/o	bladder, sac
glomerul/o	little ball, glomerulus
hemat/o	blood
hydr/o	water
lith/o	stone
nephr/o	kidney
py/o	pus
pyel/o	renal pelvis
ren/o	kidney
spadias/o	rip, tear
sten/o	narrow
ur/o	urine
ureter/o	ureter
urethr/o	urethra

Suffix	Definition
-al	pertaining to
-cele	hernia, swelling, protrusion
-emia	condition of blood
-iasis	condition of
-ic	pertaining to
-itis	inflammation
-megaly	abnormally large
-oma	tumor
-osis	condition of
-pathy	disease
-ptosis	drooping
-sis	state of
-uresis	urination
-uria	pertaining to urine, urination

KEY TERMS A–Z

acute kidney injury

11.22 A rapid-onset disease of the kidneys resulting in a failure to produce urine is known as **acute kidney injury (AKI)**. Formerly called *acute renal failure*, _____ _____ _____ is usually caused by physical injury, septic shock, severe dehydration, or surgical complications, and is regarded as a recoverable condition.

cystitis
siss TYE tiss

11.23 The combining form for bladder is *cyst/o*. An inflammation of the urinary bladder is called _____. The constructed form of this term is cyst/itis. It is usually caused by a bacterial infection that travels up the urethra. An infection of the urinary bladder and the urethra is called **urethrocystitis** (yoo REE throh siss TYE tiss), with the following word parts: urethr/o/cyst/itis.

cystocele
SISS toh seel

11.24 Because the suffix *-cele* means "hernia, swelling, protrusion," a herniation of the urinary bladder is called a **cystocele**. In females, the protrusion pushes into the adjacent vagina. The term _____ is a constructed term: cyst/o/cele.

cystolith
SISS toh lith

11.25 A _____ is a stone, or calculus, in the urinary bladder. If it is too large to pass through the urethra, medical intervention is required to eliminate it. The constructed form of this term is cyst/o/lith.

end-stage kidney disease

11.26 Failure of both kidneys to form urine from any cause is a life-threatening condition called **end-stage kidney disease (ESKD)**. Also called **renal failure**, development of _____-

_____ _____ _____

produces symptoms of nausea, lethargy, itching, mental confusion, and fluid retention (edema). To prevent death, the medical team must develop an aggressive course of action, such as hemodialysis and, if possible, kidney transplant.

enuresis
ehn yoo REE siss

11.27 An involuntary release of urine, which usually occurs due to a lack of bladder control among children or older adults, is known as **enuresis**. When this occurs during sleep, it is known as **nocturnal** _____, or bedwetting. The constructed form of this term is en/uresis.

epispadias
EP ih SPAY dee ass

11.28 A congenital defect resulting in the abnormal positioning of the urinary meatus is known as **epispadias** (■ Figure 11.5). In males, the meatus opens on the dorsal (upper) surface of the penis, and in females the meatus opens dorsal to the clitoris. _____ is a constructed term with two word parts, epi/spadias, which literally means "a rip or tear upon."

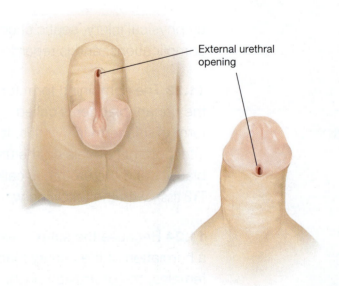

External urethral opening

■ **Figure 11.5**
Epispadias and hypospadias. In the male, epispadias is an abnormally placed opening of the urethra on the dorsal side of the penis (left), and in hypospadias, the opening is on the underside (ventral) of the penis (right).

glomerulonephritis
gloh MAIR yoo loh neh
FRYE tiss

11.29 A glomerulus is a ball of specialized capillaries within a kidney nephron (the term *glomerulus* means "little ball"). Any disease of the glomeruli is called a **glomerulonephropathy** (gloh MAIR yoo loh neh FROH path ee), which is a constructed term with two combining forms and a suffix: glomerul/o/nephr/o/pathy. An example is inflammation of the glomeruli, which is known as _____. It is either an autoimmune disease resulting from an attack on glomeruli by the body's own white blood cells, or it may be caused by a bacterial infection. The constructed form of this term is glomerul/o/nephr/itis.

hydronephrosis
HIGH droh neh FROH siss

11.30 The production of urine by the kidneys is a physiological process that is continual throughout your lifetime. If the exit of urine out of the kidneys becomes blocked by an obstruction in a ureter, the urine will back up to cause distension of the renal pelvis. This condition is known as **hydronephrosis** and is illustrated in ■ Figure 11.6. The term _____ includes four word parts: hydr/o/nephr/osis. Recall that *hydr/o* means "water," which refers to the fluid (urine) that becomes blocked from its normal passage in this condition.

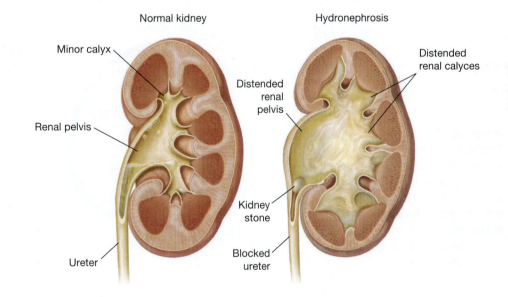

Normal kidney   Hydronephrosis

Minor calyx

Distended renal calyces

Distended renal pelvis

Renal pelvis

Kidney stone

Ureter

Blocked ureter

■ **Figure 11.6**
Hydronephrosis. Normal kidney (left) and kidney with hydronephrosis (right) are compared. Note the distension (swelling) of the renal pelvis. In this illustration, the distension was caused by the constriction of the ureter, causing urine to back up in the renal pelvis.

hypospadias
HIGH poh SPAY dee ass

11.31 You learned in Frame 11.28 that epispadias is a congenital defect in which the urinary meatus has shifted dorsally. In **hypospadias**, the change in location of the urinary meatus is ventral (see Figure 11.5). In males, it opens on the underside of the penis, and in females the meatus is within the vagina. _____ is a constructed term written hypo/spadias, which literally means "a rip or tear below."

incontinence
in KON tih nens

11.32 The inability to control urination is called **urinary** _____. In **stress incontinence**, an involuntary discharge of urine occurs during a cough, sneeze, or strained movement.

nephritis
neh FRYE tiss

11.33 One combining form for kidney is _nephr/o_, and it is found in many terms describing a kidney disease or procedure. For example, inflammation of a kidney is known as **nephritis**. _____ may be caused by an autoimmune response (attack by the body's own white blood cells) or an allergic reaction to certain medications; it may also be called **interstitial nephritis**. It is a constructed term with two word parts, nephr/itis.

nephroblastoma
NEFF roh blass TOH mah

11.34 A **nephroblastoma** is a tumor originating from kidney tissue that includes developing embryonic cells (■ Figure 11.7). It is also called **Wilms' tumor** after the 19th-century German physician who published the first description of the disease. _____ is a constructed term, nephr/o/blast/oma.

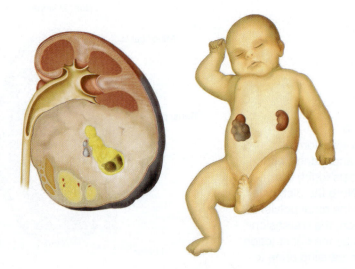

■ **Figure 11.7**
Nephroblastoma. A sectioned kidney reveals the presence of a very large tumor, which arose from fetal cells during development. A newborn with nephroblastoma is illustrated to show the location and relative size of the tumor.

nephrolithiasis
NEFF roh lith EYE ah siss

11.35 The presence of one or more stones, or calculi, within a kidney is called **nephrolithiasis**. The constructed form of this term is nephr/o/lith/iasis. An alternate term for _____ is **renal calculi** (REE nal * KAL kyoo lye) and is further described in ■ Figure 11.8.

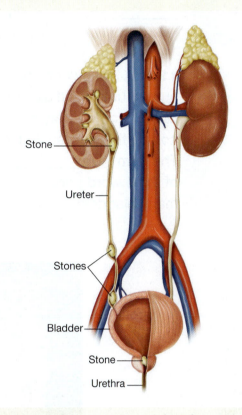

■ **Figure 11.8**
Nephrolithiasis. Stones, or calculi, may form in several areas within the urinary tract. When they form in the kidney, they usually arise within the renal pelvis to form the condition nephrolithiasis. Kidney stones may dislocate to form obstructions in the ureter, urinary bladder, or urethra, usually at their junctions.

Stone
Ureter
Stones
Bladder
Stone
Urethra

nephroma
neff ROH mah

11.36 A general term for a tumor arising from kidney tissue is _____. This constructed term has two word parts, nephr/oma.

nephromegaly
neff roh MEG ah lee

11.37 The suffix -*megaly* means "abnormally large." An abnormal enlargement of one or both kidneys is called _____. The word parts of this term can be shown as nephr/o/megaly.

nephropathy
neh-FROP-ah-thee

11.38 A severe condition of a kidney that leads to end-stage kidney disease (Frame 11.26) is generally called **nephropathy**. There are two major forms: diabetic nephropathy, resulting from unmanaged diabetes mellitus, and hypertensive nephropathy, resulting from unmanaged chronic hypertension (high blood pressure). A third form that is not as common is drug-induced nephropathy, which may be caused by certain over-the-counter drugs (such as ibuprofen), lab procedures (such as x-rays), and prescription medicines. According to the National Institutes of Health (NIH), approximately 26 million Americans suffer from a form of nephropathy. The term _____ is a constructed term, created when the combining form that means "kidney," *nephr/o*, is combined with the suffix -*pathy*, which means "disease."

nephroptosis
neff ropp TOH siss

11.39 The condition of a downward displacement ("drooping") of a kidney is known as **nephroptosis**. The constructed form of this term is nephr/o/ptosis. It occurs when the kidney is no longer held in its proper position against the posterior abdominal wall. _____ is commonly called **floating kidney**.

polycystic
PALL ee SISS tik

11.40 A kidney condition characterized by the presence of numerous cysts (fluid-filled capsules) occupying much of the kidney tissue is called **polycystic kidney disease**. The cysts replace normal tissue, resulting in a loss of kidney function (■ Figure 11.9). The term _____ is a constructed term composed of three word parts, poly/cyst/ic, and literally means "pertaining to many bladders."

■ **Figure 11.9**
Polycystic kidney disease. Notice the presence of numerous fluid-filled sacs, or cysts, in these kidneys, which were removed from a patient who died of renal failure. *Source: Courtesy of Dr. Edwin P. Ewing, Public Health Image Library, Centers for Disease Control and Prevention, Atlanta, GA.*

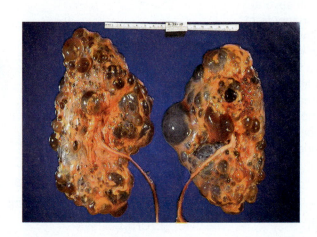

pyelitis
PYE eh LYE tiss

11.41 The combining form for renal pelvis is *pyel/o*. Inflammation of the renal pelvis is called _____. It is usually caused by a bacterial infection. The constructed form of this term is pyel/itis.

pyelonephritis
PYE eh loh neh FRYE tiss

11.42 A serious inflammatory condition of one or both kidneys is called **pyelonephritis**. The constructed form of _____ is pyel/o/nephr/itis. Pyelonephritis is usually caused by an infection involving the common intestinal bacterium *Escherichia coli* (*E .coli*), resulting from a urinary tract infection (Frame 11.49) that has been left untreated. This life-threatening condition often results in bacteremia (the presence of bacteria in the blood). Its chronic form leads to kidney failure.

strictures STRIK cherz	**11.43** A condition of abnormal narrowing is known as a **stricture**. Examples of urinary _____ include **ureteral stricture**, in which the ureter is narrowed; **urethral stricture**, in which the urethra is narrowed; and **ureterovesical stricture**, in which the junction of the ureter and bladder is narrowed. Because the medical term *stenosis* also refers to an abnormal narrowing, it may be used as an alternative term to *stricture* in each of these terms. An example term is **ureterostenosis** (yoo REE ter oh steh NOH siss), which is a ureteral stricture, or narrowing. The constructed form of this term is ureter/o/sten/osis.
uremia yoo REE mee ah	**11.44** In the condition **uremia**, an excess of urea and other nitrogenous wastes are present in the blood. The constructed form of this term is ur/emia. _____ is caused by failure of the kidneys to remove urea and is associated with renal insufficiency or renal failure.

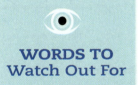

WORDS TO Watch Out For

Hematuria versus Uremia

Here is a pair of opposites. The term *hematuria* is a sign of any condition in which urine contains blood or red blood cells. On the other hand, the term *uremia* refers to a condition in which the blood contains urine (actually an excess of urea and other nitrogenous wastes), so its primary sign is azotemia (Frame 11.10). Uremia is often the result of advanced kidney disease.

ureteritis yoo REE ter EYE tiss	**11.45** The ureters are the paired narrow tubes that transport urine from the kidneys to the urinary bladder. Inflammation of a ureter is called _____ and is often the result of a bacterial infection. This constructed form of this term is ureter/itis.
ureterocele yoo REE ter oh seel	**11.46** A herniated ureter is called a **ureterocele**. The constructed form of _____ is ureter/o/cele.
ureterolithiasis yoo REE ter oh lith EYE ah siss	**11.47** The presence of one or more stones, or calculi, within a ureter is called **ureterolithiasis**. The constructed form of _____ includes a combining form *and* a word root and is written ureter/o/lith/iasis.

urinary retention

YOO rih nair ee * ree TEN shun

11.48 The abnormal accumulation of urine within the urinary bladder is called **urinary retention**. The condition of _____ _____ results from an inability to void, or urinate.

urinary tract infection

YOO rih nair ee * trakt * in FEK shun

11.49 Commonly called by its abbreviation of **UTI**, a _____ _____ _____ is an infection of urinary organs, usually the urethra and urinary bladder (called a *lower urinary tract infection*; a less common form involves the ureters and kidneys and is called an *upper urinary tract infection*). The symptoms include lumbar or abdominal pain, dysuria (Frame 11.13), and a sense of urgency to urinate, while common signs include bacteriuria (Frame 11.11), pyuria (Frame 11.21), and sometimes hematuria (Frame 11.15) (■ Figure 11.10). A UTI is more common in females and is often caused by *E. coli* bacteria.

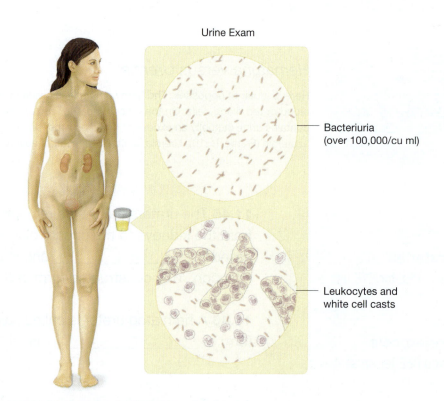

Urine Exam

Bacteriuria (over 100,000/cu ml)

Leukocytes and white cell casts

■ **Figure 11.10**
Urinary tract infection. A UTI is characterized by fever, lumbar or abdominal pain, and pain or burning during urination. A diagnosis may be confirmed in a urine exam that reveals the presence of bacteria (bacteriuria) and white blood cells (pyuria).

PRACTICE: Diseases and Disorders of the Urinary System

The Right Match

Match the term on the left with the correct definition on the right.

_____	1. cystocele	a.	condition of excess urea in the blood
_____	2. cystolith	b.	protrusion of the urinary bladder
_____	3. nephritis	c.	stone(s) in the urinary bladder
_____	4. nephromegaly	d.	urinary meatus opens on the underside of the penis
_____	5. uremia	e.	inflammation of a kidney
_____	6. hypospadias	f.	enlargement of a kidney
_____	7. polycystic kidney disease	g.	a condition of stones in the kidneys
_____	8. renal calculi	h.	involuntary discharge of urine
_____	9. urinary incontinence	i.	a condition of many cysts within a kidney
_____	10. urinary retention	j.	abnormal accumulation of urine in the bladder
_____	11. stricture	k.	a condition in which kidney function ceases
_____	12. acute kidney injury	l.	condition of abnormal narrowing

Linkup

Link the word parts in the list to create the terms that match the definitions. You may use word parts more than once. Remember to add combining vowels when needed and that some terms do not use any combining vowel. The first one is completed as an example.

Combining Form	Suffix
cyst/o	-itis
glomerul/o	-oma
hydr/o	-osis
lith/o	-iasis
nephr/o	
pyel/o	

Definition	Term
1. inflammation of the urinary bladder	*cystitis*
2. inflammation of the glomeruli	_____
3. inflammation of the renal pelvis and the nephrons	_____
4. presence of one or more stones within a kidney	_____
5. condition of blockage of urine (water) in the kidney	_____
6. tumor that arises from kidney tissue	_____
7. inflammation of the renal pelvis	_____

Treatments, Procedures, and Devices of the Urinary System

Review some of the word parts that commonly apply to the treatments, procedures, and devices of the urinary system and are covered in the following section. Note that the word parts are color-coded to help you identify them: prefixes are yellow, combining forms are red, and suffixes are blue.

Prefix	Definition
dia-	through

Combining Form	Definition
cyst/o	bladder, sac
hemat/o, hem/o	blood
lith/o	stone
meat/o	opening, passage
nephr/o	kidney
peritone/o	to stretch over, peritoneum
pyel/o	renal pelvis
ren/o	kidney
son/o	sound
tom/o	to cut
ureter/o	ureter
urethr/o	urethra
ur/o, urin/o	urine
vesic/o	bladder

Suffix	Definition
-al	pertaining to
-ectomy	surgical excision, removal
-gram	a record or image
-graphy	recording process
-logy	study or science of
-lysis	loosen, dissolve
-pexy	surgical fixation, suspension
-plasty	surgical repair
-rrhaphy	suturing
-scopy	process of viewing
-stomy	surgical creation of an opening
-tomy	incision, to cut
-tripsy	surgical crushing

KEY TERMS A–Z

blood urea nitrogen
blud * yoo REE ah

11.50 A clinical lab test that measures urea concentration in a sample of blood as an indicator of kidney function is **blood urea nitrogen**. Abbreviated **BUN**, elevated values of _____ _____ _____ for an extended length of time support a diagnosis of end-stage kidney disease (Frame 11.26).

creatinine
kree ATT ih neen

11.51 The protein **creatinine** is a normal component of urine and is a by-product of muscle metabolism. It may be measured in a urine sample. Elevated levels of _____ indicate a problem during kidney filtration, suggesting kidney disease.

cystectomy
(siss TEK toh mee)

11.52 Because the combining form *cyst/o* means "bladder, sac" and the suffix *-ectomy* means "surgical excision, removal," the surgical removal of the urinary bladder is called _____. The constructed form of this term is cyst/ectomy.

cystogram
SISS toh gram

11.53 An x-ray procedure producing an image of the urinary bladder with injection of a contrast medium or dye is called **cystography** (siss TOG rah fee). This constructed term is written cyst/o/graphy. The x-ray image is called a _____ (■ Figure 11.11). If the procedure includes the ureters, it is called a **cystoureterography** (SISS toh yoo REE ter OG rah fee), and the image obtained is a **cystoureterogram** (SISS toh yoo REE ter oh gram). The constructed form of the term *cystoureterography* is cyst/o/ureter/o/graphy. If the procedure includes the urethra, it is a **cystourethrography** (SISS toh yoo reeth ROG rah fee), and the image is a **cystourethrogram** (SISS toh yoo REE throh gram). The constructed form of the term is cyst/o/urethr/o/gram. In a **voiding** _____ (**VCUG**), x-rays are taken before, during, and after urination to observe bladder function.

cystourethrogram

■ **Figure 11.11**
Cystogram. A cystogram is an x-ray photograph of the pelvic cavity to examine the urinary bladder (visible in white in this example). The round shape of the bladder shown here is due to its maximum volume of stored urine (the bladder flattens when empty).
Source: Santibhavank P/Shutterstock.

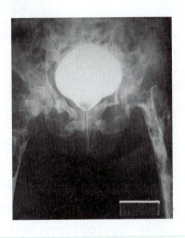

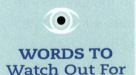

WORDS TO Watch Out For

-graphy or -gram?
Remember that the suffix *-graphy* means "a recording process," whereas the suffix *-gram* means "a record or image." In each of these procedures, switching the suffix from *-graphy* to *-gram* creates the term that refers to the *record* that is a result of the *recording process*.

cystolithotomy
siss toh lith OTT oh mee
cyst/o/lith/o/tomy

11.54 A procedure in which an incision is made through the urinary bladder wall to remove a stone is called _____. The constructed form of this term includes five word parts: _____/___/_____/___/_____.

cystoplasty
SISS toh plass tee

11.55 Surgical repair of the urinary bladder is a procedure called _____. The constructed form of this term is cyst/o/plasty, which reveals three word parts.

cystorrhaphy
sist OR ah fee

11.56 Suturing the urinary bladder wall is a procedure called _____. The constructed form of the term is cyst/o/rrhaphy, which literally means "suturing bladder."

cystoscopy

siss TOSS koh pee

11.57 A procedure using a modified endoscope to view the interior of the urinary bladder is known as _____. The instrument is inserted through the urinary meatus and urethra to enter the bladder cavity (■ Figure 11.12). The constructed form of this term is cyst/o/scopy. The **cystoscope** may also be used as a surgical instrument.

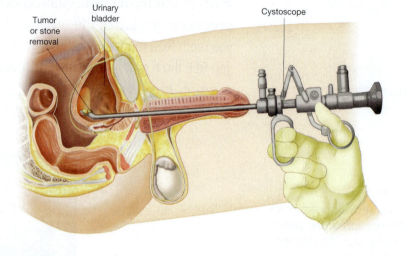

■ **Figure 11.12**
Cystoscopy. In this procedure, a specialized endoscope with a rigid tube, known as a cystoscope, is used to view the internal environment of the urinary bladder. As shown, the cystoscope may be outfitted to include surgical devices to remove tumors or stones.

cystostomy

siss TOSS toh mee

11.58 Recall that the suffix -*stomy* means "surgical creation of an opening." The surgical creation of an artificial opening into the urinary bladder is a procedure called _____. The most common application of this procedure is a **suprapubic cystostomy**, in which the incision is made just above the pubic bone and a catheter (see Frame 11.85) is inserted through the skin to the urinary bladder (■ Figure 11.13). The catheter provides an alternate exit passageway for urine if the normal passageway through the urethra is blocked or the urethra is surgically removed. Cystostomy is a constructed term, cyst/o/stomy, and suprapubic is supra/pub/ic.

■ **Figure 11.13**
Cystostomy. An artificial opening is made through the urinary bladder wall during this procedure. The suprapubic cystostomy, illustrated here, includes the insertion of a catheter and a urine collection bag. It allows the bladder to drain of urine when an obstruction to normal urinary flow is present, such as a blockage in the urethra from calculi, congenital defects, swelling of the prostate (BPH), or cancer.

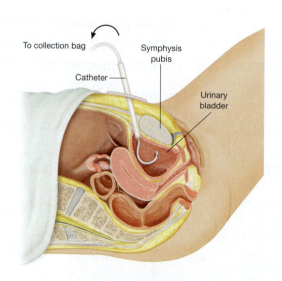

cystotomy siss TOTT oh mee	**11.59** The suffix *-tomy* means "incision" or "to cut." Therefore, the term _____ refers to an incision through the urinary bladder wall. It is also called **vesicotomy** (VESS ih KOTT oh mee) because both *cyst* and *vesic* are word roots meaning "bladder."
fulguration full guh RAY shun	**11.60** A surgical procedure that destroys living tissue with an electric current is called **fulguration**. _____ is commonly used to remove tumors and polyps from the interior wall of the urinary bladder.

(?) Did You KNOW

FULGURATION

Fulguration is derived from the Latin word *fulguratio*, which means "flash of lightning."

hemodialysis HEE moh dye AL ih siss	**11.61** The general term **dialysis** is a constructed word composed of two word parts: dia/lysis. It means "dissolving through" and refers to the movement of substances across a permeable membrane during the process of filtration. Also, *hem/o* is a combining form that means "blood." Combining these word parts forms the term _____, which is a procedure that pushes a patient's blood through permeable membranes within an instrument (■ Figure 11.14). It is performed to artificially remove nitrogenous wastes and excess ions that accumulate during normal body metabolism, temporarily replacing the function of kidney filtration for patients with kidney disease or kidney failure. *Hemodialysis* is a constructed term with four word parts: hem/o/dia/lysis.

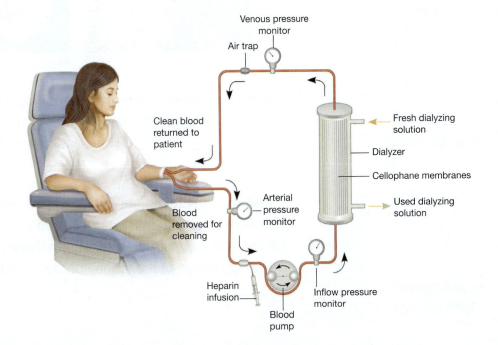

■ **Figure 11.14**
Hemodialysis. The process of hemodialysis replaces the kidney function of blood filtration by forcing blood from the patient through cellophane membranes, as shown in this schematic.

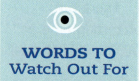

WORDS TO Watch Out For

A Misplaced Prefix?

Most prefixes appear in the very beginning of a term, but in the term *hemodialysis*, note that the prefix *dia-* appears after the combining form *hem/o*.

lithotripsy
LITH oh trip see

11.62 The suffix *-tripsy* means "surgical crushing." A surgical technique that applies concentrated sound waves to pulverize or dissolve stones into smaller pieces that may then pass with urine through the urethra is called _____. The constructed form of this term is lith/o/tripsy/. In the popular procedure **extracorporeal shock wave lithotripsy (ESWL)**, ultrasonic energy from an instrument outside of the body (hence the term *extracorporeal*, which means "pertaining to outside the body") is directed onto stones that are otherwise too large to pass through the urethra, pulverizing the stones into tiny particles that can pass with urine flow (■ Figure 11.15). It is a noninvasive technique and thereby avoids the risks of surgery.

■ **Figure 11.15**
Lithotripsy. (a) ESWL uses fluoroscopy (above the patient) to view progress. The stones are pulverized by ultrasonic shock waves from below the patient.
Photo Source: Carolina K. Smith MD/Shutterstock.
(b) Illustration of lithotripsy, during (left) and after (right) the procedure.
Source: AlexonIne/Shutterstock.

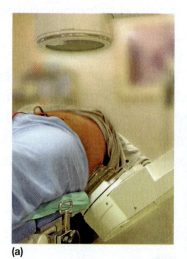
(a)

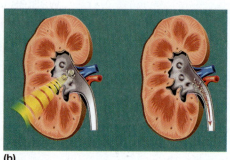
(b)

nephrectomy
neh FREK toh mee

11.63 Recall that one of the combining forms for kidney is *nephr/o*. A surgical procedure that removes a kidney is called _____. The constructed form of this term is nephr/ectomy.

nephrogram
NEFF roh gram

11.64 An x-ray technique producing an image of a kidney after injection of a contrast medium or dye is called **nephrography** (neh FROG rah fee). It is a constructed term with three word parts: nephr/o/graphy. The x-ray image of the kidney obtained in this procedure is called a _____.

nephrology neff ROL oh jee	**11.65** The medical field that studies and treats disorders associated with the kidneys is called _____. This constructed term is nephr/o/logy. A physician specializing in this field is a **nephrologist** (neff ROL oh jist).
nephrolysis neh FRALL ih siss	**11.66** The suffix -lysis means "loosen, dissolve." Combining it with the combining form for kidney, nephr/o, forms the constructed term _____. It is a surgical procedure during which abnormal adhesions are removed from a kidney, loosening the organ. The constructed form of this term is nephr/o/lysis.
nephropexy NEFF roh pek see	**11.67** The suffix that means "surgical fixation, suspension" is -pexy. Surgical fixation of a kidney is sometimes necessary if the kidney is abnormally loose within the abdominal cavity, such as in the condition nephroptosis or floating kidney (Frame 11.39). The procedure is called _____, and the constructed form of this term is nephr/o/pexy.
nephroscopy neh FROSS koh pee	**11.68** Remember that the suffix -scopy means "process of viewing." Therefore, visual examination of a kidney's interior may be performed in the procedure known as _____, during which a modified fiber-optic endoscope called a **nephroscope** (NEFF roh skope) is used.
nephrosonography neff roh son OG rah fee	**11.69** An ultrasound procedure that provides an image of a kidney for diagnostic analysis is known as **nephrosonography**. _____ is a constructed term that contains five word parts, nephr/o/son/o/graphy.
nephrostomy neff ROSS toh mee nephr/o/stomy	**11.70** A procedure that surgically creates an opening through the body wall and into a kidney is called a _____. It is usually established to allow a catheter to be inserted from the exterior to the renal pelvis for urine drainage and is also called a **pyelostomy** (PYE ell OSS toh mee). The constructed form of nephrostomy is _____/__/_____, and the term pyelostomy is pyel/o/stomy.

nephrotomogram
NEH froh toh moh gram

11.71 A diagnostic procedure that images the kidney with sectional x-rays to observe internal details of kidney structure is known as **nephrotomography** (NEH froh toh MOG rah fee). The suffix that means "a record or image" is *-gram*, so the image obtained from this procedure is a _____. *Nephrotomography* is a constructed term with five word parts: nephr/o/tom/o/graphy, which literally means "recording process of cut kidney."

peritoneal dialysis
pair ih TOH nee al * dye
AL ih siss

11.72 You learned about hemodialysis in Frame 11.61. A similar procedure is **peritoneal dialysis**, which also processes fluids and electrolytes by artificial filtration as a cleansing treatment to compensate for kidney failure. Thus, _____ _____ removes toxins and other wastes as a replacement for kidney function. In contrast to hemodialysis, peritoneal dialysis processes fluids from the peritoneal cavity rather than directly from the bloodstream. The constructed form of this term is peritone/al dia/lysis.

pyelogram
PYE ell oh gram

11.73 A **pyelogram** is an x-ray image of the renal pelvis. It is a useful diagnostic tool that is often used to examine kidney-related disorders. In obtaining an image called a **retrograde** _____, the procedure involves injection of contrast medium into the ureter using a cystoscope. As the x-ray is taken, it moves in a direction opposite from the norm (retrograde means "opposite of normal"). Retrograde pyelogram is abbreviated **RP**, and an example is shown in ■ Figure 11.16. In an **intravenous pyelogram**, iodine is used as the contrast medium and is injected into the bloodstream. It is abbreviated **IVP**.

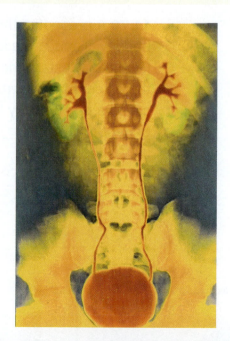

■ **Figure 11.16**
Retrograde pyelogram. A contrast medium is injected into the ureter using a cystoscope, and the x-ray moves in a direction opposite from the norm, producing the image that is shown. It serves to highlight the internal features of the renal pelvis and ureters.
Source: CNRI/Science Source.

pyelolithotomy
pye ell oh lith OTT oh mee

11.74 A kidney stone may sometimes form within the renal pelvis. A surgery performed to remove the stone from the renal pelvis involves an incision into the kidney and is called a **pyelolithotomy**. The constructed form of the term _____ is pyel/o/lith/o/tomy, which literally means "to cut stone from renal pelvis."

pyeloplasty
PYE ell oh PLASS tee

11.75 The suffix that means "surgical repair" is *-plasty*. Surgical repair of the renal pelvis is a procedure called _____. The constructed form of this term is pyel/o/plasty.

renal transplant

11.76 The replacement of a dysfunctional kidney with a donor kidney is a surgery called _____ _____ (■ Figure 11.17). The donated kidney is often provided by a close relative with a similar genetic makeup to reduce the risk of organ rejection. Unless the failed kidney is a source of infection or is cancerous, the surgical team may leave it in the body (the illustration shows it removed, indicating that the failed kidney was a potential source of disease in this case).

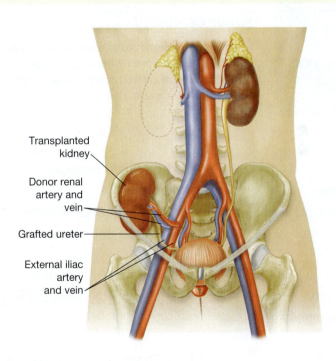

Transplanted kidney

Donor renal artery and vein

Grafted ureter

External iliac artery and vein

■ **Figure 11.17**
Renal transplant. A transplanted kidney is placed within the pelvic cavity below the location of the kidney requiring replacement.

renography
ree NOG rah fee

11.77 An examination that uses nuclear medicine by IV (intravenous) injection of radioactive material into the patient's kidneys is called **renography**. The radioactive materials highlight internal details of the kidney during the _____. The constructed form of this term is ren/o/graphy. The record is called a **renogram** (REE noh gram).

specific gravity	**11.78** The measurement of the density of substances in a liquid compared to water is called **specific gravity (SG)**. The _____ _____ of a urine sample helps to reveal the efficiency of renal filtration and the reabsorption of water.
ureterectomy yoo REE ter EK toh mee	**11.79** The suffix that means "surgical excision, removal" is *-ectomy*. The surgical removal of a ureter is called _____. The constructed form of this term is ureter/ectomy.
ureterostomy yoo REE ter OSS toh mee **ureterotomy** yoo ree ter OTT oh mee	**11.80** The surgical creation of an external opening from the ureter to the body surface is called _____. It is performed to provide an alternate exit route for urine that bypasses the urethra. The procedure includes an incision into the wall of the ureter, called _____. Both terms are constructed of three word parts: ureter/o/stomy, and ureter/o/tomy.

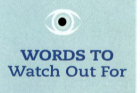

WORDS TO Watch Out For

-stomy or -tomy?

The suffix *-stomy* means "surgical creation of an opening," whereas *-tomy* means "incision, to cut." The two suffixes represent two different surgical techniques. In general, an incision is a cut through tissue, whereas the surgical creation of an opening establishes an artificial window into the body, usually for the drainage of fluids or waste. Can you see how the small addition of an *s* makes a big difference in meaning?

urethropexy yoo REE throh pek see	**11.81** Surgical fixation of the urethra is a procedure called **urethropexy**. A _____ is often performed to correct stress incontinence (Frame 11.32). It is a constructed term, as shown when it is written urethr/o/pexy.
urethroplasty yoo REE throh plass tee	**11.82** Surgical repair of the urethra is a procedure called _____. This constructed term is urethr/o/plasty.
urethrostomy yoo REE THROSS toh mee **urethrotomy** yoo ree THROTT oh mee	**11.83** The surgical creation of an opening through the urethra is called _____. It is performed to provide an alternate exit route for urine. The procedure includes an incision into the wall of the urethra, called _____. Both terms are constructed of three word parts: urethr/o/stomy, and urethr/o/tomy.

11.84 A combination of clinical lab tests that are performed on a urine specimen is called **urinalysis** (▪ Figure 11.18). The term _____ is a constructed term with two word parts, shown as urin/alysis, in which *alysis* is a shortened form of the word *analysis* to make the term easier to pronounce. Urinalysis literally means "analysis of urine." Abbreviated **UA**, it provides information for diagnostic purposes on the quality and composition of urine, including specific gravity; creatinine, glucose, and protein levels; and the abnormal presence of red blood cells, white blood cells, and pus.

urinalysis

YOO rin AL ih siss

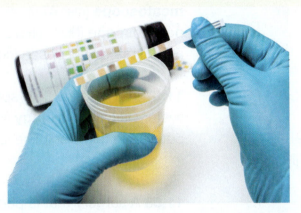

▪ **Figure 11.18**
Urinalysis. During a simple urinalysis, a stick with colored blocks is dipped into a urine specimen. Color changes in the blocks are noted and compared to a known standard.
Source: Alexander Raths/ Shutterstock.

11.85 A **catheter** is a flexible tube that is inserted into an opening of the body to transport fluids in or out. A **urinary catheter** is usually inserted through the urethra to enter the urinary bladder and is often used to drain urine from a patient who is immobile. The process of inserting the urinary catheter is called _____ _____. It is illustrated in ▪ Figure 11.19.

urinary catheterization

YOO rih nair ee * KATH eh ter ih ZAY shun

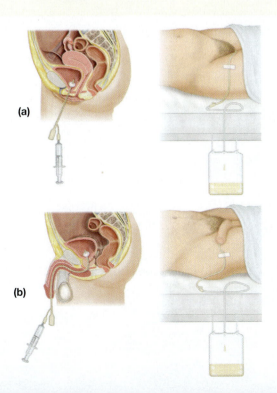

(a)

(b)

▪ **Figure 11.19**
Urinary catheterization. The procedure involves the insertion of a flexible tube, or catheter, through the urethra and into the urinary bladder. Voiding occurs through the catheter and is collected in a plastic bag adjacent to the patient. (a) Catheterization of a female patient. (b) Catheterization of a male patient.

Did You KNOW

CATHETER

The term *catheter* is from the Greek word *katheter*, which means "to send down," so named because it is a flexible tube that lets urine down from the urinary bladder.

urinary endoscopy YOO rih nair ee * ehn DOSS koh pee	**11.86** The procedural use of an endoscope to observe internal structures of the urinary system is generally known as _____ _____. A specialized endoscope is associated with each urinary organ, including a **meatoscope** (mee AT oh skope) for inserting into the urinary meatus, a **nephroscope** (NEFF roh skope) for viewing a kidney, and a **cystoscope** (SISS toh skope) for observing the interior of the urinary bladder.
urologist yoo RAHL oh jist	**11.87** The medical field specializing in disorders of the urinary system is called **urology** (yoo RAHL oh jee). A physician who treats patients in this discipline is called a _____.
vesicourethral vess ih koh yoo REE thral	**11.88** A surgery that is performed to stabilize the position of the urinary bladder is called **vesicourethral suspension**. The term _____ contains four word parts: vesic/o/urethr/al. It is performed to treat stress incontinence (Frame 11.32).

PRACTICE: Treatments, Procedures, and Devices of the Urinary System

Break the Chain

Analyze these medical terms:

   a) Separate each term into its word parts; each word part is labeled for you (**p** = prefix, **r** = root, **cf** = combining form, and **s** = suffix).

   b) For the Bonus Question, write the requested definition in the blank that follows.

1. a) cystography   _____/___/_____
                               cf   s

    b) *Bonus Question*: What is the definition of the suffix? _____

2. a) cystolithotomy   _____/___/_____/___/_____
                               cf   cf   s

    b) *Bonus Question*: What is the definition of the suffix? _____

3. a) lithotripsy   _____/___/_____
                               cf   s

    b) *Bonus Question*: What is the definition of the combining form? _____

4. a) hemodialysis   _____/___/_____/_____
                               cf   p   s

    b) *Bonus Question*: What is the definition of the prefix? _____

5. a) cystorrhaphy   _____/___/_____
                               cf   s

    b) *Bonus Question*: Does this term contain a prefix? _____

6. a) nephrolysis   _____/___/_____
                               cf   s

    b) *Bonus Question*: What is the definition of the suffix? _____

7. a) nephrogram   _____/___/_____
                               cf   s

    b) *Bonus Question*: What is the meaning of the suffix? _____

8. a) nephrotomography   _____/___/_____/___/_____
                               cf   cf   s

    b) *Bonus Question*: What is the definition of the *first* combining form? _____

9. a) ureterostomy   _____/___/_____
                               cf   s

    b) *Bonus Question*: What is the definition of the suffix? _____

The Right Match

Match the term on the left with the correct definition on the right.

_____	1. urinalysis	a.	removal of a kidney
_____	2. extracorporeal shock wave lithotripsy	b.	creates a new opening through the renal pelvis to the outside
_____	3. nephrectomy	c.	stabilizes the position of the urinary bladder
_____	4. nephrostomy	d.	evaluates urine composition
_____	5. vesicourethral suspension	e.	technique that uses ultrasonic energy to crush stones
_____	6. fulguration	f.	test for protein levels in a urine sample
_____	7. renal transplant	g.	test for water concentration in urine
_____	8. blood urea nitrogen	h.	electric current that kills unwanted tissue
_____	9. peritoneal dialysis	i.	test for urea in the blood
_____	10. creatinine	j.	insertion of a tube to drain urine
_____	11. specific gravity	k.	surgical procedure replacing a diseased kidney
_____	12. urinary catheter	l.	blood filtration using the peritoneal cavity

Abbreviations of the Urinary System

The abbreviations that are associated with the urinary system are summarized here. Study these abbreviations and review them in the exercise that follows.

Abbreviation	Definition	Abbreviation	Definition
AKI	acute kidney injury	IVP	intravenous pyelogram
BUN	blood urea nitrogen	RP	retrograde pyelogram
cath	catheter, catheterization	SG	specific gravity
ESKD	end-stage kidney disease	UA	urinalysis
ESWL	extracorporeal shock wave lithotripsy	UTI	urinary tract infection
HD	hemodialysis	VCUG	voiding cystourethrogram

PRACTICE: Abbreviations

Fill in the blanks with the abbreviation or the complete medical term.

Abbreviation	Medical Term
1. UA	_____
2. _____	retrograde pyelogram
3. cath	_____
4. _____	voiding cystourethrogram
5. IVP	_____
6. _____	urinary tract infection
7. HD	_____
8. _____	end-stage kidney disease
9. SG	_____
10. _____	acute kidney injury
11. ESWL	_____
12. _____	blood urea nitrogen

CHAPTER REVIEW

Word Building

Construct medical terms from the following meanings. (Some are built from word parts, some are not.) The first question has been completed as an example.

1. inability to pass urine
    _____ **an**uria

2. presence of bacteria in the urine
    bacteri _____

3. presence of a stone in the bladder
    _____lith

4. inflammation of a kidney
    nephr _____

5. presence of blood in the urine
    _____uria

6. protrusion of a ureter
    uretero _____

7. involuntary release of urine
    _____uresis

8. presence of stones in the kidney
    nephro _____

9. fixation of an abnormally mobile kidney
    nephro _____

10. surgical creation of an opening into the renal pelvis
    _____stomy

11. surgical repair of the urethra
    urethro _____

12. incision into the ureter wall
    uretero _____

13. x-ray image of the urinary bladder
    cysto _____

14. x-ray technique imaging a kidney
    nephro _____

15. x-ray image of the renal pelvis with iodine
    intravenous _____gram

16. an endoscope modified to view a kidney
    _____scope

17. lab test measuring urea in the blood
    blood urea _____(BUN)

18. urine test that includes multiple parameters
    urin _____

Define the Combining Form

In the space provided, write the definition of the combining form, followed by one example of the combining form used to build a medical term in Chapter 11.

	Definition	**Use in a Term**
1. ur/o	_____	_____
2. pyr/o	_____	_____
3. ren/o	_____	_____
4. pyel/o	_____	_____
5. cyst/o	_____	_____
6. nephr/o	_____	_____
7. sten/o	_____	_____
8. ureter/o	_____	_____

Complete the Labels

Complete the blank labels in ■ Figures 11.20 and ■ 11.21 by writing the labels in the spaces provided.

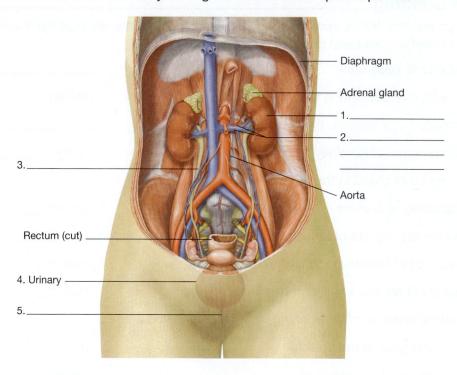

Figure 11.20
Organs of the urinary system.

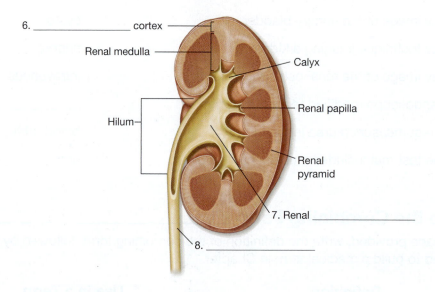

Figure 11.21
The kidney.

1. _____

2. _____

3. _____

4. _____

5. _____

6. _____

7. _____

8. _____

MEDICAL REPORT EXERCISES

Sylvia Hernandez-Brown

Read the following medical report, then answer the questions that follow.

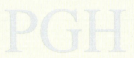

PEARSON GENERAL HOSPITAL

5500 University Avenue, Metropolis, New York
Phone: (211) 594-4000 • Fax (211) 594-4001

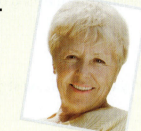

Medical Consultation: Urology

Date: 08/12/2017

Patient: Sylvia Hernandez-Brown

Patient ID: 123456

Dob: 5/20/1954   **Age**: 63   **Sex**: Female

Allergies: NKDA

Provider: Joshua Ryan, MD

Subjective:

"I have pain in my lower back on both sides all of the time for the past 3 months and getting worse lately. I also tire more easily than in the past. I feel achy, like I have the flu, and don't feel much like eating."

63 y/o female, is 40 lbs overweight and has had type 2 DM for 10 years, using oral glucophage (metformin) 1,000 mg/day. She has visited the clinic four times during the past 5 years with mild UTIs, successfully treated with antibiotics.

Objective:

Vital Signs: **T**: 100.2°F; **P**: 81; **R**: 22; **BP**: 145/105

Ht: 5'4"

Wt: 165 lb

General Appearance: Skin with pallor, mild diaphoresis. Mild edema of the face around the eyes and neck.

Heart: Rate at 81 bpm. Heart sounds with auscultation appear normal.

Lungs: Clear without signs of disease.

AbD: Bowel sounds normal all four quadrants.

MS: Joints and muscles symmetric. No swelling, masses, or deformity.

Lab: Blood positive for urea. Urinalysis with albumin high, mild hematuria.

Assessment:

Uremia, albuminuria, hematuria. Nephrotomography and nephroscopy confirm bilateral polycystic kidney disease resulting in ESKD.

Plan:

Admit STAT for hemodialysis; repeat twice weekly. Place on waiting list for renal transplant.

Photo Source: Gravicapa/Shutterstock.

Comprehension Questions

1. What patient complaints point to the kidneys as the source of the disease? _____

_____

_____

2. Describe the meaning of the term *nephrotomography*. _____

_____

_____

3. Why would a urologist order dialysis for a patient prior to renal transplant surgery? _____

_____

_____

Case Study Questions

The following Case Study provides further discussion regarding the patient in the medical report. Fill in the blanks with the correct terms. Choose your answers from the following list of terms. (Note that some terms may be used more than once.)

albuminuria	nephromegaly	polycystic kidney	renal transplant
hematuria	nephroscopy	disease	urinalysis
hemodialysis	nephrotomography	pyelonephritis	

A 63-year-old female, Sylvia Hernandez-Brown, was admitted to urology by her general practitioner following

a physical exam that included blood tests revealing abnormally high levels of urea in the blood. A generalized

test of urine composition, or (a) _____, revealed elevated levels of albumin, a symptom known

as (b) _____, and the presence of red blood cells in the urine, or (c) _____.

Following diagnostic exams that included an x-ray technique imaging the kidney by sections called

(d) _____, and an endoscopic evaluation of the kidney known as (e) _____,

the attending physician concluded a diagnosis of enlargement of both kidneys, or (f) _____,

caused by multiple cysts, or (g) _____ _____ _____, which

had resulted in inflammation of the renal pelvis and nephrons, or (h) _____, and renal failure.

Artificial filtration of the blood, or (i) _____, was ordered, due to a growing insufficiency to

reduce blood metabolites (metabolic wastes). The patient was placed on a waiting list for a replacement

kidney or a (j) _____ _____.

Del Hamilton

For a greater challenge, read the following medical report and answer the critical thinking questions that follow from the information in the chapter.

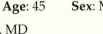

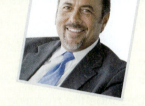

PEARSON GENERAL HOSPITAL

5500 University Avenue, Metropolis, New York
Phone: (211) 594-4000 • Fax (211) 594-4001

Medical Consultation: Urology   **Date**: 10/19/2017

Patient: Del Hamilton   **Patient ID**: 123456

Dob: 3/10/1972   **Age**: 45   **Sex**: Male   **Allergies**: NKDA

Provider: Karl Moss, MD

Subjective:

"I feel pain in the lower back that radiates to the left side, which comes and goes. It's been bothering me for about 2 months. I'm also experiencing pain when I urinate, with a reduced urine flow, which has been making me get up several times a night to go."

45 y/o male with complaints of dysuria, oliguria, and nocturia for the past 2 months. History shows type 2 DM for 2 years when obese at 270 lbs, but says he has recently lost 80 lbs on a high-protein diet. He is on oral metformin 1,500 mg/day. Father was diagnosed at 62 y/o with renal calculi and treated successfully with lithotripsy.

Objective:

Vital Signs: **T**: 98.6°F; **P**: 80; **R**: 21; **BP**: 132/90

Ht: 5'10"

Wt: 190 lb

General Appearance: Skin color healthy with no masses or discolorations.

Heart: Rate at 80 bpm. Heart sounds with auscultation appear normal.

Lungs: Clear without signs of disease.

AbD: Bowel sounds normal all four quadrants.

MS: Joints and muscles symmetric. No swelling, masses, or deformity.

Lab: Retrograde pyelogram positive for pelvic calculi, confirmed by nephrosonography.

Assessment:

Renal calculi in right renal pelvis; mild pyelonephritis

Plan:

Oral antibiotic therapy 2 weeks. Schedule for ESWL in 2 weeks. Referral to Nutrition for weight loss education.

Photo Source: Monkey Business Images/Shutterstock.

Comprehension Questions

1. What conditions other than the one diagnosed might have caused the reported symptoms?

_____

_____

_____

2. Do you think the prediagnosed condition of type 2 DM contributed to the condition of renal calculi?

_____

_____

_____

3. Describe the meaning of the terms *renal calculi* and *pyelonephritis*. _____

_____

_____

Case Study Questions

The following case study provides further discussion regarding the patient in the medical report. Fill in the blanks with the correct terms, using information in this chapter.

Del Hamilton, a 45-year-old male, was admitted to the hospital after presenting himself to the emergency

department in acute distress. He complained of intermittent pain in the left lumbar region, radiating to the

left flank. He also complained of pain and difficulty voiding, a symptom called (k) _____, with

the sensation of the need to void at night, known as (l) _____, which interrupted his sleep.

A generalized lab test of his urine sample, called a (m) _____, revealed no abnormalities.

A review of his family history revealed stones in the renal pelvis, called (n) _____. The

attending physician referred the patient to a (o) _____. The specialist in treating urinary

disorders, called a (p) _____, immediately prepared the patient for diagnostics that

included an x-ray technique that images the renal pelvis with an injected contrast medium, known as a

(q) _____ _____, followed with an endoscopic evaluation of the kidney called

a (r) _____. Both exams revealed the presence of stones in the renal pelvis, or renal calculi.

The stones were pulverized successfully using the (s) _____ procedure and passed the

next day.

MyLab Medical Terminology™

MyLab Medical Terminology is a premium online homework management system that includes a host of features to help you study. Registered users will find:

- A multitude of quizzes and activities built within the MyLab platform
- Powerful tools that track and analyze your results—allowing you to create a personalized learning experience
- Videos and audio pronunciations to help enrich your progress
- Streaming lesson presentations (Guided Lectures) and self-paced learning modules
- A space where you and your instructors can view and manage your assignments

gamete
GAMM eet

obstetrics
ob STET riks

12.2 The general function of the reproductive system is the creation of offspring, which occurs when the male gamete (sperm) unites successfully with a female _____ (ovum). The resulting fertilized egg is the origin of a new human life.

Once a new life has been conceived, the developing embryo enters into the segment of life called **prenatal** (pree NAY tal) **development**, which includes the changes in body form that occur throughout the mother's pregnancy until birth. The clinical field of **obstetrics** is focused on this period of life. _____ is often referred to by its abbreviation, **OB**. An **obstetrician** supports the mother during pregnancy, childbirth, and during the first month or so after childbirth.

12.3 Review the anatomy of the male and female reproductive systems by studying ■ Figure 12.1 and ■ Figure 12.2. Also, notice the anatomical changes that occur within a woman's body with a full-term pregnancy, shown in ■ Figure 12.3.

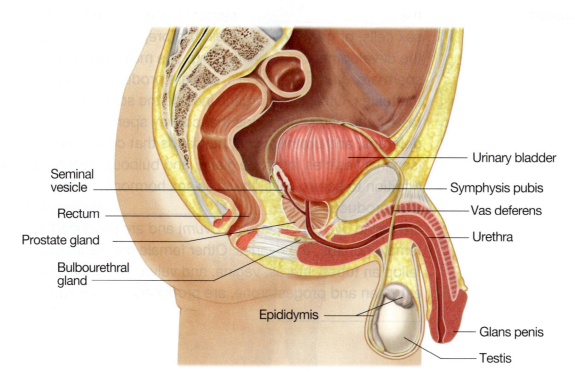

Seminal vesicle

Rectum

Prostate gland

Bulbourethral gland

Epididymis

Urinary bladder

Symphysis pubis

Vas deferens

Urethra

Glans penis

Testis

■ **Figure 12.1**
The male reproductive system.

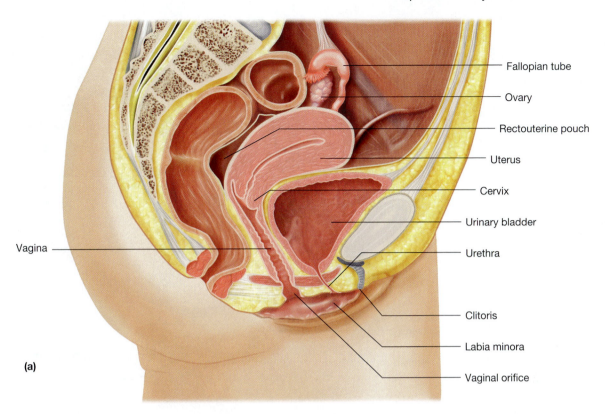

Fallopian tube

Ovary

Rectouterine pouch

Uterus

Cervix

Urinary bladder

Urethra

Clitoris

Labia minora

Vaginal orifice

Vagina

(a)

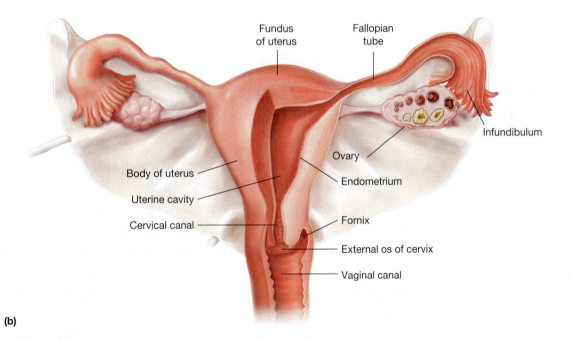

Fundus
of uterus

Fallopian
tube

Infundibulum

Ovary

Endometrium

Body of uterus

Uterine cavity

Fornix

Cervical canal

External os of cervix

Vaginal canal

(b)

■ **Figure 12.2**
The female reproductive system. (a) Sagittal section through the pelvis. (b) Top view of pelvic organs.

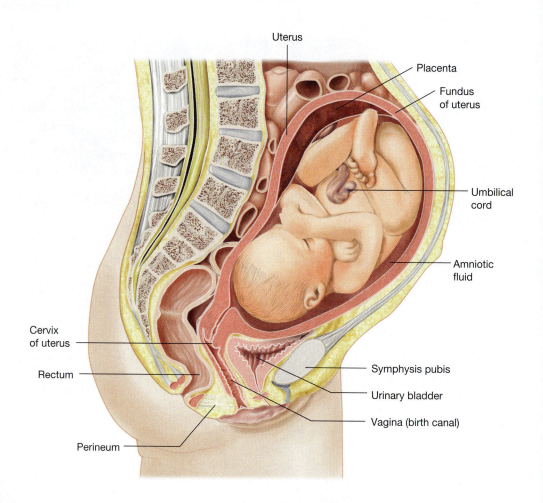

Uterus
Placenta
Fundus of uterus
Umbilical cord
Amniotic fluid
Cervix of uterus
Rectum
Perineum
Symphysis pubis
Urinary bladder
Vagina (birth canal)

■ **Figure 12.3**
A normal full-term pregnancy.

Medical Terms for the Reproductive System and Obstetrics

reproductive

urologist
  yoo RAHL oh jist
gynecology
  GYE neh KALL oh jee

12.4 The medical field of **reproductive medicine** manages the health care of both the male and female _____ systems. Because the male urethra is responsible for transporting both urine and semen, diseases of the male reproductive system are usually treated within the field of **urology** (yoo RAHL oh jee) by a _____. Diseases of the female reproductive system are generally treated by a physician called a **gynecologist** (gye neh KAHL oh jist), who specializes in the field of _____. In both sexes, reproductive diseases are often diagnosed initially during a physical examination. The diseases that require confirmation or an internal evaluation may be further analyzed using the noninvasive procedures of MRI, CT scan, or ultrasound imaging.

pathogens

sexually transmitted

12.5 The reproductive systems of the male and female are subject to infections, tumors, injury, endocrine disorders, and inherited diseases. For many people, the most common threat to health is the exposure to _____ during sexual contact. Although the reproductive tract is lined with a protective mucous membrane, certain bacteria, viruses, fungi, and protozoa can gain entry into the bloodstream directly or by way of breaks in the mucosal lining. Once established, these pathogens may spread throughout the body. Most _____ _____ **infections (STIs)**, formerly called *sexually transmitted diseases (STDs)* or *venereal diseases*, infect the body in this manner. Thus, STIs are infections acquired during intimate physical contact that occurs during sexual intercourse or other sexual activities. The most common forms of STIs are described in this chapter.

12.6 In the following sections, you will study the prefixes, combining forms, and suffixes that combine to build the medical terms of the reproductive system and obstetrics.

Signs and Symptoms of the Male Reproductive System

Here are the word parts that commonly apply to the signs and symptoms of the male reproductive system and are covered in the following section. Note that the word parts are color-coded to help you identify them: prefixes are yellow, combining forms are red, and suffixes are blue.

Prefix	Definition
a-	*without, absence of*

Combining Form	Definition
balan/o	*glans penis*
olig/o	*few in number*
orchi/o, orchid/o	*testis*
prostat/o	*prostate gland*
sperm/o	*seed, sperm*
test/o	*testis*
urethr/o	*urethra*
zo/o	*animal, living*

Suffix	Definition
-algia	*condition of pain*
-ia	*condition of*
-itis	*inflammation*
-rrhea	*discharge*

KEY TERMS A–Z

aspermia
ah SPER mee ah

12.7 Normally, male semen is a mixture of sperm cells and glandular secretions (from the prostate gland, seminal vesicles, and bulbourethral glands) released during ejaculation. In some cases, the fluid released during an ejaculation is a watery fluid that lacks sperm. This abnormality establishes a sign of male infertility and is known as _____. The constructed form of this term is a/sperm/ia, which literally means "condition of without seed."

azoospermia AY zoh oh SPER mee ah a/zo/o/sperm/ia	**12.8** The absence of living sperm in semen is called **azoospermia** and is another sign of infertility. The term _____ literally means "condition of without living seed." This constructed term has five word parts and is shown as __/____/__/_____/____.
balanorrhea BAL ah noh REE ah	**12.9** The combining form for the distal end of the penis, known as the glans penis, is *balan/o*. Recall that the suffix *-rrhea* means "discharge." Therefore, an abnormal condition of discharge from the glans is called _____, which is a symptom of the sexually transmitted infection called *gonorrhea* (Frame 12.133). Balanorrhea is a constructed term, balan/o/rrhea.
chancres SHANG kerz	**12.10** The sexually transmitted infection syphilis (Frame 12.136) may be diagnosed by the presence of small ulcers on the skin or mucous membranes, which are called **chancres**. The term _____ is a French word meaning "cancer," although syphilitic chancres are not a form of cancer.
oligospermia all ih goh SPER mee ah	**12.11** An abnormally low sperm count is the most common sign of male infertility. Combining the word part that means "few in number," *olig/o*, with the word parts meaning "condition of sperm," the term that results is the condition _____. It is a constructed term that can be represented as olig/o/sperm/ia.
papilloma pap ih LOH mah	**12.12 Papillomas** are wartlike lesions on the skin and mucous membranes. A _____ is a sign of infection by the sexually transmitted human papillomavirus (Frame 12.135), abbreviated **HPV**, and the lesions are commonly called **genital warts**. HPV infection is preventable with vaccination and the use of condoms in protected sex.
prostatitis pross tah TYE tiss	**12.13** Inflammation of the prostate gland is called _____. It is usually a sign of either BPH (Frame 12.20) or prostate cancer (Frame 12.28). This constructed term is prostat/itis.
prostatorrhea PROSS tah toh REE ah	**12.14** An abnormal discharge from the prostate gland is known as _____. This is a constructed term, prostat/o/rrhea.
testalgia test ALL jee ah	**12.15** A suffix that means "condition of pain" is *-algia*. The condition of testicular pain is known as _____, which is written test/algia. It is also known as **orchialgia** (OR kee ALL jee ah) and **orchidalgia** (OR kid ALL jee ah) because *test/o*, *orchi/o*, and *orchid/o* are each combining forms that mean "testis."

urethritis

yoo ree THRYE tiss

12.16 Inflammation of the urethra is called _____.
It is a symptom of an irritation of the urethra, usually resulting from
a sexually transmitted infection or a urinary tract infection (UTI). The
constructed form of this term reveals two word parts: urethr/itis.

PRACTICE: Signs and Symptoms of the Male Reproductive System

The Right Match

Match the term on the left with the correct definition on the right.

_____ 1. chancres

_____ 2. balanorrhea

_____ 3. prostatitis

_____ 4. papillomas

_____ 5. azoospermia

a. discharge from the glans penis

b. inflammation of the prostate gland

c. absence of living sperm in semen

d. small ulcers as a sign of syphilis

e. wartlike lesions

Break the Chain

Analyze these medical terms:

a) Separate each term into its word parts; each word part is labeled for you (**p** = prefix, **r** = root,
cf = combining form, and **s** = suffix).

b) For the Bonus Question, write the requested definition in the blank that follows.

The first set has been completed as an example.

1. a) prostatorrhea   **_prostat/o/rrhea_**

                                    cf   s

    b) *Bonus Question*: What is the definition of the suffix? **_discharge_** _____

2. a) oligospermia   _____/___/_____/_____

                                    cf   r   s

    b) *Bonus Question*: What is the definition of the combining form? _____

3. a) testalgia   _____/_____

                                    r   s

    b) *Bonus Question*: What is the definition of the word root? _____

4. a) urethritis   _____/_____

                                    r   s

    b) *Bonus Question*: What is the definition of the suffix? _____

5. a) aspermia   _____/_____/_____

                                    p   r   s

    b) *Bonus Question*: What is the definition of the prefix? _____

epididymitis
ep ih did ih MY tiss

12.22 Inflammation of the epididymis is a condition called _____. The constructed form of this term is written epididym/itis. Recall that *orchi* means "testis." Therefore, when the epididymis and one or both testes are inflamed, the condition is known as **orchiepididymitis** (OR kee ep ih did ih MY tiss), which contains three word parts: orchi/epididym/itis. If the inflammation is limited to one or more testes, the term becomes **orchitis** (or KYE tiss). To observe its word part construction, it can be shown as orch/itis, and if the epididymis is included, orch/i/epididym/itis.

erectile dysfunction
ee REK tile * diss FUNK shun

12.23 Many men experience **erectile dysfunction** at some time in their life, which is the inability to achieve an erection sufficient to perform sexual intercourse. The term _____ _____ is abbreviated **ED** and is also known as **impotence** (IM poh tens). The word *impotent* is a Latin word that means "powerless." Failing health, certain drugs, fatigue, circulatory disorders, and diabetes mellitus can cause ED.

hydrocele
HIGH droh seel

12.24 Injury is the most frequent cause of **hydrocele**, which is a swelling of the scrotum caused by fluid accumulation. _____ is a constructed term containing three word parts, which are revealed when it is shown as hydr/o/cele.

Peyronie disease
pay ROHN ee

12.25 A hardness, or induration, of the erectile tissue within the penis is a condition known as **Peyronie disease**. _____ _____ can cause erectile dysfunction (Frame 12.23), especially if the induration is greater on one side to cause a curvature of the penis.

phimosis
figh MOH siss

12.26 A narrowing of the urethral opening sometimes occurs when the prepuce (foreskin) covers the distal end of the glans penis. It is a congenital condition known as **phimosis**, which is a Greek word that means "muzzling." When it interferes with urination, _____ is surgically corrected by removal of the prepuce in a circumcision (Frame 12.34). If the glans penis becomes strangulated, the condition is called **paraphimosis** (PAIR ah figh MOH siss) and must be surgically corrected immediately to avoid complications.

priapism
PRY ah pizm

12.27 Priapism is an abnormally persistent erection of the penis, often accompanied by pain and tenderness. The most common cause of _____ is a drug overdose. The term is derived from the Latin word *priapus*, which is a Roman scarecrow figure with an erect penis.

prostate cancer

PROSS tayt * KANN ser

12.28 The prostate gland is subject to a form of cancer commonly known as _____. Also called **prostatic carcinoma** (pro STAT ik * kar sih NOH mah), it increases the size of the prostate before it spreads into the pelvic region and beyond. Prostate cancer can often be felt as a hard nodule on the prostate during a digital rectal exam (Frame 12.35). The American Cancer Society predicts about 26,730 deaths from prostate cancer in 2017, and the average age at the time of diagnosis is roughly 66 years. Prostate cancer is illustrated in ■ Figure 12.6.

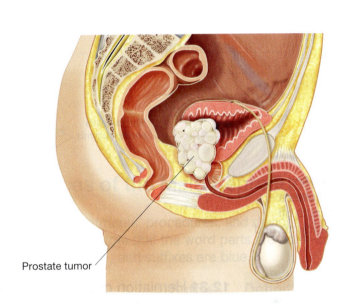

Prostate tumor

■ **Figure 12.6**

Prostate cancer. In this example, a large mass has grown into the urinary bladder. Most forms of prostate cancer are highly metastatic, sending tumor cells to the pelvic area and beyond, where they may form secondary tumor sites.

testicular carcinoma

tess TIK yoo ler * kar sih NOH mah

12.29 A cancer originating from the testis is known as _____. Its occurrence and mortality rate is highest among the 20- to 40-year-old age group. The most common form is called **seminoma** (sem ih NOH mah), which arises from sperm-forming cells and metastasizes to nearby lymph nodes. Although it strikes only 1 in 263 males, testicular carcinoma is the most common cancer diagnosis among young American men, with 8,850 new cases and 410 deaths expected in 2017, according to the American Cancer Society.

balanoplasty
BAL ah noh plass tee

12.33 The suffix that means "surgical repair" is *-plasty*. The surgical repair of the glans penis is therefore called _____.
The constructed form of this term is balan/o/plasty.

12.34 A common, routine procedure in many parts of the world is the removal of the prepuce. Known as **circumcision** after the circular cut that is made around the base of the glans penis, it is usually performed within hours after birth. Studies indicate the procedure reduces the risk of penile infections and sexually transmitted infections, which led the American Academy of Pediatrics (AAP) to release their official position in 2012, in which they state " . . . the health benefits of newborn circumcision outweigh the risks." Alternate procedures of _____ are illustrated in ■ Figure 12.8.

circumcision
ser kum SIH zhun

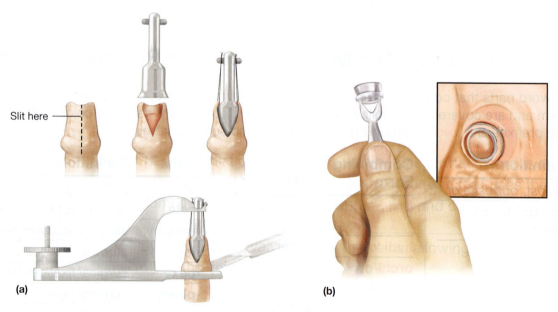

Slit here

(a)   (b)

■ **Figure 12.8**
Circumcision. Alternate procedures may be used with the common goal of removing the prepuce from the penis. (a) Use of the Yellen clamp, in which a cone is inserted over the glans and clamped in place, followed by the excision of the prepuce. (b) Use of the PlastiBell, which is inserted over the glans and the prepuce cut away. The plastic rim remains in place for 3–4 days until healing occurs, then falls away.

digital rectal examination

12.35 A **digital rectal examination** is a physical exam that involves the insertion of a finger into the rectum to feel the size and shape of the prostate gland through the wall of the rectum (■ Figure 12.9). A _____ _____ _____ is used to screen the patient for BPH (Frame 12.20) and prostate cancer (Frame 12.28), and is abbreviated **DRE**.

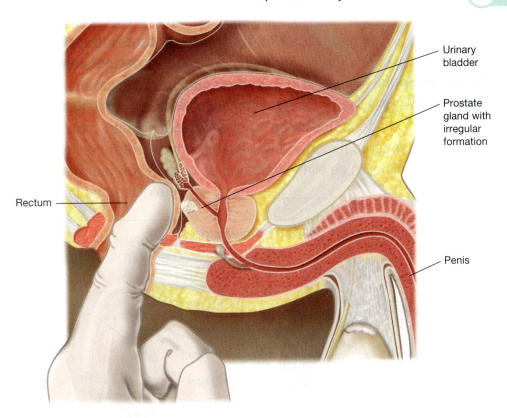

Urinary bladder

Prostate gland with irregular formation

Rectum

Penis

■ Figure 12.9
Digital rectal exam (DRE). The physician's index finger is inserted into the rectum and pressed against the prostate gland as a test for BPH and prostate cancer.

hydrocelectomy
HIGH droh see LEK toh mee

orchiectomy
OR kee EK toh mee

orchidopexy
OR kid oh PEK see

orchidoplasty
OR kid oh PLASS tee

orchid/o/tomy

12.36 Recall that the suffix *-ectomy* means "surgical excision, removal." The surgical removal of a **hydrocele** (Frame 12.24) is a procedure called _____. The constructed form of this term is written hydr/o/cel/ectomy.

12.37 The surgical removal of a testis is called _____ or, less commonly, **orchidectomy**. It may be required as treatment for testicular carcinoma (Frame 12.29). A bilateral **orchidectomy** is commonly called **castration** (kass TRAY shun). The term *castration* is derived from the Latin *castratio*, which means "a knife, instrument that cuts."

12.38 Surgical fixation of a testis is sometimes required to draw an undescended testis into the scrotum. The procedure is called _____, or **orchiopexy**, because the suffix *-pexy* means "surgical fixation, suspension." The constructed form of **orchidopexy** reveals three word parts: orchid/o/pexy.

12.39 A general term for a surgical repair of a testis is _____, or **orchioplasty**. An incision into the testis is a form of **orchidoplasty** and is called **orchidotomy** (OR kid OTT oh mee). The constructed form of the term *orchidotomy* reveals three word parts: _____/__/_____. Similar to other terms of the testis, an alternate term for orchidotomy is **orchiotomy** (OR kee OTT oh mee).

vasectomy

vas EK toh mee

12.45 A male can elect to become **sterile**, or unable to produce and ejaculate sperm, by undergoing a **vasectomy**. This constructed term literally means "surgical removal of vessel," where the "vessel" is the vas deferens. It is a simple, quick procedure in which the vas deferens is severed to block the flow of sperm during ejaculation (■ Figure 12.12). A _____ does not affect a man's ability to ejaculate (the ejaculated fluid is spermless semen) or his experience of sexual pleasure. *Vasectomy* is a constructed term with two word parts: vas/ectomy.

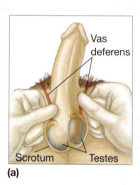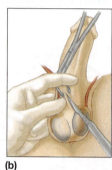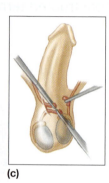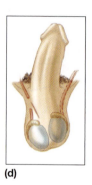

(a) (b) (c) (d)

■ **Figure 12.12**

Vasectomy. (a) Vas deferens is located within the spermatic cord on both sides. (b) A small incision is made through the scrotum, and an instrument is inserted that gently separates the vas deferens from other tissues of the spermatic cord. Once separated, the vas deferens is pulled out gently. (c) The vas deferens is cut and the exposed ends cauterized to close them. (d) The vas deferens is returned to the spermatic cord, tucked back into the scrotum, and a single suture closes the incision. The vas deferens on the other side is then cut in a duplicate procedure.

vasovasostomy

VAS oh vah SOSS toh mee

12.46 A surgery to reverse a vasectomy is known as a **vasovasostomy**. This constructed term uses the combining form for "vessel" twice and contains five word parts, as shown in vas/o/vas/o/stomy. A _____ involves the temporary creation of artificial openings and reconnection of the severed ends of the vas deferens to restore fertility.

vesiculectomy

veh SIK yoo LEK toh mee

12.47 A procedure to remove the seminal vesicles, which are male glands that contribute to the formation of semen, is called a _____. The constructed form of this term is vesicul/ectomy.

PRACTICE: Treatments, Procedures, and Devices of the Male Reproductive System

The Right Match

Match the term on the left with the correct definition on the right.

_____ 1. anti-impotence therapy

_____ 2. circumcision

_____ 3. penile implant

_____ 4. prostate-specific antigen

_____ 5. urology

_____ 6. vasectomy

_____ 7. prostatectomy

_____ 8. TURP

_____ 9. balanoplasty

a. the removal of the prepuce

b. blood protein that is measured in the PSA test

c. a collection of therapies that address erectile dysfunction

d. department that treats urinary tract problems

e. surgical insertion of a prosthesis to correct erectile dysfunction

f. surgical repair of the prepuce

g. elective form of male sterilization

h. surgical removal of the prostate gland

i. minimally invasive treatment of BPH

Break the Chain

Analyze these medical terms:

a) Separate each term into its word parts; each word part is labeled for you (**p** = prefix, **r** = root, **cf** = combining form, and **s** = suffix).

b) For the Bonus Question, write the requested definition in the blank that follows.

1. a) vasectomy   _____/_____
                              r   s

   b) *Bonus Question*: Which vessel does the word root refer to in this procedural term? _____

2. a) hydrocelectomy   _____/___/_____/_____
                                    cf   s   s

   b) *Bonus Question*: What is the definition of the *first* suffix? _____

3. a) orchidopexy   _____/___/_____
                                    cf   s

   b) *Bonus Question*: What is the definition of the combining form? _____

4. a) prostatectomy   _____/_____
                              r   s

   b) *Bonus Question*: What is the definition of the suffix? _____

5. a) vasovasostomy   _____/___/_____/___/_____
                                    cf   cf   s

   b) *Bonus Question*: What is the definition of the suffix? _____

oligomenorrhea ALL ih goh men oh REE ah	**12.57** An abnormally reduced discharge during menstruation may also be a sign of reproductive disease. It is called _____. The constructed form reveals two combining forms, as you can see in olig/o/men/o/rrhea.
pyosalpinx pye oh SAL pinks	**12.58** The combining form that means "pus" is *py/o*, and the combining form for fallopian tube is *salping/o*. As you read in the Words to Watch Out For box, when *salping/o* is used as a suffix, it is changed to -*salpinx*. Therefore, the discharge of pus from a fallopian tube is called _____. It is a sign of an infection. The constructed form is py/o/salpinx.

PRACTICE: Signs and Symptoms of the Female Reproductive System

Linkup

Link the word parts in the list to create the terms that match the definitions. You may use word parts more than once. Remember to add combining vowels when needed and that some terms do not use any combining vowel.

Prefix	Combining Form	Suffix
a-	colp/o	-algia
	hemat/o	-dynia
	hydr/o	-rrhagia
	leuk/o	-rrhea
	mast/o	-salpinx
	men/o	
	metr/o	
	salping/o	

Definition	Term
1. absence of menstrual discharge in a woman of childbearing age	_____
2. vaginal pain	_____
3. condition of pain in the breast	_____
4. profuse discharge during menstruation	_____
5. blood in a fallopian tube	_____
6. abnormally reduced menstrual	_____
7. discharge	_____
8. abnormal bleeding between periods	_____
9. white or yellow vaginal discharge	_____
10. abnormal pain during menstruation fluid accumulation within a fallopian tube	_____

Diseases and Disorders of the Female Reproductive System

Review some of the word parts that commonly apply to the diseases and disorders of the female reproductive system and are covered in the following section. Note that the word parts are color-coded to help you identify them: prefixes are yellow, combining forms are red, and suffixes are blue.

Prefix	Definition
a-	*without, absence of*
poly-	*excessive, over, many*
pre-	*to come before*

Combining Form	Definition
cervic/o	*neck, cervix*
colp/o	*vagina*
cyst/o	*bladder, sac*
fibr/o	*fiber*
hyster/o	*uterus*
lei/o	*smooth*
mast/o	*breast*
metr/i, metr/o	*uterus*
my/o	*muscle*
oophor/o	*ovary*
ovar/o	*ovary*
rect/o	*rectum*
salping/o	*trumpet, fallopian tube*
vagin/o	*sheath, vagina*
vesic/o	*bladder*
vulv/o	*vulva*

Suffix	Definition
-al	*pertaining to*
-atresia	*closure or absence of a normal body opening*
-cele	*hernia, swelling, protrusion*
-ia	*condition of*
-ic	*pertaining to*
-itis	*inflammation*
-oma	*tumor*
-osis	*condition of*
-pathy	*disease*
-ptosis	*drooping*
-s	*plural*

KEY TERMS A–Z

amastia
  ay MASS tee ah

poly/mast/ia

12.59 Recall that a combining form for breast is *mast/o*. The term that means "condition of without breast" is _____. Although the areola and nipple are present, the lack of breast tissue (mainly adipose tissue) results in this condition. In the condition **polymastia** (pahl ee MASS tee ah), the individual has more than two elevated areas on the chest or abdomen with areola and nipple. The constructed form of this term is _____/_____/___.

breast cancer

12.60 A malignant tumor arising from breast tissue is known as _____ _____. The most common form is called **infiltrating ductal carcinoma**, abbreviated **IDC** (■ Figure 12.13). According to the National Cancer Institute (a branch of the National Institutes of Health), with 252,710 new cases of breast cancer and 40,610 deaths expected in 2017, breast cancer is the second leading mortal cancer among women (lung cancer is first).

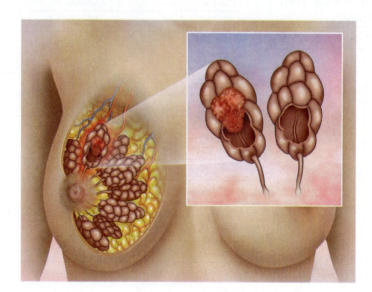

■ **Figure 12.13**
Breast cancer. Notice the tumor growing within a lactiferous gland (in red), a form of breast cancer called *infiltrating ductal carcinoma*.
Source: Alexilusmedical/ Shutterstock.

carcinoma in situ
  kar sih NOH mah * in *
  SIGH tyoo

12.61 In some women, cells of the cervix may undergo an abnormal change in a process called *dysplasia*, in which the cells begin to divide more rapidly to produce oddly shaped cells. The changing cells increase the risk of developing into a noninvasive form of precancer called **carcinoma in situ (CIS) of the cervix** (■ Figure 12.14). Although _____ _____ _____ of the cervix is not cervical cancer, it poses an elevated risk of developing into cancer.

■ **Figure 12.14**
Carcinoma in situ (CIS) of the cervix. Photograph of the cervix as seen during a gynecological exam. The reddish tissue is inflamed and indicative of carcinoma in situ of the cervix.
Source: Courtesy of the Centers for Disease Control and Prevention.

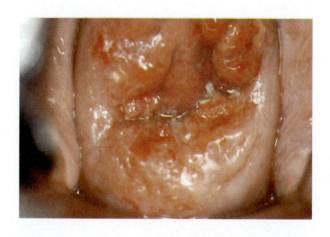

Did You KNOW

IN SITU

The term *in situ* (pronounced in * SIGH tyoo) is a Latin phrase that literally means "in site." Its use in modern medicine refers to confinement to a site of origin. *Carcinoma in situ* describes a tumor that is confined to its organ of origin, rather than a metastatic tumor in a secondary site. For example, a tumor that originates and remains in the cervix is *in situ*, while a tumor that originates from the cervix but sheds cells to other organs such as the lungs or stomach is metastatic (or malignant).

cervical cancer
SER vih kal * KANN ser

12.62 A malignant tumor of the cervix is known as _____ _____ (■ Figure 12.15). The most common form is a squamous cell carcinoma, arising from the epithelial cells lining the opening into the uterus. It is called **cervical intraepithelial neoplasia** (SER vih kal * in trah ep ih THEE lee al * nee oh PLAY zee ah), or **CIN**. A smaller percentage, about 20%, are adenocarcinomas, arising from the underlying glandular tissue. According to the National Cancer Institute, in 2016 an estimated 12,990 women were diagnosed and 4,120 deaths were reported. Because human papillomavirus (HPV; Frame 12.136) has been found to be the primary cause of CIN, it is hoped that the vaccines against HPV, Gardasil and Cervarix, will reduce the incidences of cervical cancer in the future.

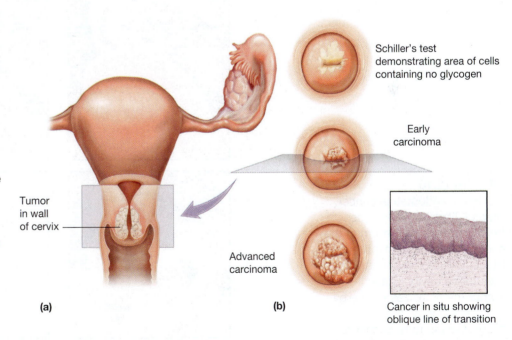

■ Figure 12.15
Cervical cancer (a) Top view of the uterus showing the presence of a tumor in the wall of the cervix. (b) Three successive stages in the development of cervical cancer, as seen through a gynecological exam. The inset shows a histological exam revealing the tumor and how it differs from normal tissue that borders it.

Schiller's test demonstrating area of cells containing no glycogen

Early carcinoma

Tumor in wall of cervix

Advanced carcinoma

(a)

(b)

Cancer in situ showing oblique line of transition

cervicitis
SER vih SIGH tiss

endo/cervic/itis

12.63 Inflammation of the cervix is a condition known as _____. The constructed form of this term is written cervic/itis. The most common form of cervicitis occurs when the inner lining of the cervix becomes inflamed. It is called **endocervicitis** (EHN doh ser vih SIGH tiss) because the prefix *endo-* means "within." Write the constructed form of this term here: _____/_____/_____.

cystocele
SISS toh seel

12.64 A protrusion of the urinary bladder against the wall of the vagina may occur if the attachments between the two organs weaken. It is called a **cystocele**, which is a constructed term with two word parts: cyst/o/cele. A large _____ may affect urinary bladder function. Similarly, a **rectocele** (REK toh seel) is a protrusion of the rectum against the wall of the vagina. The constructed form of this term is rect/o/cele.

endometrial cancer
ehn doh MEE tree al *
KANN ser

12.65 A malignant tumor arising from the endometrial tissue lining the uterus is called _____ _____. The four stages of endometrial cancer are illustrated in ■ Figure 12.16. Most endometrial cancers arise from the glandular cells of the endometrium and are therefore called adenocarcinomas (you might recall from Chapter 5 that *aden/o* means "gland"). According to the National Cancer Institute, 60,050 new cases and 10,470 deaths from endometrial cancer were reported in 2016.

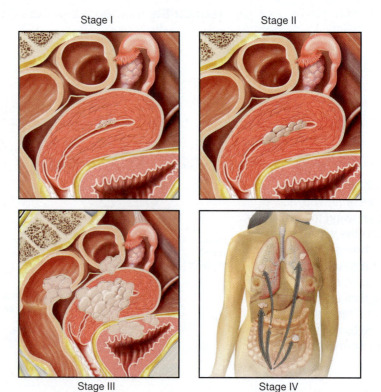

Stage I   Stage II

Stage III   Stage IV

■ **Figure 12.16**
Stages of endometrial cancer. Stage I: Mutated cells arise from glandular epithelium of the endometrium to form a tumor. Stage II: Tumor expands within the uterine cavity. Stage III: Tumor metastasizes to nearby organs. Stage IV: Metastasis progresses to form secondary tumors throughout the body.

endometriosis
EHN doh mee tree OH siss

12.66 The abnormal growth of endometrial tissue may occur throughout areas of the pelvic cavity, including the external walls of the uterus, fallopian tubes, urinary bladder, and even on the peritoneum. The condition is called **endometriosis**. This constructed term has four word parts: endo/metr/i/osis. It literally means "condition of within the uterus." Because endometrial tissue responds to hormonal changes by undergoing the cyclic bleeding and proliferation of menstruation, the unwanted tissue located outside the uterus that forms in _____ performs in the same manner, resulting in scarring, adhesions, and pelvic pain.

endometritis
EHN doh meh TRY tiss

12.67 Inflammation of the endometrium is a condition called _____. It is usually caused by bacterial infection. The constructed form of this term reveals three word parts: endo/metr/itis.

fibrocystic breast disease
figh broh SISS tik

12.68 In the condition **fibrocystic breast disease (FBD)**, one or more benign, fibrous cysts develop within the breast. _____ _____ _____ is an inherited condition that has no known association with breast cancer. The term *fibrocystic* is a constructed term with four word parts: fibr/o/cyst/ic.

fistulas
FISS tyoo lahs

12.69 In Latin, *fistula* means "pipe or flute." In medicine, a **fistula** is an abnormal tube-like passage from one organ or cavity to another (■ Figure 12.17). Two major types of vaginal _____ may occur. A **rectovaginal** (rek toh VAJ ih nal) **fistula** occurs between the vagina and rectum, and a **vesicovaginal** (vess ih koh VAJ ih nal) **fistula** is located between the urinary bladder and the vagina.

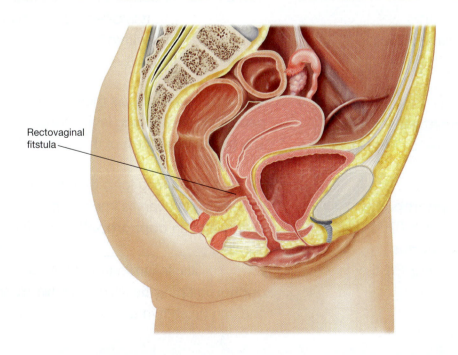

Rectovaginal fitstula

■ **Figure 12.17**
Rectovaginal fistula; an abnormal passageway between the rectum and vagina.

hysteratresia
hiss ter ah TREE zee ah

12.70 The suffix *-atresia* means "closure or absence of a normal body opening." Adding this suffix to the word root for uterus forms the term _____, which means a closure of the uterus. The closure results in an abnormal obstruction within the uterine canal that may interfere with childbirth. The constructed form of this term is hyster/atresia.

leiomyoma
lye oh my OH mah

12.71 The muscular wall of the uterus is the origin of benign tumors known as **leiomyomas**. Also known as **fibroid tumors** or **fibroids** because of their tough, fibrous structure, their presence can produce abnormal pain during menstruation (■ Figure 12.18). _____ is a constructed term with four word parts: lei/o/my/oma, which literally means "tumor of smooth muscle."

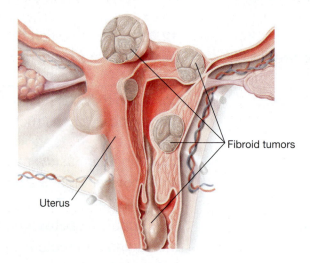

Fibroid tumors

Uterus

■ **Figure 12.18**
Fibroid tumors, or leiomyomas. Fibroids develop from the muscular wall of the uterus to form a variety of hard, round benign structures.

mastitis
mass TYE tiss

12.72 Inflammation of the breast is a condition known as _____. It is often caused by bacterial infection of the lactiferous ducts within breast tissue. The constructed form of this term is mast/itis.

mastoptosis
mass top TOH siss

12.73 The suffix *-ptosis* means "drooping." A breast that is abnormally pendulous or drooping is the condition known as _____. The constructed form of this term is mast/o/ptosis.

oophoropathy
oh OF or OPP ah thee
oophoritis
oh OF or EYE tiss

12.74 A combining form that means "ovary" is *oophor/o*. Any disease of an ovary is known as _____. An example of an **oophoropathy** is inflammation of an ovary, which is called _____. The constructed form of this term is oophor/itis. Inflammation of an ovary and fallopian tube is called **oophorosalpingitis** (oh OF or sal pin JYE tiss). This term is also constructed and can be shown as oophor/o/salping/itis to reveal its four word parts.

ovarian cancer

oh VAIR ee an * KANN ser

12.75 Aside from breast cancer (Frame 12.60), the most lethal form of reproductive cancer in women is **ovarian cancer**. Older women and women who have not given birth are at higher risk, and there is some evidence for a genetic link. The incidences of _____ _____ in 2016 included 22,280 new cases and 14,240 deaths, according to the National Cancer Institute.

ovarian cyst

oh VAIR ee an * sist

12.76 A cyst is a fluid-filled sac that forms within the body from mutated cells. An _____ _____ is a cyst on an ovary that is usually benign and asymptomatic, although in some cases it may cause pelvic pain and dysmenorrhea (Frame 12.50). A related and more serious disease of the ovaries is called **polycystic ovary syndrome (PCOS)**. Numerous ovarian cysts often develop in this condition, sometimes increasing the size of the ovary dramatically (see ■ Figure 12.19). _____ _____ _____ is a hormonal disturbance resulting from the excessive production of androgens, which are masculinizing hormones produced by the adrenal glands. The disorder is characterized by lack of ovulation (called _anovulation_), amenorrhea (Frame 12.48), infertility, and hirsutism (masculine hair growth). PCOS is extremely common, affecting roughly 1 in 10 women of childbearing age. If cyst development spreads into the fallopian tube, the condition is called **parovarian cyst** (par oh VAIR ee an * sist).

polycystic ovary syndrome

PALL ee SISS tik *OH var ee*SIN drohm

■ **Figure 12.19**
Polycystic ovary syndrome. Surgical removal of an ovary afflicted with polycystic ovary syndrome. The ovary is visible as the fist-sized mass during its removal from the pelvic cavity. Its size is abnormally enlarged, about 10 times the size of a normal ovary, and it has numerous cysts protruding from its outer wall.
Source: Chaikom/Shutterstock.

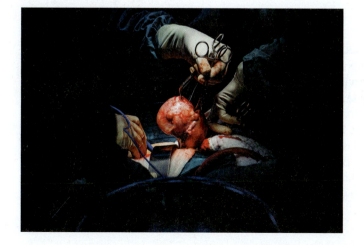

pelvic inflammatory disease	**12.77** An inflammation involving some or all of the female organs within the pelvic cavity is called **pelvic inflammatory disease**, abbreviated **PID**. It is often accompanied by pelvic pain and is usually caused by a bacterial infection originating from an STI that spreads from other organs. Complications of _____ _____ _____ include obstruction of the fallopian tubes and infertility.
premenstrual syndrome pre MEN stroo al * SIN drohm	**12.78 Premenstrual syndrome** is a collection of symptoms—including nervous tension, irritability, breast pain (mastalgia; Frame 12.54), edema, and headache—which usually occur during the 10 days preceding menstruation. _____ _____ is abbreviated **PMS**.
prolapsed uterus	**12.79** The uterus is suspended in the pelvic cavity by ligaments. If these ligaments weaken, often due to a congenital deformity or trauma, the uterus may become displaced to droop downward into the vagina. The condition is called **prolapsed uterus**, and in some cases it may even fall completely within the vagina (■ Figure 12.20). Another term for _____ _____ is **hysteroptosis** (HISS ter op TOH siss), which is a constructed term with three word parts: hyster/o/ptosis.

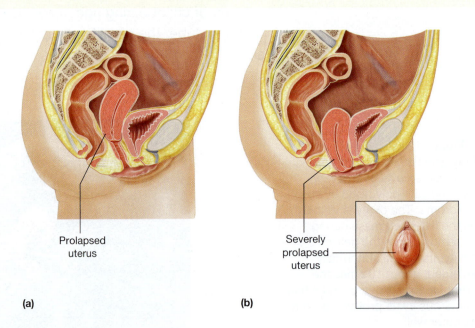

■ **Figure 12.20**
Prolapsed uterus. (a) A prolapse is the abnormal drop of the uterus into the vagina, representing the most common type of uterine displacement. It is usually caused by weakened uterine ligaments. (b) A severely prolapsed uterus may extend through the vaginal orifice, as shown.

(a)   Prolapsed uterus

(b)   Severely prolapsed uterus

salpingitis sal pin JYE tiss	**12.80** Inflammation of a fallopian tube is called _____. The constructed form of this term is salping/itis. It is usually caused by bacterial infection and is often associated with PID (Frame 12.77).

salpingocele sal PING goh seel	**12.81** A protrusion, or herniation, of a fallopian tube wall is known as _____. The constructed form is salping/o/cele, revealing its three word parts.
vaginitis vaj ih NYE tiss	**12.82** Inflammation of the vagina is known as _____. Because *colp/o* is an alternate combining form for vagina, it is also called **colpitis** (kol PYE tiss). In a common form known as **atrophic vaginitis** (ay TROH fik * vaj ih NYE tiss), the usual symptoms of redness and swelling are accompanied by thinning of the vaginal wall and loss of moisture, usually due to a depletion of estrogen, and is common among postmenopausal women.
vulvitis vul VYE tiss vulv/o/vagin/itis	**12.83** Inflammation of the external genitals, or vulva, is called _____. When the vagina is also inflamed, the condition is known as **vulvovaginitis** (VUL voh vaj ih NYE tiss). The constructed form of this term reveals four word parts and is written _____/__/_____/____.

PRACTICE: Diseases and Disorders of the Female Reproductive System

The Right Match

Match the term on the left with the correct definition on the right.

_____ 1. breast cancer

_____ 2. carcinoma in situ

_____ 3. cervical cancer

_____ 4. fibrocystic breast disease

_____ 5. fistula

_____ 6. ovarian cancer

_____ 7. ovarian cyst

_____ 8. pelvic inflammatory disease

_____ 9. premenstrual syndrome

_____ 10. prolapsed uterus

a. a malignant tumor of the cervix

b. the most common form is infiltrating ductal carcinoma

c. cancer in site

d. a common form of reproductive cancer in women

e. a condition in which one or more benign, fibrous cysts develop within the breast

f. an abnormal passage from one hollow organ to another

g. inflammation that involves some or all of the female organs within the pelvic cavity

h. displacement of the uterus into the vagina

i. a fluid-filled sac on an ovary

j. collection of symptoms that occur during the 10 days preceding menstruation

Break the Chain

Analyze these medical terms:

- a) Separate each term into its word parts; each word part is labeled for you (**p** = prefix, **r** = root, **cf** = combining form, and **s** = suffix).
- b) For the Bonus Question, write the requested words or definition in the blank that follows.

1. a) vulvitis   _____/_____
                          r   s

   b) *Bonus Question*: What is the definition of the word root? _____

2. a) salpingocele   _____/___/_____
                               cf   s

   b) *Bonus Question*: What anatomical part does the combining form refer to? _____

3. a) amastia   _____/_____/_____
                        p   r   s

   b) *Bonus Question*: What is the definition of the word root? _____

4. a) endometriosis   _____/_____/___/_____
                                p   cf   s

   b) *Bonus Question*: What is the definition of the prefix? _____

5. a) leiomyoma   _____/___/_____/_____
                           cf   r   s

   b) *Bonus Question*: What is the definition of the combining form? _____

Treatments, Procedures, and Devices of the Female Reproductive System

Here are the word parts that commonly apply to the treatments, procedures, and devices of the female reproductive system and are covered in the following section. Note that the word parts are color-coded to help you identify them: prefixes are yellow, combining forms are red, and suffixes are blue.

Prefix	Definition
endo-	within
trans-	through, across, beyond

Combining Form	Definition
cervic/o	neck, cervix
colp/o	vagina
episi/o	vulva
gyn/o, gynec/o	woman
hyster/o	uterus
lapar/o	abdomen
mamm/o	breast
mast/o	breast
metr/i	uterus
oophor/o	ovary
path/o	disease
salping/o	trumpet, fallopian tube
son/o	sound
vagin/o	sheath, vagina
vulv/o	vulva

Suffix	Definition
-al	pertaining to
-ectomy	surgical excision, removal
-gram	a record or image
-graphy	recording process
-ic	pertaining to
-logist	one who studies
-logy	study or science of
-pexy	surgical fixation, suspension
-plasty	surgical repair
-rrhaphy	suturing
-scopy	process of viewing
-stomy	surgical creation of an opening

KEY TERMS A–Z

biopsy
BYE op see

12.84 A minor surgical procedure that involves the surgical extraction of tissue for microscopic analysis is called a _____. Abbreviated **bx** or **Bx**, the sample may be removed from any tissue including the cervix, endometrium, or breast. Any one of several procedures may be used to extract a tissue sample, including scraping (curettage), aspiration, or excision. (■ Figure 12.21).

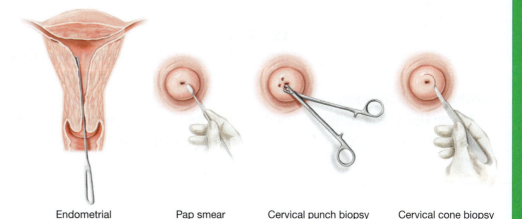

■ **Figure 12.21**
Biopsy. Various forms of gynecological biopsy are shown.

Endometrial curretage   Pap smear   Cervical punch biopsy   Cervical cone biopsy

cervical conization

cervicectomy
SER vih SEK toh mee

12.85 To remove precancerous or cancerous tissue from the cervix, the anterior part of the cervix can be removed in a **cervical conization** (SER vih kal * koh nih ZAY shun). In this procedure, a cone-shaped section of the cervix is removed as a common treatment for precancerous conditions. A _____ _____ is often performed with an electrical wire loop, called a **LEEP**, which is an acronym for "loop electrosurgical excision procedure." If the cancer is developed, the cervix may be removed in a _____. The constructed form of this term is cervic/ectomy.

colpectomy
kol PEK toh mee

12.86 Recall that a word root for vagina is *colp*. Removal of the vagina is a surgery called a _____, or alternatively called **vaginectomy** (VAJ ih NEK toh mee).

colpoplasty
KOL poh plass tee
colporrhaphy
kol POR ah fee

colp/o/scopy

12.87 Surgical repair of the vagina is a procedure called _____. This constructed term includes three word parts: colp/o/plasty. A colpoplasty often includes suturing the wall of the vagina in a procedure called _____. Also a constructed term, it may be shown with its three word parts as colp/o/rrhaphy. Both procedures often follow an endoscopic evaluation of the vagina, called a **colposcopy**. Write the constructed form of this term here: _____/__/_____.

dilation and curettage
dye LAY shun * and * koo reh TAZH

12.88 A common procedure that is used for both diagnostic and treatment purposes is called **dilation and curettage**, abbreviated **D&C**. During a _____ _____ _____, the cervix is dilated to permit the insertion of a spoon-shaped instrument called a **curette**, which is used to scrape the lining of the endometrium (see Figure 12.21). It is often performed to control bleeding, obtain a tissue sample for biopsy, or remove polyps.

endometrial ablation
ehn doh MEE tree al * ahb LAY shun

12.89 If the endometrium requires more treatment than can be provided by a D&C, an **endometrial ablation** may be applied. The term *ablation* means "surgical removal of tissue." In an _____ _____, lasers, electricity, or heat may be used to destroy the endometrium, followed by suction to remove the dead tissue.

gynecology
GYE neh KOL oh jee

12.90 Two combining forms that mean "woman" are *gynec/o* and *gyn/o*. The branch of medicine focusing on women is known as _____, abbreviated **GYN**. The constructed form of this term is gynec/o/logy. Frequently, a physician known as an **obstetrician-gynecologist** combines these two areas of expertise; this is abbreviated **OB/GYN**. Also, the study of diseases that afflict women is known as _____. As a constructed term, it includes two combining forms: gyn/o/path/o/logy. A physician specializing in this field of medicine is called a **gynopathologist** (GYE no path ALL oh jist). Show the five word parts of this term: ___/___/___/___/_____.

gynopathology
GYE no path ALL oh jee

gyn/o/path/o/logist

hormone replacement therapy

12.91 As a common therapy for hormonal management, **hormone replacement therapy**, abbreviated **HRT**, can be very effective in correcting disrupted menstrual and ovarian cycles. In _____ _____ _____, the hormones estrogen and progesterone are frequently prescribed in pill form. It is also the most effective means of **female contraception** for the prevention of unwanted pregnancy.

hysterectomy
HISS teh REK toh mee

12.92 The surgical removal of the uterus is commonly called _____. The surgery may include surrounding structures with their corresponding terminology, as shown in ■ Figure 12.22. This constructed term includes two word parts: hyster/ectomy.

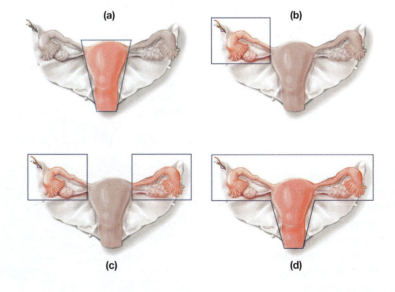

(a)   (b)

(c)   (d)

■ **Figure 12.22**
Alternative forms of surgeries involving the uterus, ovaries, and fallopian tubes. The solid lines indicate excision. (a) Hysterectomy. (b) Right salpingo-oophorectomy. (c) Bilateral salpingo-oophorectomy. (d) Bilateral hysterosalpingo-oophorectomy, or panhysterectomy.

hysteropexy

HISS ter oh PEK see

12.93 The surgical procedure that may be used to correct the position of prolapsed uterus (Frame 12.79) by strengthening its connections to the abdominal wall is called _____. The constructed form of this term is hyster/o/pexy and means "surgical fixation of the uterus."

WORDS TO Watch Out For

-pexy or -plasty?

The meanings of these two suffixes both relate to surgery—but they are very different forms of surgery. Remember that *-pexy* means "surgical *fixation, suspension*," and *-plasty* means "surgical *repair*." One way to remember the meaning of *-pexy* is that it uses an *x*, as does the word *fixation* in its definition. Similarly, a way to remember the meaning of *-plasty* is that it uses a *p*, as does the word *repair* in its definition.

hysteroscopy

HISS ter OSS koh pee

laparoscopy

lap ahr OSS koh pee

12.94 A noninvasive diagnostic technique that uses a modified endoscope, called a **hysteroscope** (HISS ter oh skope), to evaluate the uterine cavity is called _____. It contains three word parts, as you can see in hyster/o/scopy. To evaluate the external appearance of the uterus and other organs of the pelvic cavity, a **laparoscope** (LAP ahr oh skope) is inserted through a small incision in the lower abdominal wall during a _____. The procedure is shown in ■ Figure 12.23. This is also a constructed term, shown as lapar/o/scopy (the word root *lapar* means "abdomen").

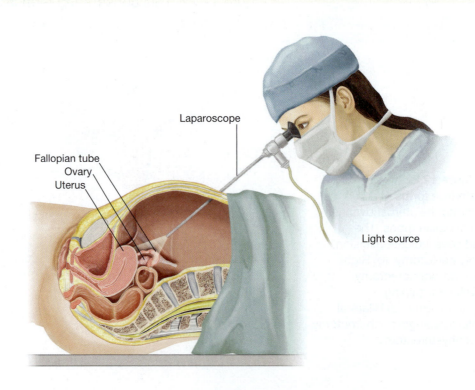

Laparoscope

Fallopian tube
Ovary
Uterus

Light source

■ **Figure 12.23**
Laparoscopy. A lighted endoscope specialized for insertion into the abdomen, called a *laparoscope*, is used to view reproductive organs. The laparoscope may also be outfitted with surgical devices for excision of structures.

mammography

mam OG rah fee

12.95 An x-ray procedure that produces an x-ray image of a breast, called a **mammogram**, is called _____. The procedure and a mammogram are shown in ■ Figure 12.24. The procedure is an early screening for breast cancer. The term **mammography** is a constructed word: mamm/o/graphy.

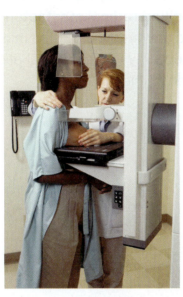 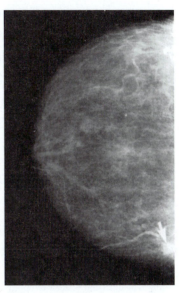

(a)　　　　　　　　　　　　　(b)

■ **Figure 12.24**
Mammography. (a) A healthcare professional assists the patient to ensure the breast is placed ideally for the x-ray. *Source: Keith Brofsky/Photo-disc/Getty Images.*
(b) A mammogram. A tumor is visible in this mammogram, indicated by the arrow in the lower right corner. *Source: Courtesy of Dr. Dwight Kaufman, National Institutes of Health, National Cancer Institute Visuals Online, Bethesda, MD.*

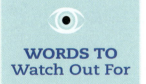

WORDS TO Watch Out For

-graph, *-graphy*, or *-gram*?

Remember that the suffix *-y* means "process of." Thus, because the suffix *-graph* means "instrument for recording," the suffix *-graphy* means "recording process." In a slightly different twist, the suffix *-gram* means "a record or image." In each of these suffixes, switching the ending creates the term used for recording information.

mammoplasty

MAM moh PLASS tee

12.96 The surgical repair of one or both breasts is called a _____. It involves either the enlargement or reduction of breast size or, in some cases, removal of a tumor. Mammoplasty is also an important reconstructive procedure for women who have had a mastectomy (Frame 12.97).

mastectomy

mass TEK toh mee

12.97 In addition to the combining form *mamm/o*, the combining form *mast/o* also means "breast." Thus, a procedure involving the removal of breast tissue is a _____ (■ Figure 12.25). In a **simple mastectomy**, one entire breast is removed while leaving underlying muscles and lymph nodes intact. In a **radical mastectomy** (or *Halsted mastectomy*), the entire affected breast is removed along with muscles and lymph nodes of the chest. In a **modified radical mastectomy**, the affected breast and lymph nodes are removed but the muscles are left intact. Finally, a **lumpectomy** is the removal of the cancerous lesions only, which conserves the breast.

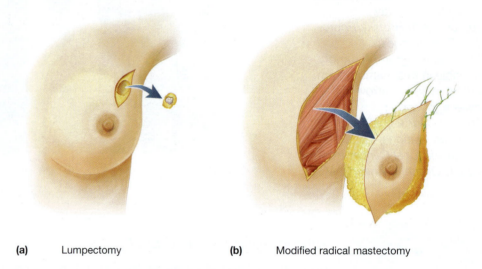

■ **Figure 12.25**
Breast surgery. Surgical removal of all or part of the breast is a treatment against the spread of breast cancer.

(a)   Lumpectomy   (b)   Modified radical mastectomy

oophorectomy

oh OF oh REK toh mee

12.98 Surgical removal of an ovary is performed in an _____. Its two word parts are shown in oophor/ectomy.

Pap smear

12.99 A common diagnostic procedure that screens for precancerous cervical dysplasia and cervical cancer is known as the **Papanicolaou smear** (pap an IK oh lau * smeer), commonly called a _____ _____. It involves the gentle scraping of cells from the cervix and vagina followed by their microscopic examination (■ Figure 12.26).

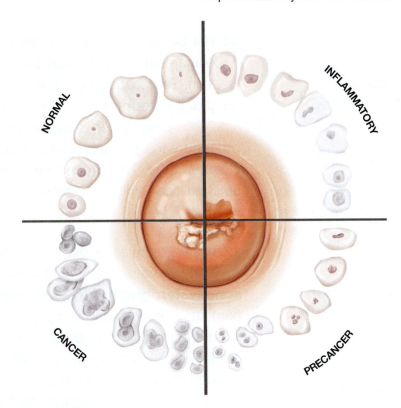

NORMAL

INFLAMMATORY

CANCER

PRECANCER

■ **Figure 12.26**
Pap smear. Cells of the cervix (shown in the center) change in appearance as they progress through the stages of cervical cancer, as shown in this diagram. During the Pap smear, cells are obtained from the cervix in a cervical biopsy and studied under a microscope for changes. Based on the appearance of cells, a diagnosis can be made.

? **Did You KNOW**

PAPANICOLAOU SMEAR

Named after Dr. George Papanicolaou, an anatomist and cytologist, the Pap smear is a screening test for cervical cancer that has made early detection possible. The American Cancer Society recommends annual tests at ages 20 and 21, followed by tests at 3-year intervals throughout later years.

---

salpingectomy
SAL pin JEK toh mee

salping/o/- oophor/ectomy

12.100 The surgical removal of a fallopian tube is performed in a procedure called a _____. The constructed form of this term is salping/ectomy. If an ovary is also removed, the procedure is called a **salpingo-oophorectomy** (sal ping goh oh OF oh REK toh mee). Also a constructed term, it includes four word parts: _____/__-_____/_____.

👁 WORDS TO Watch Out For

The *O*'s in Salpingo-oophorectomy

When two combining forms are joined together to form a term, the first combining form keeps its combining vowel, even if the second begins with a vowel. Thus, in the term *salpingo-oophorectomy*, the combining form *salping/o* retains its combining vowel. In this long term, the hyphen is included to distinguish between the two adjacent combining forms and to make pronunciation easier. This makes for a lot of *o*'s, so be careful when you spell this term.

salpingopexy
sal PING oh PEK see

salping/o/stomy

12.101 Surgical fixation of a fallopian tube may become necessary if the ligaments that support the tube within the pelvic cavity weaken. The procedure is called _____. This constructed term includes three word parts, as you can see in salping/o/pexy. Often, a **salpingopexy** is accompanied by a procedure to open a blocked fallopian tube or to drain fluid from an inflamed tube. This procedure is called a **salpingostomy** (SAL ping GOSS toh mee), which can be shown with its word parts separated as _____/__/_____.

sonohysterography
son oh HIST er OG rah fee

12.102 A noninvasive diagnostic procedure that uses ultrasound waves to visualize the uterus within the pelvic cavity is called **sonohysterography**. The constructed term _____ contains five word parts, represented as son/o/hyster/o/graphy. In the diagnostic procedure known as **transvaginal sonography** (trans VAJ ih nal * son OG rah fee) (**TVS**), an ultrasound probe is inserted through the vagina to record images of the uterine cavity and fallopian tubes. The constructed form of these terms is trans/vagin/al son/o/graphy. In addition to its use for observing tumors or cysts, it is used to monitor pregnancy.

tubal ligation
TOO bal * lye GAY shun

12.103 The most common form of female sterilization as a contraceptive measure is called **tubal ligation**, during which the fallopian tubes are severed and closed to prevent the migration of sperm upward into the tubes (■ Figure 12.27). The term _____ _____ includes the word that means "to tie up," *ligate*. Recently, in an effort to minimize the invasiveness of surgery, ligation is sometimes replaced by the use of clamps to close the fallopian tubes during endoscopic surgery.

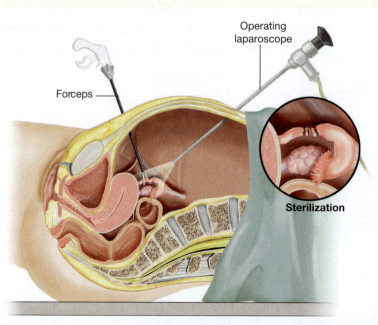

Operating laparoscope

Forceps

Sterilization

■ **Figure 12.27**
Tubal ligation. To minimize the size of the incisions necessary, laparoscopic surgery may be used to enter the abdominal cavity through a small incision, cut the fallopian tubes, and ligate (tie off) or clamp.

vaginal speculum VAJ ih nal * SPEK yoo lum	**12.104** A **vaginal speculum** is an instrument used during a gynecological exam. A _____ _____ is used to open the vaginal orifice wide enough to permit visual examination of the vagina and cervix.
vulvectomy vuhl VEK toh mee	**12.105** The surgical removal of the vulva is called a _____. The constructed form of this term is vulv/ectomy.

PRACTICE: Treatments, Procedures, and Devices of the Female Reproductive System

The Right Match

Match the term on the left with the correct definition on the right.

_____ 1. biopsy

_____ 2. dilation and curettage

_____ 3. cervical conization

_____ 4. Papanicolaou smear

_____ 5. hormone replacement therapy

_____ 6. transvaginal sonography

_____ 7. endometrial ablation

_____ 8. tubal ligation

_____ 9. vaginal speculum

a. removal of the anterior part of the cervix

b. severs and closes the fallopian tubes to prevent migration of sperm

c. common therapy for hormone imbalances

d. destroys the endometrium with a laser

e. a procedure in which the cervix is dilated and a curette is inserted to scrape the endometrium

f. instrument that opens the vaginal orifice to permit visual examination

g. records images of the uterine cavity and fallopian tubes

h. microscopic examination of cells scraped from the cervix and vagina

i. surgical extraction of tissue for microscopic analysis

Linkup

Link the word parts in the list to create the terms that match the definitions. You may use word parts more than once. Remember to add combining vowels when needed and that some terms do not use any combining vowel.

Combining Form	Suffix
colp/o	-ectomy
gynec/o	-gram
hyster/o	-logy
mamm/o	-pexy
oophor/o	-plasty
salping/o	-rrhaphy
vulv/o	

Definition	Term
1. surgical removal of the vulva	_____
2. surgical repair of the vagina	_____
3. branch of medicine that focuses on women	_____
4. surgical removal of the uterus	_____
5. suturing the wall of the vagina	_____
6. surgical fixation of the uterus	_____
7. x-ray image of a breast	_____
8. surgical removal of an ovary	_____
9. surgical removal of a fallopian tube	_____

Signs and Symptoms of Obstetrics

Here are the word parts that commonly apply to the signs and symptoms of obstetrics and are covered in the following section. Note that the word parts are color-coded to help you identify them: prefixes are yellow, combining forms are red, and suffixes are blue.

Prefix	Definition	Combining Form	Definition	Suffix	Definition
dys-	bad, abnormal, painful, difficult	amni/o	amnion	-cyesis	pregnancy
hyper-	excessive, abnormally high, above	cyes/o	pregnancy	-emesis	vomiting
		gravid/o	pregnancy	-ia	condition of
poly-	excessive, over, many	hydr/o	water	-rrhea	discharge
		lact/o	milk	-s	plural
		pseud/o	false		
		toc/o	birth		

KEY TERMS A–Z

amniorrhea
AM nee oh REE ah

12.106 Recall that the suffix *-rrhea* means "discharge." The abnormal discharge of amniotic fluid is a sign of a ruptured amniotic sac. The sign is called _____. This constructed term includes three word parts: amni/o/rrhea.

dystocia
diss TOH see ah

12.107 The combining form for birth is *toc/o*. When the prefix *dys-* and the suffix *-ia* are added, the new term is _____ and means "condition of difficult labor." The constructed form is shown as dys/toc/ia.

hyperemesis gravidarum
HIGH per EM eh siss * grav ih DAR um

12.108 The symptom of severe nausea and emesis (vomiting) during pregnancy is called **hyperemesis gravidarum**. The term literally means "excessive vomiting when pregnant." _____ _____ can cause severe dehydration in the mother and fetus if left untreated.

lactorrhea
LAK toh REE ah

12.109 An abnormal, spontaneous discharge of milk usually between nursings or after weaning is known as _____. This constructed term contains three word parts, shown as lact/o/rrhea.

polyhydramnios
PALL ee high DRAM nee ohs

12.110 An excessive production of amniotic fluid during fetal development is called **polyhydramnios**. If left untreated, _____ can cause unwanted pressure on the fetus that can disturb development. The term is constructed of 5 word parts, shown as poly/hydr/amni/o/s.

pseudocyesis
SOO doh sigh EE siss

12.111 A sensation of being pregnant when a true pregnancy does not exist is called **pseudocyesis**, which literally means "false pregnancy." The constructed form of _____ is pseud/o/cyesis.

PRACTICE: Signs and Symptoms of Obstetrics

Break the Chain

Analyze these medical terms:

a) Separate each term into its word parts; each word part is labeled for you (**p** = prefix, **r** = root, **cf** = combining form, and **s** = suffix).

b) For the Bonus Question, write the requested definition in the blank that follows.

1. a) dystocia   _____/_____/_____
                   p   r   s

   b) *Bonus Question*: What is the definition of the suffix? _____

2. a) hyperemesis   _____/_____
                   p   s

   b) *Bonus Question*: What is the definition of the prefix? _____

3. a) pseudocyesis   _____/___/_____
                   cf   s

   b) *Bonus Question*: What is the definition of the combining form? _____

4. a) polyhydramnios   _____/_____/_____/___/_____
                   p   r   cf   s

   b) *Bonus Question*: What is the definition of the combining form? _____

5. a) lactorrhea   _____/___/_____
                   cf   s

   b) *Bonus Question*: What is the definition of the suffix? _____

6. a) amniorrhea   _____/___/_____
                   cf   s

   b) *Bonus Question*: What is the definition of the suffix? _____

Diseases and Disorders of Obstetrics

Here are the word parts that commonly apply to the diseases and disorders of obstetrics and are covered in the following section. Note that the word parts are color-coded to help you identify them: prefixes are yellow, combining forms are red, and suffixes are blue.

Combining Form	Definition	Combining Form	Definition	Suffix	Definition
blast/o	germ, bud, developing cell	fet/o	fetus	-al	pertaining to
		plasm/o	form	-osis	condition of
erythr/o	red	tox/o	poison	-sis	state of

KEY TERMS A–Z

abruptio placentae
  ah BRUP shee oh * plah
  SEN tee

12.112 The premature separation of the placenta from the uterine wall is called **abruptio placentae**. This Latin word means "abrupt (loss) of placenta." _____ _____ results in either a miscarriage, stillbirth, or premature birth and is illustrated in ■ Figure 12.28.

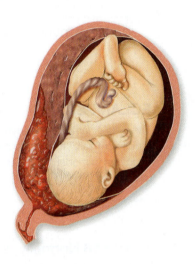

■ **Figure 12.28**
Abruptio placentae. The placenta becomes prematurely detached from the uterine wall.

breech presentation

12.113 An abnormal childbirth in which the buttocks, feet, or knees appear through the birth canal first is commonly called a **breech presentation**. A _____ _____ is relatively common and places the child at risk due to an increased risk of complications during birth.

congenital anomaly
  kon JENN ih tal * ah NOM
  ah lee

12.114 A **congenital anomaly** is an abnormality present at birth. As an example, **cleft palate** is a failure of the roof of the mouth to close during prenatal development. Another _____ _____ is **esophageal atresia** (eh sof ah JEE al * ah TREE zhe ah), in which the child is born with an absence of part of the esophagus. This constructed term literally means "closure of the esophagus." A severe, relatively common congenital anomaly is **Down syndrome**. Also called *trisomy 21* to identify the chromosome number that contains the defective genes, it is an abnormality present at birth and characterized by mental retardation, glossomegaly (enlarged tongue), stubby fingers, and a fold over the eyelids.

eclampsia
eh KLAMP see ah

12.115 A circulatory disorder that places a pregnant woman and her child at risk is called **pregnancy-induced hypertension (PIH)**, or **preeclampsia** (pree eh KLAMP see ah). It is characterized by high blood pressure, proteinuria (protein in the urine), and edema, all due to toxemia (toxins in the bloodstream) during pregnancy. In some women, it may progress to the more dangerous condition known as _____, in which the high blood pressure worsens to cause convulsions and possibly coma and death.

? Did You KNOW

ECLAMPSIA

The term *eclampsia* is derived from the Greek word *eclampsis*, which means "to shine forth rapidly or flash." It refers to a sudden development and was chosen to be used for this condition in modern times because of the sudden onset of convulsions that often marks the disease.

ectopic pregnancy
ek TOP ik * PREG nan see

12.116 Normally, about 8 days after fertilization the zygote will implant into the inner lining of the uterus. However, in some cases the zygote may implant in other tissues, such as the fallopian tube lining or even the peritoneum, and from there proceed through embryonic and fetal development (■ Figure 12.29). The term *ectopic* means "out of place." Therefore, a pregnancy occurring outside the uterus is called _____ _____.

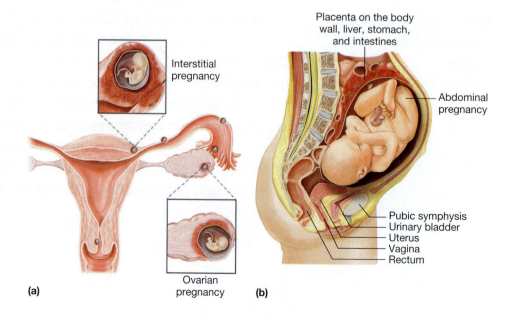

■ Figure 12.29
Ectopic pregnancies. (a) An ectopic pregnancy may occur in any of the locations shown. Interstitial pregnancy is the most common, with implantation occurring near the union of a fallopian tube and uterus. If the pregnancy is not terminated, it will destroy the fallopian tube and cause blood loss. An ovarian pregnancy has the unfortunate result of destroying the ovary. (b) An abdominal pregnancy is shown at full term. Note that the fetus is surrounded by the amniotic sac, but outside the uterus.

erythroblastosis fetalis

eh RITH roh blass TOH siss *

fee TAL iss

12.117 A condition of neonates, or newborns, in which red blood cells are destroyed due to an incompatibility between the mother's blood and baby's blood is called **erythroblastosis fetalis**. It occurs when the mother has RH- blood and has previously had an RH+ child (■ Figure 12.30). The term _____ _____ is constructed as erythr/o/blast/osis fetalis and means "condition of fetal development of red (cells)." It is also called **hemolytic disease of the newborn**.

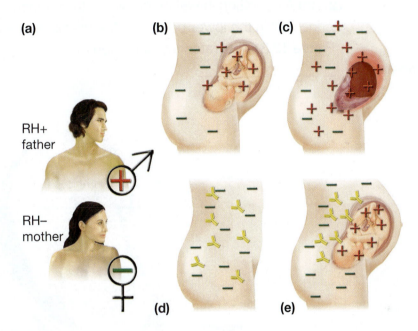

■ **Figure 12.30**
Erythroblastosis fetalis. (a) The condition occurs with an RH+ father and RH– mother. (b) First pregnancy with an RH+ fetus stimulates the mother's blood to form antibodies against the fetal blood. (c) As the placenta separates during birth, the mother is further exposed to the RH+ blood, increasing her blood's reaction against it. (d) The mother carries antibodies against the RH+ blood. (e) In a subsequent pregnancy with an RH+ fetus, the mother's antibodies attack the RH+ blood of the fetus, causing hemolysis of the fetal red blood cells, resulting in the disease that can kill the child.

fetal alcohol syndrome

12.118 A neonatal condition caused by excessive alcohol consumption by the mother during pregnancy is known as **fetal alcohol syndrome**, or **FAS**. _____ _____ _____ often causes brain dysfunction and growth abnormalities that usually afflict the child throughout life. Because it causes a range of physical and mental defects, it is also called **fetal alcohol spectrum disorder (FASD)**.

neonatal respiratory distress syndrome

12.119 A lung disorder of neonates, particularly premature infants, in which certain cells of the lungs fail to mature at birth to cause lung collapse that can result in suffocation is called **neonatal respiratory distress syndrome**. Abbreviated **NRDS**, it is also called **respiratory distress syndrome of the newborn**. The condition of _____ _____ _____ _____ may be managed by placing monitors around the baby that trigger when breathing has stopped during the sleep cycle.

placenta previa
   plah SEN tah * PREE vee ah

12.120 A condition in which the placenta is abnormally attached to the uterine wall in the lower portion of the uterus is called **placenta previa**. ■ Figure 12.31 illustrates the condition of _____ _____.

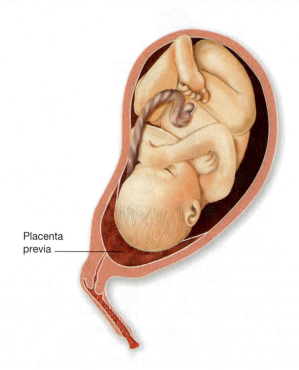

Placenta previa

■ **Figure 12.31**
Placenta previa. The condition is caused by the development of the placenta over the cervical canal, creating an occlusion of the birth canal.

toxoplasmosis
   TAHK soh plaz MOH siss

12.121 Caused by the protozoan *Toxoplasma gondii*, the disease _____ may be contracted by exposure to animal feces, most commonly from household cats. This constructed term is written tox/o/plasm/osis and means "condition of toxic form." It is a danger to pregnant women because the protozoa are capable of crossing the placental barrier to infect the fetus and cause birth defects.

PRACTICE: Diseases and Disorders of Obstetrics

The Right Match

Match the term on the left with the correct definition on the right.

_____ 1. congenital anomaly

_____ 2. breech presentation

_____ 3. eclampsia

_____ 4. abruptio placentae

_____ 5. ectopic pregnancy

_____ 6. fetal alcohol syndrome

_____ 7. neonatal respiratory distress syndrome

_____ 8. placenta previa

a. severely high blood pressure in the pregnant woman

b. brain dysfunction and growth abnormalities caused by excessive alcohol consumption by the mother during pregnancy

c. abnormality present at birth

d. placenta is abnormally located

e. lung disorder of neonates

f. abnormal birth position in which the buttocks, feet, or knees appear through the birth canal first

g. pregnancy that occurs outside the uterus

h. premature separation of the placenta from the uterine wall

Treatments, Procedures, and Devices of Obstetrics

Here are the word parts that commonly apply to the treatments, procedures, and devices of obstetrics and are covered in the following section. Note that the word parts are color-coded to help you identify them: prefixes are yellow, combining forms are red, and suffixes are blue.

Prefix	Definition
epi-	*upon, over, above, on top*

Combining Form	Definition
abort/o	*miscarry*
amni/o	*amnion*
dur/o	*hard*
episi/o	*vulva*
fet/o	*fetus*
obstetr/o	*midwife*

Suffix	Definition
-al	*pertaining to*
-centesis	*surgical puncture*
-ic	*pertaining to*
-ician	*one who practices*
-metry	*measurement, process of measuring*
-tomy	*incision, to cut*

KEY TERMS A–Z

abortion
ah BOR shun

12.122 A term derived from the Latin word *aborto*, which means "miscarry," is **abortion**. It is the termination of pregnancy by expulsion of the embryo or fetus from the uterus. A natural expulsion is called a **miscarriage** or **spontaneous abortion (SAB)**. An _____ induced by surgery or drugs is called a **therapeutic abortion (TAB)**. A drug that induces TAB is called an **abortifacient** (ah BOR tih FAY shent).

amniocentesis
AM nee oh sehn TEE siss

12.123 A procedure that involves penetration of the amnion with a syringe and aspiration of a small amount of amniotic fluid for analysis is known as **amniocentesis**. The constructed form of this term is amni/o/centesis. _____ literally means "surgical puncture of amnion." It is shown in ■ Figure 12.32.

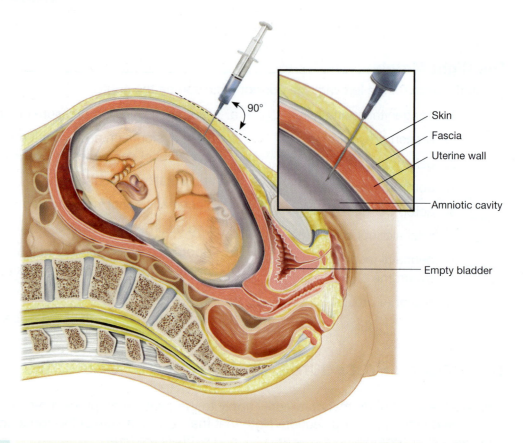

90°

Skin

Fascia

Uterine wall

Amniotic cavity

Empty bladder

■ **Figure 12.32**
Amniocentesis. In this procedure, amniotic fluid is aspirated with a syringe that is inserted through the abdominal wall, uterine wall, and amnion.

cesarean section
seh ZAIR ee an * SEK shun

12.124 As an alternative to the nonsurgical birth of a child through the birth canal, birthing can be accomplished surgically by making an incision through the abdomen and uterus. This procedure is called _____ _____; it is abbreviated **C-section**.

? Did You KNOW

CESAREAN SECTION

The Latin word *caesar* literally means "to cut." Because of the Latin meaning of the word, it is believed that the term *cesarean section* was first used to describe this surgical alternative to vaginal birth during ancient Roman times. At one time it was thought that Julius Caesar was given the name "Caesar" because his origin was from such a birth, but that is now known to be false. During Roman times, physicians lacked the skills and knowledge to perform the operation without killing the mother; it was performed only if the mother had died while pregnant in an effort to save the child. His mother survived his birth, so the origin of the Caesar name remains a mystery.

contraception
kon trah SEP shun

12.125 The term **contraception** literally means "against conception," or prevention of birth. It is the use of devices and drugs to prevent fertilization, implantation of a fertilized egg, or both. The most effective _____ is surgical sterilization, including the vasectomy in males (Frame 12.45) and tubal ligation in females (Frame 12.103). The most popular method is the birth control pill, taken orally by females to block ovulation. Other methods include condoms, diaphragms, and intrauterine devices (IUDs).

epidural

episiotomy
eh peez ee OTT oh mee

fetometry
fee TOM eh tree

12.126 To reduce pain during childbirth, a patient may request an _____ **block**, during which an anesthetic is injected into the epidural space of the vertebral column to block sensation from the pelvic region. _Epidural_ is a constructed term, shown as epi/dur/al. Another elective treatment may be made in an effort to prevent tearing of the vulva and perineum during childbirth. This procedure involves an incision through these tissues to widen the vaginal opening and is called **episiotomy**. _____ is a constructed term, episi/o/tomy.

12.127 A procedure that measures the size of a fetus is called _____. This constructed term is fet/o/metry and means "fetal measurement." It is performed using ultrasound technology on the pregnant mother in a technique known as **obstetrical sonography** (ob STET rih kal * son OG rah fee), which is shown in ■ Figure 12.33.

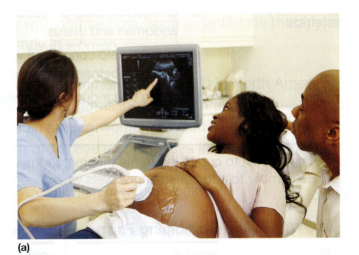

(a)

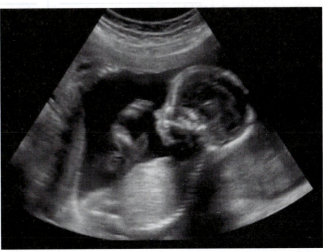

(b)

■ **Figure 12.33**
Obstetrical sonography and fetometry. (a) The procedure is performed in a clinical setting. The instrumentation includes a monitor, control panel, and ultrasound probe. _Source: Monkey Business Images/ Shutterstock_. (b) The fetometry is obtained by measuring the size of the fetal head and other parts of the fetal body from the image on the monitor. _Source: GagliardiImages/Shutterstock_.

hepatitis B	**12.134** Hepatitis is an inflammatory disease of the liver that has many different forms that are categorized as types A through E. In _____, commonly called **hep B**, the cause is a virus (known as **HBV**) that is primarily transmitted via blood exchange, often through blood transfusions or sharing IV needles. It may also be acquired through sexual exchange of body fluids. Hep B causes liver damage that can lead to liver failure and death. (Recall from Chapter 10 that *hepatitis* is a constructed term, hepat/itis: *hepat/o* means "liver" and *-itis* means "inflammation.")
human papillomavirus	**12.135** The **human papillomavirus**, or **HPV**, is a virus that is extremely common in the human population and is transmitted during intercourse. In some people, _____ _____ forms the symptom of papillomas or genital warts, which are transient vesicles on the penis or within the vagina. It is well established that HPV is the primary cause of cervical cancer (Frame 12.62) and elevates the risk of several other types of cancers.
syphilis SIFF ih liss	**12.136** An STI that is caused by a bacterium called a *spirochete* (*Treponema pallidum*) is known as **syphilis**. It is transmitted by sexual contact and usually first appears as red, painless pustules on the skin that erode to form small ulcers known as **chancres** (SHANG kerz) (Frame 12.10). If left untreated, _____ can result in mental confusion, organ destruction, and death. The term *syphilis* is named after the main character in a poem written in 1530 about a shepherd afflicted with this dreaded disease.
trichomoniasis TRIK oh moh NYE ah siss	**12.137** An STI caused by the protozoan *Trichomonas*, which is an amoeba-like single-celled organism, is called _____. It is spread by sexual contact and infects both women and men. In women, the sexually transmitted form is called *Trichomonas vaginalis* and causes vaginal swelling and pain. In men, the urethra and prostate gland become infected, causing inflammation and pelvic pain.

PRACTICE: Sexually Transmitted Infections (STIs)

The Right Match

Match the term on the left with the correct definition on the right.

_____ 1. chlamydia

_____ 2. genital herpes

_____ 3. acquired immuno deficiency syndrome

_____ 4. hepatitis B

_____ 5. human papillomavirus

_____ 6. syphilis

_____ 7. gonorrhea

_____ 8. trichomoniasis

_____ 9. candidiasis

a. extremely common STI that causes genital warts in some people and may also increase risk of cervical cancer

b. caused by a bacterium called a spirochete

c. the most common bacterial STI in North America; symptoms include urethritis and inflammation of the conjunctiva

d. characterized by skin and mucous membrane irritation; can lead to endocarditis and septicemia

e. a bacterial infection that produces ulcerlike lesions on the mucous membranes and skin of the genital region and urethral discharge

f. results from infection with the human immunodeficiency virus (HIV)

g. infection caused by a protozoan that causes inflammation of the urethra and prostate and pelvic pain

h. a form of an inflammatory disease of the liver caused by a virus that is sexually transmitted

i. characterized by periodic outbreaks of ulcerlike sores on the genital and anorectal skin and mucous membranes

Abbreviations of the Reproductive System and Obstetrics

The abbreviations associated with the reproductive system and obstetrics are summarized here. Study these abbreviations and review them in the exercise that follows.

Abbreviation	Definition
AIDS	acquired immunodeficiency syndrome
BPH	benign prostatic hyperplasia
Bx, bx	biopsy
CIN	cervical intraepithelial neoplasia
CIS	carcinoma in situ
C-section	cesarean section
D&C	dilation and curettage
DRE	digital rectal exam
ED	erectile dysfunction
FAS	fetal alcohol syndrome
FASD	fetal alcohol spectrum disorder
FBD	fibrocystic breast disease
GYN	gynecology
HBV	hepatitis B virus
HIV	human immunodeficiency virus
HPV	human papillomavirus
HRT	hormone replacement therapy
HSV-2	herpes simplex virus type 2

Abbreviation	Definition
IDC	infiltrating ductal carcinoma
LEEP	loop electrosurgical excision procedure
NRDS	neonatal respiratory distress syndrome
OB	obstetrics
OB/GYN	obstetrics/gynecology
Pap smear (test)	Papanicolaou smear (or test)
PID	pelvic inflammatory disease
PIH	pregnancy-induced hypertension
PMS	premenstrual syndrome
PCOS	polycystic ovary syndrome
PSA	prostate-specific antigen
SAB	spontaneous abortion
STI	sexually transmitted infection
TAB	therapeutic abortion
TURP	transurethral resection of the prostate
TVS	transvaginal sonography

PRACTICE: Abbreviations

Fill in the blanks with the abbreviation or the complete medical term.

Abbreviation	Medical Term
1. PSA	_____
2. _____	sexually transmitted infection
3. HIV	_____
4. _____	transurethral resection of the prostate
5. BPH	_____
6. _____	acquired immunodeficiency syndrome
7. _____	hepatitis B virus
8. HSV-2	_____
9. _____	digital rectal exam
10. HPV	_____
11. _____	cervical intraepithelial neoplasia
12. D&C	_____
13. _____	carcinoma in situ
14. HRT	_____
15. _____	neonatal respiratory distress syndrome
16. PMS	_____
17. _____	therapeutic abortion
18. PCOS	_____
19. _____	pelvic inflammatory disease
20. TVS	_____
21. _____	gynecology
22. Bx	_____
23. _____	Papanicolaou smear
24. ED	_____
25. _____	fibrocystic breast disease
26. OB	_____
27. _____	cesarean section
28. OB/GYN	_____
29. _____	spontaneous abortion
30. PIH	_____
31. _____	fetal alcohol syndrome
32. IDC	_____

CHAPTER REVIEW

Word Building ⎯⎯⎯⎯⎯⎯⎯⎯⎯⎯⎯⎯⎯⎯⎯⎯⎯⎯⎯⎯⎯⎯

Construct medical terms from the following meanings. (Some are built from word parts, some are not.)
The first question has been completed as an example.

1. absence of one or both testes ⎯⎯⎯⎯⎯⎯⎯⎯⎯**an**orchism

2. cancer originating from a testis testicular carcin⎯⎯⎯⎯⎯⎯⎯⎯⎯

3. abnormally persistent erection ⎯⎯⎯⎯⎯⎯⎯⎯⎯ism

4. constriction of the prepuce ⎯⎯⎯⎯⎯⎯⎯⎯⎯mosis

5. excision of the prepuce circum⎯⎯⎯⎯⎯⎯⎯⎯⎯

6. an STI that causes liver inflammation ⎯⎯⎯⎯⎯⎯⎯⎯⎯B

7. incision into a testis ⎯⎯⎯⎯⎯⎯⎯⎯⎯tomy

8. condition of an undescended testis ⎯⎯⎯⎯⎯⎯⎯⎯⎯orchidism

9. condition of abnormally few sperm ⎯⎯⎯⎯⎯⎯⎯⎯⎯spermia

10. inflammation of a testis orch⎯⎯⎯⎯⎯⎯⎯⎯⎯

11. herniation of veins in the spermatic cord ⎯⎯⎯⎯⎯⎯⎯⎯⎯cele

12. absence of menstrual discharge ⎯⎯⎯⎯⎯⎯⎯⎯⎯menorrhea

13. white or yellow discharge from the uterus ⎯⎯⎯⎯⎯⎯⎯⎯⎯rrhea

14. condition of pain in the breast ⎯⎯⎯⎯⎯⎯⎯⎯⎯algia

15. profuse bleeding during menstruation meno⎯⎯⎯⎯⎯⎯⎯⎯⎯

16. abnormally reduced bleeding during menstruation ⎯⎯⎯⎯⎯⎯⎯⎯⎯menorrhea

17. spread of endometrial tissue into the pelvic organs endometri⎯⎯⎯⎯⎯⎯⎯⎯⎯

18. inflammation of the cervix ⎯⎯⎯⎯⎯⎯⎯⎯⎯itis

Define the Combining Form ⎯⎯⎯⎯⎯⎯⎯⎯⎯⎯⎯⎯⎯⎯⎯⎯⎯⎯

In the space provided, write the definition of the combining form, followed by one example of the combining
form used to build a medical term in Chapter 12.

	Definition	**Use in a Term**
1. balan/o	⎯⎯⎯⎯⎯⎯⎯⎯⎯⎯⎯	⎯⎯⎯⎯⎯⎯⎯⎯⎯⎯⎯
2. orchi/o	⎯⎯⎯⎯⎯⎯⎯⎯⎯⎯⎯	⎯⎯⎯⎯⎯⎯⎯⎯⎯⎯⎯
3. test/o	⎯⎯⎯⎯⎯⎯⎯⎯⎯⎯⎯	⎯⎯⎯⎯⎯⎯⎯⎯⎯⎯⎯
4. sperm/o	⎯⎯⎯⎯⎯⎯⎯⎯⎯⎯⎯	⎯⎯⎯⎯⎯⎯⎯⎯⎯⎯⎯
5. colp/o	⎯⎯⎯⎯⎯⎯⎯⎯⎯⎯⎯	⎯⎯⎯⎯⎯⎯⎯⎯⎯⎯⎯
6. mamm/o	⎯⎯⎯⎯⎯⎯⎯⎯⎯⎯⎯	⎯⎯⎯⎯⎯⎯⎯⎯⎯⎯⎯
7. metr/o	⎯⎯⎯⎯⎯⎯⎯⎯⎯⎯⎯	⎯⎯⎯⎯⎯⎯⎯⎯⎯⎯⎯
8. salping/o	⎯⎯⎯⎯⎯⎯⎯⎯⎯⎯⎯	⎯⎯⎯⎯⎯⎯⎯⎯⎯⎯⎯
9. cyes/o	⎯⎯⎯⎯⎯⎯⎯⎯⎯⎯⎯	⎯⎯⎯⎯⎯⎯⎯⎯⎯⎯⎯
10. toc/o		

Complete the Labels

Complete the blank labels in ■ Figures 12.34 and 12.35 by writing the labels in the spaces provided.

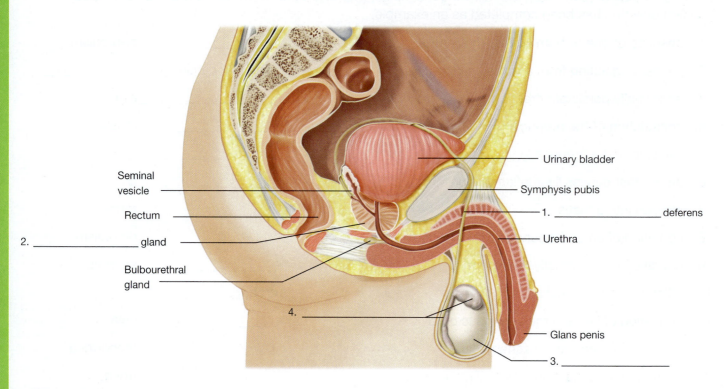

■ Figure 12.34
The male reproductive system.

1. _____

2. _____

3. _____

4. _____

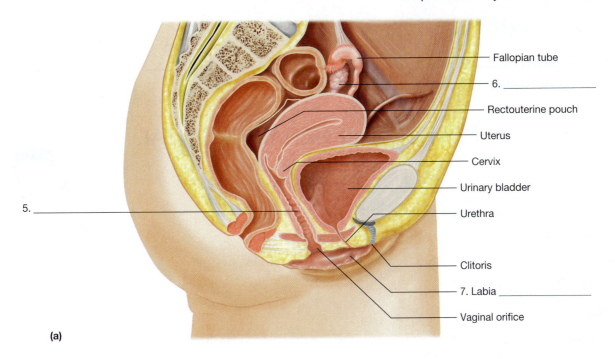

Fallopian tube

6. _____

Rectouterine pouch

Uterus

Cervix

Urinary bladder

Urethra

Clitoris

7. Labia _____

Vaginal orifice

5. _____

(a)

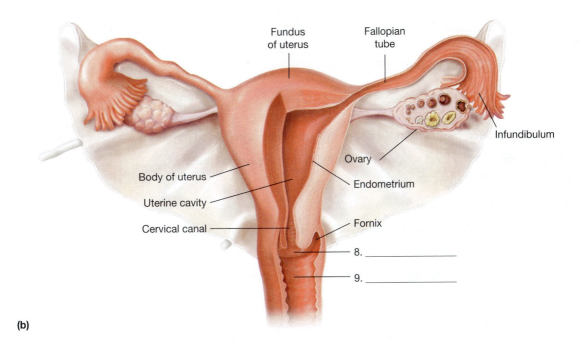

Fundus of uterus

Fallopian tube

Infundibulum

Ovary

Endometrium

Body of uterus

Uterine cavity

Fornix

Cervical canal

8. _____

9. _____

(b)

■ **Figure 12.35**
The female reproductive system. (a) Sagittal section through the pelvis. (b) Top view of the pelvic organs.

5. _____

6. _____

7. _____

8. _____

9. _____

MEDICAL REPORT EXERCISES

Marsha Williams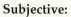

Read the following medical report, then answer the questions that follow.

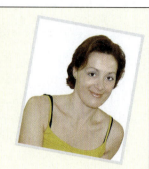

PEARSON GENERAL HOSPITAL

PGH

5500 University Avenue, Metropolis, New York
Phone: (211) 594-4000 • Fax (211) 594-4001

Medical Consultation: Gynecology   **Date**: 04/15/2017

Patient: Marsha Williams   **Patient ID**: 123456

Dob: 3/10/1972   **Age**: 45   **Sex**: Female   **Allergies**: NKDA

Provider: Jennifer Holland, MD

Subjective:

"I experience very painful, heavy periods, especially in the past 5 years. Recently, for the past 2 weeks between my last two periods, I have noticed spotty discharge."

45 y/o female is nulligravida with a history of dysmenorrhea since puberty, but she explains has increased in intensity during the past 5 years and presently complains of menorrhagia between the past two periods. A D&C was performed on 3/01/2011 but failed to correct symptoms.

Objective:

Vital Signs: **T**: 98.5°F; **P**: 74; **R**: 19; **BP**: 122/80

Ht: 5′8″

Wt: 145 lb

General Appearance: Skin with mild pallor, possible diaphoresis. No apparent masses or discolorations.

Heart: Rate at 74 bpm. Heart sounds with auscultation appear normal.

Lungs: Clear without signs of disease.

AbD: Bowel sounds normal all four quadrants.

MS: Joints and muscles symmetric. No swelling, masses, or deformity.

GYN: Erythema, mild edema present at cervical face.

Lab: Pap smear positive for anaplasia, HPV positive. Colposcopy positive for CIS.

Assessment:

CIS at anterior face of cervix

Plan:

Schedule cervical conization within 2 weeks. Biopsy, and consult with Pathology. If recommended, schedule for cervicectomy.

Photo Source: Peter Baxter/Shutterstock.

Comprehension Questions

1. Which patient complaints are consistent with the evidence? _____

_____

_____

2. Why was a Pap smear performed? _____

_____

_____

3. What is the meaning of the terms *dysmenorrhea* and *menorrhagia*? _____

_____

_____

Case Study Questions

The following Case Study provides further discussion regarding the patient in the medical report. Fill in the blanks with the correct terms. Choose your answers from the following list of terms. (Note that some terms may be used more than once.)

carcinoma in situ of the cervix	dilation and curettage	leukorrhea
cervical conization	dysmenorrhea	menorrhagia
colposcopy	HPV (human papillomavirus)	Papanicolaou (Pap) smear

A 45-year-old woman, Marsha Williams, was admitted after complaining of excessive pain during

menstruation, or (a) _____, that was often accompanied by profuse bleeding, or

(b) _____. A white discharge, or (c) _____, was also mentioned by the

patient, usually between periods. A prior treatment in which the cervix was dilated and the endometrium

scraped, called a (d) _____ _____ _____, did not eliminate

the symptoms. The woman had no prior history of reproductive disease, STI, or cancer. A scraping of the

vagina and cervix for microscopic evaluation of cells, or (e) _____ _____,

showed abnormalities of cells. Culturing the cells indicated a type of virus that produces vaginal warts,

called (f) _____, was present and may have been the source of the abnormalities. Further

evaluation of the cervix, in which a tissue sample is removed with the aid of endoscopy and known as

(g) _____, indicated a premetastatic population of mutated cells that were cancerous, a

condition called (h) _____ _____ _____ _____

_____. This finding was confirmed by a negative blood test for ovarian cancer cells. To

eliminate the possibility of metastasis, the location of the anaplastic cell population, at the end of the cervix,

was confirmed by (i) _____ before it was surgically removed in a cervicectomy procedure.

Richard Miller

For a greater challenge, read the following medical report, then answer the critical thinking questions that follow.

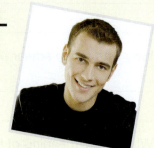

PEARSON GENERAL HOSPITAL

5500 University Avenue, Metropolis, New York
Phone: (211) 594-4000 • Fax (211) 594-4001

Medical Consultation: Urology

Patient: Richard Miller

Dob: 1/15/1995   **Age**: 22   **Sex**: Male

Provider: Samantha M. Ramapurthy, MD

Date: 06/03/2017

Patient ID: 123456

Allergies: NKDA

Subjective:

"For the past month I have been feeling pain deep in my groin area. I also experience pain during urination, and have noticed leakage from my penis."

22 y/o male has no prior history of health concerns. He reported that he has been sexually active with frequent unprotected sex in the past year. The pain he describes is scrotal and at the urinary meatus, combined with balanorrhea.

Objective:

Vital Signs: **T**: 98.8°F; **P**: 73; **R**: 20; **BP**: 119/75

Ht: 5'11"

Wt: 165 lb

General Appearance: Skin with mild pallor and diaphoresis. Palpable lump on lateral aspect of right testis, accompanied by tenderness.

Heart: Rate at 73 bpm. Heart sounds with auscultation appear normal.

Lungs: Clear without signs of disease.

AbD: Bowel sounds normal all four quadrants.

MS: Joints and muscles symmetric. No swelling, masses, or deformity.

bx: Positive for nonseminoma testicular cancer.

Lab: Blood test positive for *N. gonorrhoeae*.

MRI: Tumor present on lateral aspect of r. testis, with some swelling of l. testis.

Assessment:

Nonseminoma testicular cancer of right testis with mets to left testis; gonorrhea

Plan:

Antibiotic therapy to defeat STI. Consult Oncology; if approved, schedule bilateral orchiectomy to remove testicular cancer with inguinal lymph node dissection and exploratory into pelvic region. Follow with 6 months chemotherapy and radiation.

Photo Source: Vgstudio/Shutterstock.

Comprehension Questions

1. What evidence supports the diagnosis of testicular cancer? _____

   _____

   _____

2. How was the gonorrhea infection obtained? _____

   _____

   _____

3. What is a bilateral orchiectomy? _____

   _____

   _____

Case Study Questions
The following case study provides further discussion regarding the patient in the medical report.
Recall the terms from this chapter to fill in the blanks with the correct terms.

A 22-year-old male presented with symptoms that included abnormally few sperm in a semen sample,

called (j) _____, pain in the scrotal and perineal regions, inflammation of the right testis

and epididymis, known as (k) _____, and a palpable lump on his right testis. An evaluation

of his medical history revealed excessive discharge from the glans, called (l) _____,

caused by a concurrent infection resulting in the STI known as (m) _____. The STI

was treated with antibiotics and reported cleared. A biopsy taken from the right testis was positive for

(n) _____ cancer. The left testis also showed evidence of early metastasis, so both testes

were removed during a bilateral (o) _____ that included lymph node dissection from the

pelvic region, followed with chemotherapy and radiation therapy. Intervention proved successful: the patient

survived and is recovering from the treatment with no late-stage metastasis evident. However, the patient

is now (p) _____, or incapable of producing viable gametes.

MyLab Medical Terminology™

MyLab Medical Terminology is a premium online homework management system that includes a host of features to help you study. Registered users will find:

- A multitude of quizzes and activities built within the MyLab platform
- Powerful tools that track and analyze your results—allowing you to create a personalized learning experience
- Videos and audio pronunciations to help enrich your progress
- Streaming lesson presentations (Guided Lectures) and self-paced learning modules
- A space where you and your instructors can view and manage your assignments

Chapter 13

The Nervous System and Mental Health

∨ Learning Objectives

After completing this chapter, you will be able to:

13.1 Define and spell the word parts used to create terms for the nervous system.

13.2 Identify the major organs of the nervous system.

13.3 Break down and define common medical terms used for symptoms, diseases, disorders, procedures, treatments, and devices associated with the nervous system and mental health.

13.4 Build medical terms from the word parts associated with the nervous system and mental health.

13.5 Pronounce and spell common medical terms associated with the nervous system and mental health.

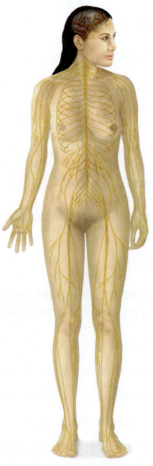

Anatomy and Physiology Terms

The following table provides the combining forms that commonly apply to the anatomy and physiology of the nervous system. Note that the combining forms are colored red to help you identify them when you see them again later in the chapter.

Combining Form	Definition
cephal/o	head
cerebell/o	little brain, cerebellum
cerebr/o	brain, cerebrum
crani/o	skull, cranium
encephal/o	brain
gangli/o	swelling, knot
mening/i, mening/o	membrane

Combining Form	Definition
myel/o	spinal cord, medulla, myelin
neur/o	nerve
phren/o	mind
psych/o	mind
radic/o, radicul/o	nerve root
vag/o	vagus nerve
ventricul/o	little belly, ventricle

nervous
NURR vuss

13.1 The _____ system is a complex part of the body that has been studied extensively, yet there is still much more to learn. It is composed of the brain, spinal cord, and nerves. Together, these important organs enable you to sense the world around you, integrate this information to form thoughts and memories, and control your body movements and many internal functions. The brain and spinal cord form the **central nervous system**, or **CNS**, and the nerves and ganglia form the **peripheral nervous system**, or **PNS**.

homeostasis

neuron

13.2 The nervous system maintains body stability, or _____, by monitoring changes in the body and initiating responses to those changes. It is able to perform this important function by its ability to perceive changes, or stimuli, and convert this information into nerve impulses. A nerve impulse begins when a nerve cell, or **neuron**, opens its membrane channels to sodium and potassium ions, resulting in a flow of these ions across the cell membrane. The flow causes a sudden change in electrical current, which flows along the _____ and is transmitted to other adjacent neurons. The result is an impulse that can travel very quickly along the nerves in your skin and elsewhere and throughout the spinal cord and brain. Neurons are supported by other cells of nervous tissue, known as **neuroglia**, which make up most of the brain and spinal cord.

13.3 Review the anatomy of the nervous system by studying
■ Figure 13.1 and ■ Figure 13.2.

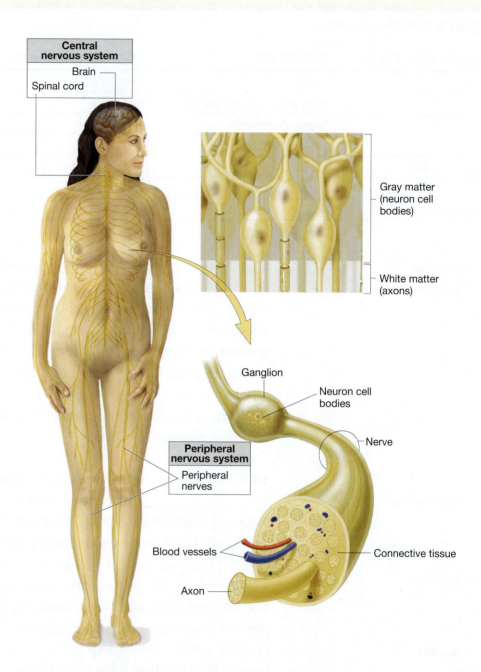

Central nervous system
Brain
Spinal cord

Gray matter (neuron cell bodies)

White matter (axons)

Ganglion

Neuron cell bodies

Nerve

Peripheral nervous system
Peripheral nerves

Blood vessels

Connective tissue

Axon

■ **Figure 13.1**
Organization of the nervous system.

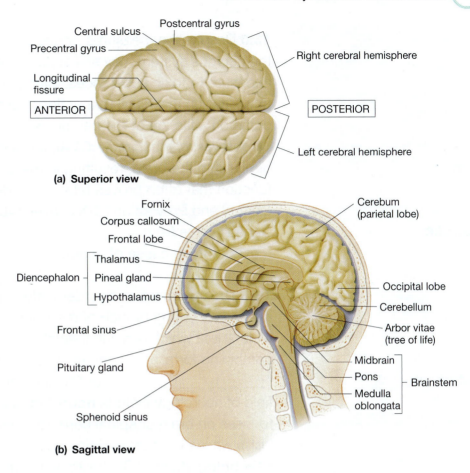

Figure 13.2
The brain. (a) Superior (top) view.
(b) Sagittal view of a sectioned
brain to reveal internal features.

Medical Terms for the Nervous System and Mental Health

nervous

blood–brain barrier

13.4 The nervous system can experience many challenges to health. The tissue making up the brain, spinal cord, and nerves, called _____ tissue, is quite delicate and easily damaged. Therefore, it requires special protective features, such as bone, meninges, and cerebrospinal fluid (CSF). Protection from pathogens circulating in the bloodstream is further assisted by a barrier between brain fluids and the blood, known as the _____–_____ _____, which keeps most bacteria, harmful cells, and many toxins from entering the nervous system. Usually, the unwanted substances that successfully penetrate the blood–brain barrier are eliminated by special neuroglial cells in the brain, called _microglia_.

brain

stroke

13.5 Despite the measures protecting the brain and spinal cord, the nervous system may still experience infectious diseases, exposure to toxic substances, injury, and inherited conditions, any of which may lead to functional losses. For example, the most common affliction of the nervous system is stroke. Also known as *cerebrovascular accident (CVA)*, it is a disruption of the normal flow of blood to the brain, resulting in the loss of _____ function that often proves fatal. According to the Centers for Disease Control and Prevention (CDC), over 140,000 lives were lost in the United States from _____ in 2016, making it the fifth most common cause of death.

study of

mind

13.6 The treatment of disorders affecting the nervous system is a relatively young branch of medicine known as **neurology** (noo RAHL oh jee), which is a subspecialty of internal medicine. The combining form *neur/o* means "nerve," and the suffix *-logy* means "_____" or "science of." Specialists within the broad field of neurology include **neurologists**, whose medical practice focuses on brain or spinal cord treatments; **psychiatrists** (sye KYE ah trists), whose medical practice addresses mental illness; and **clinical psychologists** (sye KOL oh jists), who are mental health professionals trained in the treatment of behavioral disorders. The combining form *psych/o* means "_____."

13.7 In the following sections, you will study the prefixes, combining forms, and suffixes that combine to build the medical terms of the nervous system.

Signs and Symptoms of the Nervous System

Here are the word parts that commonly apply to the signs and symptoms of the nervous system and are covered in the following section. Note that the word parts are color-coded to help you identify them: prefixes are yellow, combining forms are red, and suffixes are blue.

Prefix	Definition
a-	without, absence of
hyper-	excessive, abnormally high, above
hypo-	deficient, abnormally low, below
par-	alongside, abnormal
poly-	excessive, over, many

Combining Form	Definition
cephal/o	head
esthes/o	sensation
neur/o	nerve
phas/o	to speak

Suffix	Definition
-algesia	pain
-algia	condition of pain
-asthenia	weakness
-ia	condition of

KEY TERMS A–Z

aphasia
ah FAY zee ah

a/phas/ia

cephalalgia
seff al ALL jee ah

convulsion
kon VUHL shun

hyperalgesia
HIGH per al JEE zee ah

13.8 The combining form *phas/o* means "to speak," and the prefix *a-* means "without or absence of." Therefore, the inability to speak is known as _____. It is a clinical sign of a disease process causing the disability. The term is constructed of word parts. To highlight the word parts, aphasia can be written as ___/_____/____. It literally means "condition of without speaking." A similar word with a different meaning is **dysphasia**, which means "speech difficulty." Rather than a complete inability to speak, dysphasia is a speech or comprehension disorder resulting from a brain injury or disease. It is also a constructed term, *dys/phas/ia*.

13.9 The clinical term for a **headache**, or a generalized pain in the region of the head, includes the combining form for head, *cephal/o*, and the suffix that means "condition of pain." The term is _____. It includes two word parts, cephal/algia and literally means "condition of head pain."

? Did You **KNOW**

CEPHALALGIA

There are several forms of cephalalgia, including muscle contraction (tension) headaches resulting from sustained muscle contractions often caused by tension; cluster headaches, in which the pain is felt on one side of the head around one eye; and migraine headaches, believed to be caused by changes in the brainstem and its effects on a nerve of the face known as the *trigeminal nerve* (CN V). Migraine pain is often accompanied by extreme sensitivity to light and sound (hyperesthesia; Frame 13.12), nausea, and sometimes vomiting. Migraines were first written about in the 12th century AD, using the old French word *migraigne* that described "a blinding pain in the head."

13.10 A **convulsion** is a series of involuntary muscular spasms caused by an uncoordinated excitation of motor neurons that triggers muscle contraction. A _____ is a sign of a neurological disorder and is also called **seizure** (SEE zhur).

13.11 The symptom **hyperalgesia** is an excessive sensitivity to painful stimuli. The symptom **hypoalgesia** is a deficient sensitivity to normally painful stimuli. The constructed form of _____ is hyper/algesia, and the constructed form of *hypoalgesia* is hypo/algesia.

hyperesthesia HIGH per ess THEE zee ah	**13.12** The combining form *esthes/o* means "sensation." When the prefix *hyper-* and the suffix *-ia* are included, the term _____ is created, which means an excessive sensitivity to a stimulus, such as touch, sound, or pain. This constructed term has three word parts: hyper/esthes/ia.
neuralgia noo RAL jee ah	**13.13** The suffix *-algia* means "condition of pain." A condition of pain in a nerve is a symptom known as _____ and its constructed form is neur/algia.
neurasthenia noo ras THEE nee ah	**13.14** The suffix *-asthenia* means "weakness." When the word root *neur* is included, the clinical term is spelled _____. The symptom of neurasthenia is a generalized experience of body fatigue, which is often associated with mental depression. The constructed form of *neurasthenia* is neur/asthenia.
paresthesia par ess THEE zee ah	**13.15** The prefix *par-* means "alongside or abnormal." Combining it with the combining form for "sensation" forms the term _____. The symptom of **paresthesia** is an abnormal sensation of numbness and tingling caused by an injury to one or more nerves. Its constructed form is par/esthes/ia to identify its three word parts.
neuralgia noo RAL jee ah **polyneuralgia** pall ee noo RAL jee ah	**13.16** In Frame 13.13, you learned that _____ is a condition of pain in a nerve. A condition of pain in many nerves can be termed by adding the prefix that means "many," as in the clinical term _____. The term *polyneuralgia* is constructed of three word parts: poly/neur/algia.
syncope SIN ko pee	**13.17 Syncope** is a temporary loss of consciousness due to a sudden reduction of blood flow to the brain. _____ is often called "fainting." The term is a Greek word that means "a sudden loss of strength."

PRACTICE: Signs and Symptoms of the Nervous System

Linkup

Link the word parts in the list to create the terms that match the definitions. You may use word parts more than once. Remember to add combining vowels when needed and that some terms do not use any combining vowel. The first one is completed as an example.

Prefix	Combining Form	Suffix
a-	asthen/o	-algia
hyper-	esthes/o	-algesia
par-	neur/o	-ia
poly-	phas/o	

Definition

1. the inability to speak
2. an extreme sensitivity to painful stimuli
3. pain in many nerves
4. an excessive sensitivity to a stimulus
5. generalized body fatigue and weakness
6. pain in a nerve
7. abnormal sensation of numbness and tingling caused by nerve injury

Term

aphasia
_____
_____
_____
_____
_____
_____

The Right Match

Match the term on the left with the correct definition on the right.

_____ 1. aphasia

_____ 2. cephalalgia

_____ 3. paresthesia

_____ 4. neuralgia

_____ 5. hyperesthesia

_____ 6. neurasthenia

_____ 7. convulsion

_____ 8. syncope

a. a series of involuntary muscle spasms

b. a vague condition of fatigue

c. excessive sensitivity to a stimulus

d. a headache

e. inability to speak

f. a sudden loss of consciousness

g. abnormal sensation of numbness

h. pain in a nerve

Diseases and Disorders of the Nervous System

Here are the word parts that commonly apply to the diseases and disorders of the nervous system, which are covered in the following section. Note that the word parts are color-coded to help you identify them: prefixes are yellow, combining forms are red, and suffixes are blue.

Prefix	Definition
a-	without, absence of
epi-	upon, over, above, on top
hemi-	half
intra-	within
mono-	one
para-	alongside or abnormal
poly-	excessive, over, many
quadri-	four

Combining Form	Definition
ather/o	fatty plaque
aut/o	self
cephal/o	head
cerebell/o	little brain, cerebellum
cerebr/o	brain, cerebrum
crani/o	skull, cranium
embol/o	plug
encephal/o	brain
gli/o	glue
gnos/o	knowledge
hem/o	blood
hydr/o	water
later/o	side
mening/i, mening/o	membrane
my/o	muscle
myel/o	spinal cord, medulla, myelin
narc/o	numbness
neur/o	nerve
poli/o	gray
scler/o	hard
thromb/o	clot
vascul/o	little vessel
ventricul/o	little belly, ventricle

Suffix	Definition
-al	pertaining to
-ar	pertaining to
-cele	hernia, swelling, protrusion
-ia	condition of
-ic	pertaining to
-ism	condition or disease
-itis	inflammation
-lepsy	seizure
-malacia	softening
-oma	tumor
-osis	condition of
-pathy	disease
-plegia	paralysis
-rrhage	abnormal discharge
-troph	development
-us	pertaining to

KEY TERMS A–Z

agnosia
ahg NOH see ah

Alzheimer's disease
ALTS high merz

13.18 The combining form that means "knowledge" is *gnos/o*. The loss of the ability to interpret sensory information is a disorder known as _____, which is a constructed term that literally means "a condition without knowledge." Its constructed form is *a/gnos/ia*.

13.19 Among some individuals over the age of 40 years, the brain undergoes gradual deterioration resulting in confusion, short-term memory loss, restlessness, and cognitive losses. The disease is called _____ _____ and is abbreviated **AD**. It is a progressive terminal disease with over 5 million sufferers in the United States.

?

Did You KNOW

ALZHEIMER'S DISEASE

This disease is named after German physician Alois Alzheimer, who, in 1906, was the first to draw the connection between the symptoms and the presence of abnormal clumps of protein that form in the brains of patients who died of the disease. The clumps are now called *amyloid plaques* and *neurofibrillary tangles* in the cerebrum and are irreversible changes without a known cause or cure. Even with today's technology, these troublesome clumps of proteins are observable only at postmortem, so a diagnosis of AD is given when the behavioral deficiencies of short-term memory loss, confusion, restlessness, and cognitive losses become apparent after other conditions have been ruled out.

amyotrophic lateral sclerosis
ah my oh TROF ik * LAT er al * skleh ROH siss

13.20 A disease characterized by the progressive atrophy (loss) of muscle caused by hardening of nervous tissue on the lateral columns of the spinal cord is called **amyotrophic lateral sclerosis**. Also known as **Lou Gehrig's disease** after the professional baseball player whose experience with this disease brought it to national attention in 1939, _____ _____ _____ is abbreviated **ALS**. The constructed form of the term *amyotrophic* is a/my/o/troph/ic and literally means "pertaining to without muscle development." ALS is a progressive, terminal disease with no known cause.

autism
AHW tizm

13.21 The Greek word *autos* means "self" or "same" and is the source of the combining form *aut/o*. The disease **autism** literally means "disease of self." _____ is a developmental disorder that varies in its severity with the patient, characterized by withdrawal from outward reality and impaired development in social conduct and communication. Children with autism often avoid eye contact with others and have perseverative behaviors such as rocking back and forth for long periods of time, banging the head, and scratching the skin.

Bell's palsy
behlz * PAHL zee

13.22 In general, a **palsy** is a condition of muscular paralysis. In _____ _____, the patient suffers from paralysis of the face muscles on one side due to damage to the seventh cranial nerve (CN VII).

cerebellitis
ser eh bell EYE tiss

13.23 An inflammation of the cerebellum is called _____. Symptoms of this disease include a loss of muscle coordination and equilibrium. This constructed term can be written as cerebell/itis.

cerebral aneurysm
seh REE bral * AN yoo rizm

13.24 An **aneurysm** is a circulatory problem caused by the weakened wall of a blood vessel, resulting in a bulge in the wall that is in danger of bursting. Aneurysm is derived from the Greek word *aneurysmos*, which means "dilation." A _____ _____ affects arteries channeling blood to the brain, placing the brain at great risk of the damage that would result from a burst aneurysm (■ Figure 13.3). A burst cerebral aneurysm is one major cause of hemorrhagic stroke (Frame 13.28).

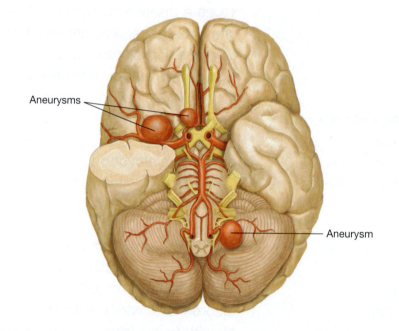

■ Figure 13.3
Cerebral aneurysm. A cerebral aneurysm is the abnormal dilation of arteries supplying the brain, which is caused by a weakening of the arterial walls. In this illustration of the ventral side of the brain, three "berry" aneurysms are revealed as the ball-like swellings of the arteries in red.

Aneurysms

Aneurysm

cerebral atherosclerosis
seh REE bral * ath er oh
skleh ROH siss

cerebral embolism
seh REE bral * EM bol izm

13.25 The disease **cerebral atherosclerosis** affects arteries supplying the brain. The term contains six word parts, which are revealed by writing the term as cerebr/al ather/o/scler/osis. In _____ _____, the vessels gradually close due to the accumulation of fatty plaques, reducing the flow of blood to the brain. This disease also increases the risk of stroke (Frame 13.28), as atherosclerotic plaques tend to break away and float downstream, causing plugs that lodge in blood vessels to cut off the blood supply completely during acute events. A moving blood clot in an artery of the brain is called a _____ _____ (seh REE bral * EM boh lizm). The condition of a stationary blood clot in an artery of the brain is known as **cerebral thrombosis**.

cerebral hemorrhage seh REE bral * HEM ohr ahj	**13.26** Recall that the term **hemorrhage** means the loss of blood, or bleeding. A _____ _____ is the condition of bleeding from blood vessels associated with the cerebrum. The constructed form of this term is cerebr/al hem/o/rrhage.
cerebral palsy seh REE bral * PAWL zee	**13.27** A condition that appears at birth or shortly afterward as a partial muscle paralysis is called **cerebral palsy (CP)**. The paralysis of _____ _____ persists throughout life and is caused by a brain lesion present at birth (known as *congenital CP*) or a brain malfunction that arises during early childhood (known as *acquired CP*). Presently, there is no treatment or cure.
cerebrovascular accident seh REE broh VASS kyoo lar * AKS ih dent	**13.28** The clinical term for a **stroke** is **cerebrovascular accident** and is abbreviated **CVA** (■ Figure 13.4). A _____ _____ occurs when the blood supply to the brain is reduced or cut off, resulting in the irreversible death of brain cells followed by losses of mental function or death. The two major forms of CVA include ischemic stroke, which may be caused by emboli (moving blood clots) or a thrombus (a lodged, stationary blood clot), and hemorrhagic stroke, in which bleeding within the cranial cavity follows an injury to blood vessels or a burst aneurysm. In some cases, a blood clot may form temporarily before it breaks apart and dissolves, resulting in a brief minor episode of ischemia to an area of the brain that is usually without permanent injury. Popularly known as a "mini stroke," it is medically called a **transient ischemic attack (TIA)** and usually lasts less than 5 minutes.

Diagnosis of Stroke

Ischemic ◄————— **Stroke** —————► Hemorrhagic

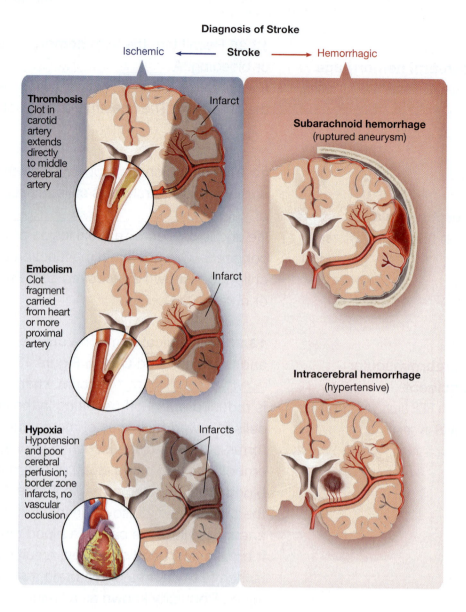

Thrombosis
Clot in carotid artery extends directly to middle cerebral artery

Infarct

Embolism
Clot fragment carried from heart or more proximal artery

Infarct

Hypoxia
Hypotension and poor cerebral perfusion; border zone infarcts, no vascular occlusion

Infarcts

Subarachnoid hemorrhage
(ruptured aneurysm)

Intracerebral hemorrhage
(hypertensive)

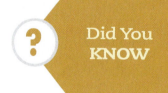

■ **Figure 13.4**
Causes of cerebrovascular accident (CVA), or stroke.

? Did You KNOW

WARNING SIGNS OF A STROKE

Although it may not be possible to completely prevent a stroke, there are warning signs that, if followed, can minimize the neural damage that might otherwise result. The popular acronym FAST includes three signs and a response:

Face: Ask the subject to smile to see if one side of the face droops.

Arms: Ask the subject to raise both arms and observe if one arm drifts downward or is immoveable.

Speech: Ask the subject to say something and listen for slurred or strange speech.

Time: If any of the signs is present, call 911 immediately. The sooner a medical response is made, the greater the chance of a full recovery.

coma
KOH mah

13.29 A **coma** is a general term describing several levels of abnormally decreased consciousness. The term _____ is derived from *koma*, the Greek word that means "deep sleep."

concussion
kon KUH shun

13.30 The Latin word that means "shaking" is *concussio*. This word has been used to create the medical term _____, which is an injury to soft tissue resulting from a blow or violent shaking. In a **cerebral concussion**, the cerebrum undergoes physical damage when it strikes against the inside wall of the cranium. A concussion is considered a minor injury, resulting in head pain, dizziness, and sometimes nausea. A more severe brain injury is called a **traumatic brain injury (TBI)**, which often involves bleeding that can result in functional losses and death. Half of all TBIs in the United States are caused by motorcycle accidents.

encephalitis
en seff ah LYE tiss

13.31 A Greek word for brain is *encephalos*, providing us with the combining form *encephal/o*, which is used in many medical terms associated with the brain. For example, the term for an inflammation of the brain is _____. The condition of encephalitis is usually caused by bacterial or viral infection and is a life-threatening condition, especially among young children. The constructed form of this term is *encephal*/itis.

encephalomalacia
en seff ah loh mah LAY she ah
encephal/o/malacia

13.32 The suffix *-malacia* means "softening." When the combining form for brain is included, the resulting term _____ is created, which refers to a softening of brain tissue. Write the constructed form of this term: _____/___/_____. Encephalomalacia is usually caused by deficient blood flow to the brain, resulting in a large-scale loss of neurons.

epilepsy
EP ih lep see

13.33 A chronic brain disorder characterized by recurrent seizures, including convulsions and temporary loss of consciousness, is the disease **epilepsy**. Each episode results from a sudden, uncontrolled burst of electrical activity in the brain. Epileptic seizures are classified as focal (partial) seizures, which are usually limited to a small area of the brain and may include unexplainable sensations and feelings, and generalized seizures, which strike both hemispheres of the brain and often involve muscle convulsions (in the severest form known as *tonic-clonic* or *grand mal*) and brief losses of consciousness. The term _____ literally means "seized upon."

? Did You KNOW

EPILEPSY

Epileptic seizures have been written about since 400 BC, when they were first described by Hippocrates in his book *Sacred Disease*. His Greek culture believed it was a punishment for offending the gods. The original meaning of the Greek word *epileptikos* is "seized upon by the gods." The misconception that epilepsy is divine punishment or a form of evil persisted until the late 19th century.

glioma
glee OH mah

13.34 A neoplasm (tumor) of glial cells is called a _____.
The term includes two word parts: gli/oma. A glioma becomes life-threatening when it crowds out functional neurons (see ■ Figure 13.5).

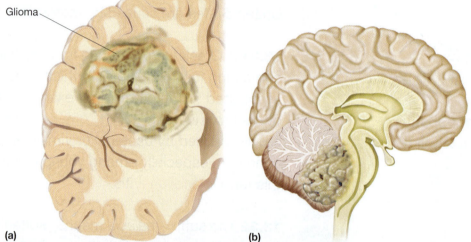

Glioma

(a)   (b)

(c)

■ **Figure 13.5**
Glioma. (a) Illustration of a large glioma (colored area) within the left cerebral hemisphere in a sectioned brain. Notice how the tumor crowds out normal brain tissue. (b) A glioma may also press against the cerebellum and brainstem, causing a loss of motor function and reflexes. (c) PET scan of a glioma (yellow mass). The red and yellow colors indicate that metabolic activity is very high, compared to normal nervous tissue in green and purple. This type of glioma is called a glioblastoma multiforme, which is a fast-growing tumor.
Photo Source: Dr. Giovanni DiChiro, Neuroimaging Section, National Institute of Neurological Disorders and Stroke.

hydrocephalus

HIGH droh SEFF ah luss

13.35 The term **hydrocephalus** literally means "head water." This constructed term includes four word parts: hydr/o/cephal/us. It is usually caused by a blockage or narrowing of one or more channels inside the brain that transport cerebrospinal fluid (CSF) between brain ventricles. Because CSF is continually produced, the result of a blockage or narrowing is a backup of watery CSF, causing the brain ventricles to fill beyond their normal capacity to damage surrounding brain tissue. When it strikes a child before the cranial sutures have sealed, it results in enlargement of the cranium. If it strikes after the cranial sutures have closed, it leads to permanent brain damage. But if diagnosed early, _____ can be surgically corrected by placement of a CSF shunt that drains the excess fluid.

meningioma

meh nin jee OH mah

13.36 The meninges are several layers of membranes surrounding the brain and spinal cord, which include the pia mater, arachnoid mater, and dura mater. The combining form *mening/i* means "membrane." Adding the suffix *-oma* forms the term _____, which is a benign tumor of the meninges usually arising from the arachnoid mater and occurring within the superior sagittal sinus on top of the brain. The constructed form of this term is mening/i/oma.

meningitis

men in JYE tiss

13.37 Adding the suffix *-itis* to the word root that means "membrane" forms the term _____, which is an inflammation of the meninges. It is usually caused by a bacterial infection that begins at the meninges surrounding the spinal cord to form **spinal meningitis**. If left untreated, it poses a risk of spreading along the meninges to the brain to cause the more serious condition, encephalitis (see Frame 13.31). The constructed form of meningitis is written mening/itis.

? Did You KNOW

MYEL/O

The combining form *myel/o* has four different meanings: "bone marrow," "spinal cord," "medulla," and "myelin." The combining form is derived from the Greek word *myelos*, which means "middle." This derivative was used to describe a "middle" structure: the medulla of the brain is in the middle between the higher brain and spinal cord, marrow lies in the middle of a bone, and myelin is in the middle of a neuron. Over time, *myel/o* was assigned separate meanings whenever its use became accepted.

narcolepsy
NAR koh lep see

neuritis
noo RYE tiss

polyneuritis
PALL ee noo RYE tiss

neuroma
noo ROH mah

13.41 A sleep disorder characterized by sudden uncontrollable episodes of sleep, attacks of paralysis, and hypnagogic hallucinations (dreams intruding into the wakeful state) is called **narcolepsy**. Because *narc/o* means "numbness" and *-lepsy* means "seizure," _____ literally means "seizure of numbness." According to the National Institutes of Health, narcolepsy is a widely underdiagnosed condition that may affect approximately 1 in 3,000 Americans.

13.42 Inflammation of a nerve is called _____. It is usually caused by a bacterial or viral infection of the connective tissue coverings surrounding a nerve, although it may also result from physical injury to the nerve. In the condition _____, many nerves at once are inflamed. The term *polyneuritis* includes three word parts: poly/neur/itis. Polyneuritis may be an early sign of increased pressure within the cranium, called **intracranial** (*intra-* = "within"; *crani/al* = "pertaining to the cranium") **pressure**.

13.43 A tumor originating from a neuron is generally called a _____. It is a benign tumor that may form on a nerve or within the brain and is shown in ■ Figure 13.8. Neuroma is a constructed term that may be written as neur/oma to reveal its two word parts.

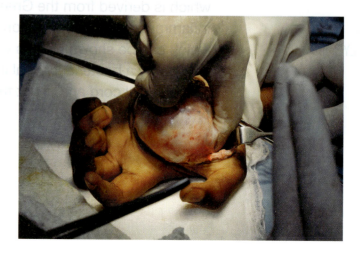

■ **Figure 13.8**
Neuroma. Surgical removal of a large neuroma from the hand of a patient in a procedure known as a *neurectomy*.
Source: Medicimage/Universal Images Group North America LLC/Alamy Stock Photo.

neuropathy
noo ROH path ee

polyneuropathy
pall ee noo ROH path ee

13.44 Damage to peripheral nerves due to any cause is called **neuropathy**, which means "disease of nerves." This constructed term may be written as neur/o/pathy. The most common form of _____ results from a reduction of blood flow to the limbs, such as occurs in diabetic neuropathy, and includes symptoms of pain, tingling, and numbness and can lead to limb amputation. If multiple areas of the body are affected, the prefix *poly-* is added to change the term to _____. The four word parts of the term *polyneuropathy* can be shown as poly/neur/o/pathy.

paraplegia
pair ah PLEE jee ah

quadriplegia
qwad rih PLEE jee ah

13.45 The suffix *-plegia* means "paralysis," or the inability to contract muscles. In _____, muscles of the legs and lower body are paralyzed. Other forms of paralysis include **monoplegia** (mon oh PLEE jee ah), in which one limb is paralyzed; **hemiplegia** (hem ee PLEE jee ah), paralysis of one arm and leg on one side of the body; and _____ (qwad rih PLEE jee ah), paralysis from the neck down including all four limbs. Note how the prefixes alter the meaning of the term: *para-* for "alongside," *mono-* for "one," *hemi-* for "half," and *quadri-* for "four."

Parkinson's disease
PARK ihn sonz

13.46 A chronic, progressive degenerative disease of the brain characterized by tremors, rigidity, and shuffling gait is called **Parkinson's disease**. The cause of _____ _____ is not yet known, although it is diagnosed in over 50,000 Americans each year. It is also called **parkinsonism** and is abbreviated **PD**.

? **Did You KNOW**

PARKINSON'S DISEASE

This tremor-producing disease was first described by English physician James Parkinson in 1817. In his publication he called it "shaking palsy" and, in Latin, *paralysis agitans*. Later, in 1877, it was referenced in French medical texts as "maladie de Parkinson," and by 1890 it was commonly called in English, "Parkinson's disease."

poliomyelitis
poh lee oh my eh LYE tiss

13.47 Caused by one of several viruses belonging to the family poliovirus, the disease **poliomyelitis** is characterized by inflammation of the gray matter of the spinal cord, sometimes resulting in paralysis or death. _____ is commonly referred to as **polio**. A vaccine for this disease has been available since 1955; soon after its discovery by Dr. Jonas Salk it was widely distributed, ending a pandemic that was destroying many lives prior to that year.

ventriculitis

vehn TRIK yoo LYE tiss

13.48 The condition of inflammation of the ventricles of the brain is known as _____. Its most common cause is a blockage of one of the channels that carry cerebrospinal fluid (CSF). The constructed form of this term is ventricul/itis. Untreated ventriculitis results in hydrocephalus (Frame 13.35).

PRACTICE: Diseases and Disorders of the Nervous System

Break the Chain

Analyze these medical terms:

a) Separate each term into its word parts; each word part is labeled for you (**p** = prefix, **r** = root, **cf** = combining form, and **s** = suffix).

b) For the Bonus Question, write the requested definition in the blank that follows.

The first set has been completed for you as an example.

1. a) agnosia
   a/gnos/ia
     p   r   s

   b) *Bonus Question:* What is the meaning of the suffix? _**condition of**_ _____

2. a) cerebellitis
   _____/_____
       r   s

   b) *Bonus Question:* What is the meaning of the word root? _____

3. a) encephalitis
   _____/_____
       r   s

   b) *Bonus Question:* What is the meaning of the word root? _____

4. a) epilepsy
   _____/_____
       p   s

   b) *Bonus Question:* What is the meaning of the suffix? _____

5. a) meningitis
   _____/_____
       r   s

   b) *Bonus Question:* What is the meaning of the suffix? _____

6. a) paraplegia
   _____/_____
       p   s

   b) *Bonus Question:* What is the meaning of the suffix? _____

7. a) neuroma
   _____/_____
       r   s

   b) *Bonus Question:* What is the meaning of the suffix? _____

8. a) neuritis
   _____/_____
       r   s

   b) *Bonus Question:* What is the definition of the word root? _____

The Right Match

Match the term on the left with the correct definition on the right.

_____ 1. encephalitis

_____ 2. coma

_____ 3. Alzheimer's disease

_____ 4. epilepsy

_____ 5. Parkinson's disease

_____ 6. amyotrophic lateral sclerosis

_____ 7. Bell's palsy

_____ 8. autism

_____ 9. concussion

_____ 10. stroke

_____ 11. cerebral palsy

a. a disease resulting in recurrent seizures

b. partial muscle paralysis caused by a brain defect

c. a disease characterized by paralysis of face muscles on one side

d. an injury to the brain resulting from a blow or violent shaking

e. decreased consciousness

f. a developmental disorder that varies in severity

g. a disease characterized by brain deterioration

h. a disease characterized by tremors and rigidity

i. a cerebrovascular accident

j. a disease characterized by progressive atrophy of muscle

k. inflammation of the brain

Treatments, Procedures, and Devices of the Nervous System

Here are the word parts that commonly apply to the treatments, procedures, and devices of the nervous system, which are covered in the following section. Note that the word parts are color-coded to help you identify them: prefixes are yellow, combining forms are red, and suffixes are blue.

Prefix	Definition
an-	without, absence of
epi-	upon, over, above, on top

Combining Form	Definition
angi/o	blood vessel
cerebr/o	brain, cerebrum
crani/o	skull, cranium
dur/o	hard
ech/o	sound
electr/o	electricity
encephal/o	brain
esthes/o	sensation
gangli/o, ganglion/o	swelling, knot
myel/o	spinal cord, medulla, myelin
neur/o	nerve
psych/o	mind
radic/o	nerve root
rhiz/o	nerve root
tom/o	to cut
vag/o	vagus nerve

Suffix	Definition
-al	pertaining to
-algesia	pain
-ectomy	surgical excision, removal
-gram	a record or image
-graphy	recording process
-ia	condition of
-iatry	treatment, specialty
-ic	pertaining to
-ist	one who specializes
-logy	study or science of
-lysis	loosen, dissolve
-plasty	surgical repair
-rrhaphy	suturing
-tome	cutting instrument
-tomy	incision, to cut

KEY TERMS A–Z

analgesic
anne ahl JEE sik

13.49 Pain management is an important part of treating many forms of disease. The most common form of pain management is the use of **analgesics**, such as aspirin, ibuprofen, and acetaminophen. The term _____ means "pertaining to without pain." Analgesics commonly used for severe pain include codeine and morphine. Because they are classified as opioid compounds, they are called **opioid** (OH pee oyd) **analgesics**.

anesthesia
anne ehs THEE zee ah

anesthetist
anne EHS the tist

13.50 The primary type of pain management that is used during surgical procedures is _____. The constructed form of the term is an/esthes/ia and means "without the condition of sensation." The anesthetic is usually a blend of narcotics designed to drop the patient into unconsciousness quickly and as risk-free as possible. It may be administered by inhalation, injection, or drip through a catheter. Anesthesia is managed by a physician called an **anesthesiologist** (anne ehs THEE zee AHL oh jist) and is often administered by a trained specialist called an _____. A **nerve block anesthesia** is an injection made into a nerve to block the conduction of impulses between the nerve and the CNS.

cerebral angiography
seh REE bral * anj ee OHG rah fee

13.51 A diagnostic procedure that reveals blood flow to the brain by x-ray photography is known as **cerebral angiography**. An example of a cerebral angiogram is provided in ■ Figure 13.9. The _____ _____ procedure can identify cerebral aneurysm (Frame 13.24) and cerebral thrombosis (Frame 13.25) and track the damage that might occur following a cerebral hemorrhage (Frame 13.26). This term may be separated into its word parts by writing it as cerebr/al angi/o/graphy.

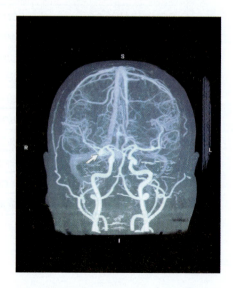

■ **Figure 13.9**
Cerebral angiography. The cerebral angiogram shown here reveals the arteries supplying the brain and branching throughout the brain. The largest white vessels are the right and left internal carotid arteries, which carry blood to the brain from the heart. The arrow points to a cerebral aneurysm.
Source: hasa/Shutterstock.

computed tomography
kom PYOO ted * toh MOG rah fee

13.52 A procedure involving the use of a computer to interpret a series of x-ray images and construct from them a three-dimensional view of the brain is known as **computed tomography**. Commonly called a **CT scan**, _____ _____ is particularly useful in diagnosing tumors, including gliomas (Frame 13.34).

craniectomy
kray nee EK toh mee

13.53 The surgical removal of part of the bony cranium is called _____. The term includes two word parts, which can be shown as crani/ectomy. A craniectomy is usually performed to remove a fractured cranial bone.

craniotomy
kray nee OTT oh mee

13.54 In the slightly less major surgery called a **craniotomy**, an incision is made through the cranium to provide surgical access to the brain. The term _____ can be written as crani/o/tomy to reveal its three word parts. The surgical knife used to perform this operation is called a **craniotome** (crani/o/tome). A craniotomy is shown in ■ Figure 13.10.

■ **Figure 13.10**
Craniotomy. An area of the brain's surface is made accessible for additional procedures by cutting through the cranial wall in a craniotomy. In this photograph, a craniotomy has been performed, setting the stage for the removal of injured or diseased parts of the brain. Here, the surgeon is preparing for the removal of the tumor (the dark mass to the left of normal brain tissue).
Source: ChaNaWiT/Shutterstock.

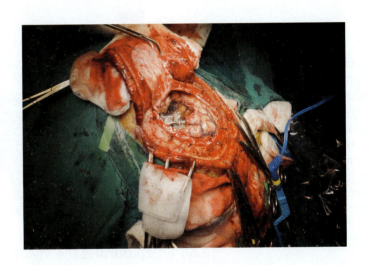

echoencephalography
ek oh en SEFF ah LOG rah fee
ech/o/encephal/o/graphy

13.55 In the procedure **echoencephalography**, ultrasound (sound wave) technology is used to record brain structures in the search for abnormalities. _____ is abbreviated **EchoEG**. Write the term with its division into five word parts here: ____/__/_____/__/_____.

effectual drug therapy

antidepressants

13.56 A general type of treatment to manage neurological disorders is known as **effectual drug therapy**. Examples of _____ _____ _____ include **antianxiety** medication that reduces patient anxiety levels, **anticonvulsants** that control convulsions occurring in diseases such as epilepsy, **antipyretics** that are effective against fever, _____ that combat depression, and **antipsychotics** that reduce hallucinations and confusion. Also, **tranquilizers** and **sedatives** are often used to calm agitated and anxious patients, whereas stronger **narcotics** produce stupor or induce sleep.

electroencephalography
ee LEK troh en SEFF ah
LOG rah fee
electr/o/
encephal/o/graphy

13.57 A diagnostic procedure that records electrical impulses of the brain to measure brain activity is called _____ and is abbreviated **EEG** (■ Figure 13.11). Write the word part construction of this term: _____/__/_____/__/_____.

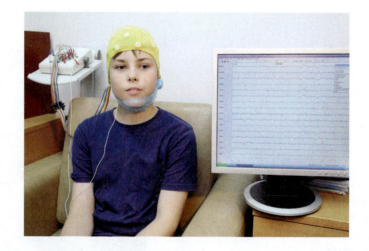

■ **Figure 13.11**
Electroencephalography (EEG). To perform the EEG, electrodes attached to the patient's head by way of a rubber helmet pick up electrical signals and convey them to a computer for analysis and printing.
Source: Pavel L Photo and Video/Shutterstock.

epidural
ep ih DUHR ahl

13.58 An **epidural** is the injection of a spinal block anesthetic into the epidural space external to the spinal cord. It is a common procedure to manage pain during painful childbirth labor or as an emergency procedure following severe trauma to the pelvic region. The term _____ is a constructed term that can be written as epi/dur/al and literally means "pertaining to on top of the dura (mater)."

evoked potential studies

13.59 A group of diagnostic tests that measures changes in brain waves during particular stimuli to determine brain function is known as **evoked potential studies**, or **EP studies**. _____ _____ _____ evaluate sight, hearing, and other senses.

ganglionectomy GANG lee on EK toh mee	**13.60** Surgical removal of a ganglion is known as _____, or **gangliectomy**. Both terms have only two word parts (ganglion/ectomy, gangli/ectomy).
lumbar puncture LUM bar * PUNK shur	**13.61** A **lumbar puncture** is the withdrawal (aspiration) of CSF from the subarachnoid space in the lumbar region of the vertebral column, where the spinal cord is absent (■ Figure 13.12). Abbreviated **LP**, a _____ _____ is performed to evaluate the composition of CSF. A lumbar puncture is commonly called a **spinal tap**.

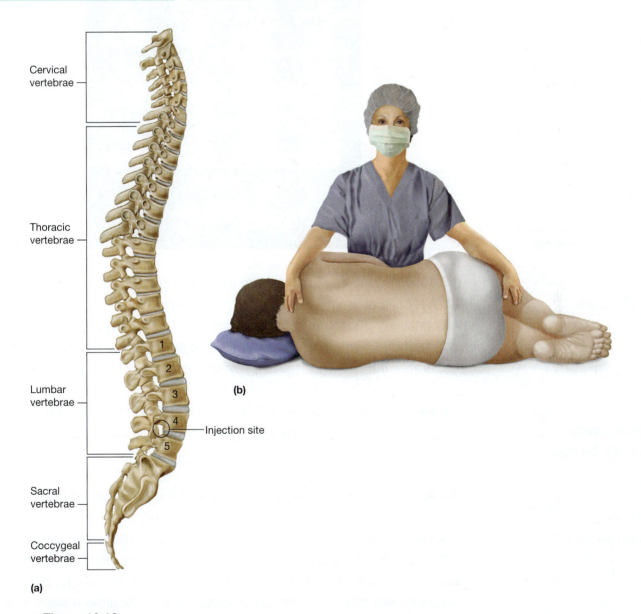

Cervical vertebrae

Thoracic vertebrae

Lumbar vertebrae

1
2
3
4 — Injection site
5

(b)

Sacral vertebrae

Coccygeal vertebrae

(a)

■ **Figure 13.12**
Lumbar puncture. Abbreviated LP, the lumbar puncture is a common procedure that withdraws cerebrospinal fluid from the lumbar region of the spinal canal for examination. Between vertebrae L4 and L5, the needle is pushed through the dura mater to enter the subarachnoid space and CSF circulation. (a) Diagram of the vertebral column to illustrate the location where the needle is inserted for the LP procedure. (b) Supporting the patient for a lumbar puncture.

magnetic resonance imaging

13.62 In the frequently used diagnostic procedure **magnetic resonance imaging**, powerful magnets are used to observe soft tissues in the body, including the brain. Abbreviated **MRI**, _____ _____ _____ is used to target brain tumors, brain trauma, MS, and other conditions (■ Figure 13.13).

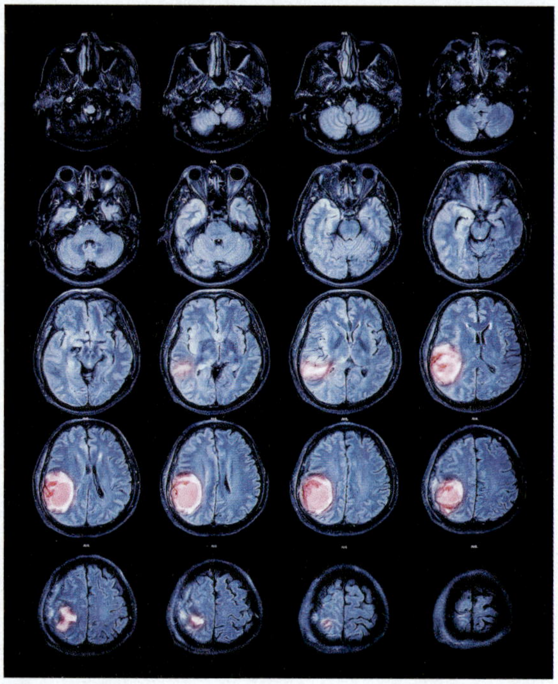

■ **Figure 13.13**
MRI of the brain. In an effort to precisely locate areas of brain injury and disease, multiple images are often recorded at different depths. In this MRI series of the head, transverse section slices through the head have been obtained to observe the precise location of a brain tumor (in pink) within the right parietal lobe.
Source: Puwadol Jaturawutthi-chai/Alamy Stock Photo.

myelogram
  MY eh loh gram

myel/o/graphy

13.63 Using the combining form for spinal cord, *myel/o*, with the suffix for a record or image, *-gram*, forms the term _____. It is an x-ray photograph of the spinal cord following injection of a contrast dye. The procedure is called **myelography**, which can be separated into its word parts by writing it as _____/__/_____.

neurectomy
  noo REK toh mee

13.64 The surgical removal of a nerve is a procedure known as _____. Its word part construction is neur/ectomy.

neurology
  noo RAHL oh jee

neurologist
  noo RAHL oh jist

13.65 The study and medical practice of the nervous system is known as _____. It is also the department of a hospital or clinic where medical procedures on the brain, spinal cord, and nerves are performed. The related term **neurologic** is an adjective associated with the general field of neurology, and a **neuroscientist** is one who participates in neurological research. A _____ is a physician who specializes in neurology, and a **neurosurgeon** is a physician who performs surgery of the brain, spinal cord, and peripheral nerves. The constructed term *neurology* may be shown as neur/o/logy to reveal its three word parts.

neurolysis noo RAHL ih siss	**13.66** The procedure of separating a nerve by removing unwanted adhesions is known as **neurolysis**. _____ can be written as neur/o/lysis. The suffix -*lysis* means "loosen or dissolve."
neuroplasty NOO roh plass tee	**13.67** The suffix -*plasty* means "surgical repair." When adding the combining form for nerve, the term becomes _____. Thus, neuroplasty is the surgical repair of a nerve. Its three word parts may be shown as neur/o/plasty.
neurorrhaphy noo ROR ah fee	**13.68** The suffix -*rrhaphy* refers to a procedure involving sutures. When adding the combining form for nerve, the term becomes _____, or neur/o/rrhaphy. It means "suture of a nerve."
neurotomy noo ROT oh mee neur/o/tomy	**13.69** Recall that the suffix -*tomy* means "incision, to cut." Adding the combining form for nerve creates the term _____, which means "incision into a nerve." Write the word part construction of this term: _____/__/_____.
positron emission tomography PAHZ ih tron * ee MISH un * toh MOG rah fee	**13.70** A scan using a radioactive chemical to provide a map of metabolically active cells within the brain is a common procedure known as _____ _____ _____. It is often called a **PET scan** and is a useful diagnostic procedure to evaluate brain function.
psychiatry sigh KIGH ah tree	**13.71** The branch of medicine that addresses disorders of the brain resulting in mental, emotional, and behavioral disturbances is known as _____. The constructed form of this term is psych/iatry, which means "treatment of the mind." A physician practicing in this field is a **psychiatrist**, who often uses **psychopharmacology**, or drug therapy targeting the brain, and **psychoanalysis**, or psychiatric therapy, to improve a patient's quality of life.
psychology sigh KALL oh jee **psychotherapy** SIGH koh THAIR ah pee	**13.72** In contrast to psychiatry, the field of _____ is not a medical specialty. It is the study of human behavior. The term *psychology* contains three word parts, psych/o/logy, which means "study or science of the mind." However, a subdiscipline within this field, known as **clinical psychology**, uses applied psychology to treat patients suffering from behavioral disorders and emotional trauma. The technique used in treating behavioral and emotional issues is called _____.

radicotomy ray dih KOT oh mee	**13.73** Recall that the suffix *-tomy* means "incision, to cut." A surgical incision into a nerve root is called _____. It is also called **rhizotomy** because a nerve root has two combining forms, *radic/o* and *rhiz/o*.
reflex testing	**13.74 Reflex testing** is a series of diagnostic tests performed to observe the body's response to touch stimuli. _____ _____ is useful in assessing stroke, head trauma, birth defects, and other neurological challenges. The tests include **deep tendon reflexes (DTR)** involving percussion at the patellar tendon and elsewhere and Babinski reflex involving stimulation of the plantar surface of the foot.
tPA	**13.75** As a treatment for stroke (Frame 13.28), a powerful chemical that dissolves blood clots in vessels supplying the brain is known as **tissue plasminogen activator**, abbreviated **tPA** (or IV tPA because it is given through an IV into the arm). If it is administered within 3 hours of a stroke, _____ may reopen blood flow to the brain in time to reduce brain injury and make a full recovery possible.
vagotomy vay GOT oh mee	**13.76** The vagus nerve (CN X) is a large cranial nerve passing from the brainstem into the thoracic and abdominal cavities. During a _____, several branches of the vagus nerve are severed to reduce acid secretion into the stomach to help prevent the reoccurrence of peptic ulcer or reduce pain from the digestive organs. The constructed form of this term is *vag/o/tomy*.

PRACTICE: Treatments, Procedures, and Devices of the Nervous System

Linkup

Link the word parts in the list to create the terms that match the definitions. You may use word parts more than once. Remember to add combining vowels when needed and that some terms do not use any combining vowel.

Prefix	Combining Form	Suffix
an-	crani/o	-ectomy
	esthes/o	-ia
	neur/o	-iatry
	psych/o	-logy
	vag/o	-rrhaphy
		-tomy

Definition

Term

1. the primary type of pain management that is used during surgical procedures _____
2. surgical removal of part of the cranium _____
3. the study and medical practice of the nervous system _____
4. a procedure in which an incision is made through the cranium to provide _____ surgical access to the brain
5. suture of a nerve _____
6. branch of medicine that addresses disorders of the brain that result in _____ mental and emotional disturbances
7. surgical severing of several branches of the vagus nerve to reduce acid _____ secretion in the stomach
8. the study of human behavior _____

The Right Match

Match the term on the left with the correct definition on the right.

_____ 1. computed tomography
_____ 2. effectual drug therapy
_____ 3. reflex testing
_____ 4. sedative
_____ 5. analgesic
_____ 6. lumbar puncture
_____ 7. vagotomy

a. the withdrawal of CSF from the spinal cord
b. agent with a calming effect
c. treatment with medications to manage neurological disorders
d. cutting the vagus nerve to reduce peptic ulcers and pain
e. a procedure that constructs a three-dimensional view of the brain
f. series of tests that observe responses to touch stimuli
g. agent that relieves pain

Mental Health Diseases and Disorders

Here are the word parts that commonly apply to mental health diseases and disorders and are covered in the following section. Note that the word parts are color-coded to help you identify them: prefixes are yellow, combining forms are red, and suffixes are blue.

Prefix	Definition	Combining Form	Definition	Suffix	Definition
bi-	two	ment/o	mind	-ia	condition of
dys-	bad, abnormal, painful, difficult	neur/o	nerve	-ic	pertaining to
		phren/o	mind	-lexia	pertaining to a word or phrase
		psych/o	mind		
		schiz/o	to divide, split	-mania	madness, frenzy
		somat/o	body	-osis	condition of
				-pathy	disease
				-phobia	fear

KEY TERMS A–Z

anxiety disorder
ang ZIGH eh tee * dihs OR der

13.77 Anxiety is the apprehension of danger, filling a person with fear over the future. An _____ _____ occurs when this mental state dominates behavior. It is usually an acute response that includes restlessness, psychological tension, tachycardia, and shortness of breath.

attention-deficit disorder

13.78 A neurological disorder characterized by short attention span and poor concentration is called **attention-deficit disorder**. Abbreviated **ADD**, _____ _____ _____ is usually associated with school-age children but can also affect adults and makes learning very difficult. A similar disorder is **attention-deficit/hyperactivity disorder**, abbreviated **ADHD**, which has the added symptom of hyperactivity, or hyperkinesia.

bipolar disorder
bye POHL ar

13.79 Bipolar literally means "pertaining to two poles." The mental disorder called _____ _____ affects the cognitive functions of the cerebrum, causing alternating periods of high energy and mental confusion (known as mania, discussed in Frame 13.82) with low energy and mental depression (■ Figure 13.14).

■ **Figure 13.14**
Bipolar disorder. The term *bipolar* means "pertaining to two poles." The individual with this form of mental disease cycles between the two extreme behaviors of high-energy mania and low-energy depression, each often lasting for days.

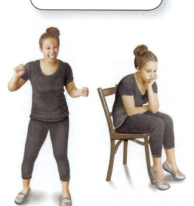

BIPOLAR DISEASE

MANIC

- Begins suddenly and escalates over several days
- Elevated mood
- Loud, rapid speech
- Grandiose statements
- Delusional thoughts
- Hyperactive

DEPRESSIVE

- Despairing
- Reduced, slow speech
- Reduced interest in pleasure
- Negative views
- Fatigue
- Loss of appetite
- Insomnia
- Suicidal thoughts

dementia
de MEN she ah

13.80 The Latin word that means "not in the mind," **dementia**, is an impairment of mental function characterized by memory loss, disorientation, and confusion. _____ is usually associated with old age and sometimes accompanies Alzheimer's disease (Frame 13.19) and Parkinson's disease (Frame 13.46).

dyslexia
dihs LEKS ee ah

13.81 Some individuals have a reading handicap that has a neurological cause, in which some letters and numbers are reversed in order by the brain. The condition is called **dyslexia**. _____ literally means "condition of difficult reading."

mania
MAE nee ah

13.82 The Greek word for madness or frenzy is *mania*. The clinical condition of _____ is an emotional disorder of abnormally high psychomotor activity, which includes excitement, a rapid movement of ideas, unstable attention, sleeplessness, and confusion between reality and imagination. Different forms of mania include the *-mania* suffix, such as **megalomania** (MEHG ah lo MAE nee ah), in which an individual believes oneself to be a person of great fame or wealth (*megalon* means "great" in Greek), and **pyromania** (PIE roh MAE nee ah), which is an obsessive fascination with fire (*pyro* in Latin means "fire").

neurosis
noo ROH siss

13.83 A **neurosis** is an emotional disorder involving a counterproductive way of dealing with mental stress. _____ is a constructed term with two word parts, shown as neur/osis.

paranoia
pahr ah NOY ah

13.84 A person experiencing persistent delusions of persecution resulting in mistrust and combativeness suffers from **paranoia**. The term _____ is derived from a Greek word meaning "abnormal mind, madness."

phobia
FOE bee ah

13.85 A **phobia** is an irrational, obsessive fear. Derived from the Greek word for fear, *phobos*, _____ is often used as a suffix (*-phobia*) when describing a particular fear. For example, fear of spiders is called **arachnophobia** because the root is from the Greek word *arachne*, which means "spider." Similarly, **agoraphobia** is the abnormal fear of public places (*agora* means "meeting place" in Greek), **acrophobia** is the abnormal fear of heights (*acro* means "peak" in Greek), and **phobophobia** is the fear of developing a phobia.

posttraumatic stress disorder	**13.86** Many individuals who have experienced a severe mental strain, physical threat or injury such as military combat or a physical assault, or emotional trauma suffer from an acute condition that includes sleeplessness, anxiety, and paranoia. The condition is called _____ _____ _____. It is abbreviated **PTSD**.
psychopathy sy KOH path ee	**13.87 Psychopathy** is a general term for a mental or emotional disorder. _____ literally means "disease of the mind." Its word parts may be shown as psych/o/pathy.
psychosis sy KO siss	**13.88** An individual suffering from a gross distortion or disorganization of their mental capacity, emotional response, and capacity to recognize reality and relate to others may be diagnosed with the disease known as **psychosis**. The most common form of _____ is schizophrenia (Frame 13.90). The constructed form of the term is psych/osis and literally means "condition of the mind."
psychosomatic SY koh soh MAT ik	**13.89** The term **psychosomatic** literally means "pertaining to mind and body." Its word parts can be shown as psych/o/somat/ic. It refers to the influence of the mind over bodily functions, especially disease. Among some people, their mind creates symptoms that suggest an illness when physical signs are absent. In others, a _____ illness can be a real physical illness resulting from mental anxiety, such as peptic ulcer and hypertension.
schizophrenia SKIZ oh FREHN ee ah schiz/o/phren/ia	**13.90** The most common form of psychosis is _____, which literally means "condition of split mind." It is characterized by delusions, hallucinations, and extensive withdrawal from other people and the outside world. There are many forms of schizophrenia, each type classified according to the experiences of the patient. Its constructed form is _____/_/_____/___.

PRACTICE: Mental Health Diseases and Disorders

The Right Match

Match the vocabulary term on the left with the correct definition on the right.

_____ 1. anxiety disorder

_____ 2. bipolar disorder

_____ 3. dementia

_____ 4. posttraumatic stress disorder

_____ 5. paranoia

_____ 6. attention-deficit disorder

a. a neurological disorder characterized by short attention span and poor concentration

b. a disorder that results from severe mental strain or emotional trauma

c. alternating periods of high energy and mental confusion (mania) with low energy and mental depression

d. persistent delusions of persecution that result in mistrust and combativeness

e. impairment of mental function characterized by memory loss, disorientation, and confusion

f. a disorder in which the mental state of apprehension and fear dominates behavior

Break the Chain

Analyze these medical terms:

   a) Separate each term into its word parts; each word part is labeled for you (**p** = prefix, **r** = root, **cf** = combining form, and **s** = suffix).

   b) For the Bonus Question, write the requested definition in the blank that follows.

1. a) dyslexia   _____/_____
                          p   s

   b) *Bonus Question:* What is the definition of the prefix? _____

2. a) neurosis   _____/_____
                          r   s

   b) *Bonus Question:* What is the definition of the word root? _____

3. a) psychopathy   _____/___/_____
                          cf   s

   b) *Bonus Question:* What is the definition of the suffix? _____

4. a) psychosis   _____/_____
                          r   s

   b) *Bonus Question:* What is the definition of the word root? _____

Abbreviations of the Nervous System and Mental Health

The abbreviations that are associated with the nervous system and mental health are summarized here. Study these abbreviations and review them in the exercise that follows.

Abbreviation	Definition
AD	Alzheimer's disease
ADD	attention-deficit disorder
ADHD	attention-deficit/hyperactivity disorder
ALS	amyotrophic lateral sclerosis
CNS	central nervous system
CP	cerebral palsy
CSF	cerebrospinal fluid
CT (CAT) scan	computed (axial) tomography scan
CVA	cerebrovascular accident (stroke)
DTR	deep tendon reflexes
EchoEG	echoencephalography

Abbreviation	Definition
EEG	electroencephalography
EP studies	evoked potential studies
LP	lumbar puncture
MRI	magnetic resonance imaging
MS	multiple sclerosis
PD	Parkinson's disease
PET	positron emission tomography
PNS	peripheral nervous system
PTSD	posttraumatic stress disorder
TBI	traumatic brain injury
TIA	transient ischemic attack
tPA	tissue plasminogen activator

PRACTICE: Abbreviations

Fill in the blanks with the abbreviation or the complete medical term.

Abbreviation	Medical Term
1. _____	evoked potential studies
2. PET	_____
3. EEG	_____
4. _____	computed tomography scan
5. MRI	_____
6. _____	Parkinson's disease
7. CP	_____
8. _____	echoencephalography
9. DTR	_____
10. _____	multiple sclerosis
11. CVA	_____
12. _____	Alzheimer's disease
13. ALS	_____
14. _____	attention-deficit disorder
15. ADHD	_____
16. _____	traumatic brain injury

CHAPTER REVIEW

Word Building

Construct medical terms from the following meanings. The first question has been completed for you as an example.

1. excessive sensitivity to painful stimuli   _____***hyper***algesia

2. a pain in the head (headache)   _____algia

3. inflammation of the cerebellum   cerebell_____

4. a disease of blood vessels in the cerebrum   _____vascular disease

5. a tumor of neuroglial cells   gli_____

6. softening of brain tissue   encephalo_____

7. nervous system disease   neuro_____

8. excessive sensitivity to a stimulus   _____esthesia

9. inflammation of the brain   _____itis

10. protrusion of the meninges   meningo_____

11. literally a "condition of many hard" areas   _____sclerosis

12. inflammation of the spinal cord   _____itis

13. literally "nerve weakness"   neur_____

14. a tumor arising from nervous tissue   neur_____

15. pain in a nerve   neur_____

16. abnormal sensation of numbness   par_____

17. paralysis on one side of the body   _____plegia

18. inflammation of many nerves   poly_____

19. a disease of the mind   _____pathy

20. paralysis of all four limbs   _____plegia

Define the Combining Form

In the space provided, write the definition of the combining form, followed by one example of the combining form used to build a medical term in Chapter 13.

	Definition	**Use in a Term**
1. mening/o	_____	_____
2. cerebr/o	_____	_____
3. encephal/o	_____	_____
4. myel/o	_____	_____
5. neur/o	_____	_____
6. esthesi/o	_____	_____
7. crani/o	_____	_____
8. gangli/o	_____	_____
9. psych/o	_____	_____
10. phasi/o	_____	_____

Complete the Labels _____

Complete the blank labels in ■ Figures 13.15 and 13.16 by writing the labels in the spaces provided.

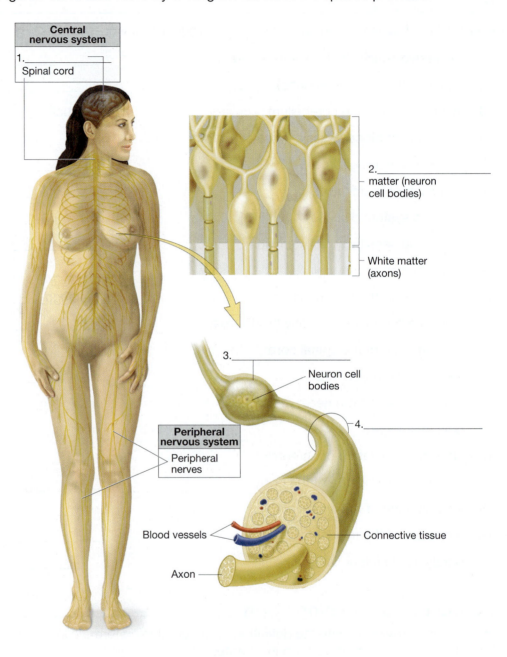

Central nervous system

1._____
Spinal cord

2._____
matter (neuron cell bodies)

White matter (axons)

3._____
Neuron cell bodies

4._____

Peripheral nervous system
Peripheral nerves

Blood vessels

Connective tissue

Axon

■ **Figure 13.15**
Organization of the nervous system.

1. _____

2. _____

3. _____

4. _____

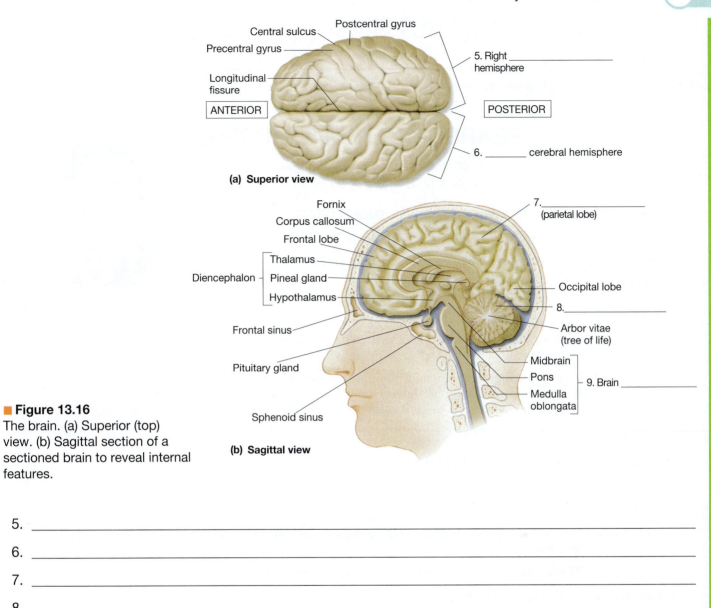

Figure 13.16
The brain. (a) Superior (top) view. (b) Sagittal section of a sectioned brain to reveal internal features.

5. _____

6. _____

7. _____

8. _____

9. _____

MEDICAL REPORT EXERCISES

Melissa Tampico

Read the following medical report, then answer the questions that follow.

PGH

PEARSON GENERAL HOSPITAL

5500 University Avenue, Metropolis, New York
Phone: (211) 594-4000 • Fax (211) 594-4001

Medical Consultation: Neurology   **Date:** 11/05/2017

Patient: Melissa Tampico   **Patient ID:** 123456

Dob: 2/11/1998   **Age:** 19   **Sex:** Female   **Allergies:** NKDA

Provider: Mark P. Simmons, MD

Subjective:

"Since a car crash I was in several weeks ago, I've been dealing with severe headaches. I also feel intermittent sharp pains running from the top of the left shoulder down the arm, with tingling sensations."

19 y/o female recently immigrated from the Philippine Islands, without a forwarding medical history. She explains that her complaints of cephalalgia, neuralgia, and polyneuritis have appeared since an automobile accident 3 weeks ago. She was not examined at the time because of health insurance concerns.

Objective:

Vital Signs: T: 98.6°F; **P:** 77; **R:** 20; **BP:** 137/90

Ht: 5′4″

Wt: 115 lb

General Appearance: Skin appears healthy, with no apparent masses or discolorations. Bruising present at top of left shoulder.

Heart: Rate at 77 bpm. Heart sounds with auscultation appear normal.

Lungs: Clear with no sign of disease.

AbD: Bowel sounds normal all four quadrants.

MS: No swelling, masses, or deformity. ROM limited 30 degrees at right shoulder.

CT: Subdural hemorrhage 1.5 mm inferior to right of squamosal suture. Confirmed by MRI without additional complications known. No internal damage to r. shoulder.

Assessment:

Traumatic brain injury with active subdural hemorrhage of right temporal lobe. Intracranial pressure is rising. Mild polyneuritis of left shoulder and arm.

Plan:

STAT craniotomy to treat subdural hemorrhage and drain fluid to reduce intracranial pressure. Treat polyneuritis with anti-inflammatory.

Photo Source: Creativa Images/Shutterstock.

Comprehension Questions

1. What patient complaint is an early indication of increasing intracranial pressure on the right side of the brain?

    _____

    _____

    _____

2. If the intracranial pressure is not relieved in time, what do you suppose might be the consequences to the patient? _____

    _____

    _____

3. Explain the meanings of the terms *neuralgia* and *cephalalgia*. _____

    _____

    _____

Case Study Questions

The following case study provides further discussion regarding the patient in the medical report. Fill in the blanks with the correct terms. Choose your answers from the following list of terms. (Note that some terms may be used more than once.)

analgesics	craniotomy	neuralgia
cephalalgia	intracranial	paresthesia
computed tomography	magnetic resonance imaging	polyneuritis

The patient, Melissa Tampico, was examined following an automobile collision. At the time of admittance

she reported symptoms of headache, or (a) _____, generalized pain in the nerves, or

(b) _____, of the right shoulder and upper arm. Physical examination showed an inflammation

of multiple nerves, or (c) _____, of the shoulder and upper arm. Anti-inflammatory

medication and pain relievers, or (d) _____, were prescribed for treatment. Two weeks after

the first exam, the patient returned with reported abnormal sensations along the left side of the body, or

(e) _____. Following a preliminary CT, or (f) _____ _____

scan, an MRI, or (g) _____ _____ _____, was ordered for a

more complete evaluation. The MRI revealed bleeding below the dura mater (subdural hemorrhage), which

was increasing the (h) _____ (within the cranium) pressure. An incision into the cranium,

or (i) _____, was performed to stop the hemorrhage and reduce the intracranial pressure.

The patient made a complete recovery.

Chapter 14

The Special Senses of Sight and Hearing

Learning Objectives

After completing this chapter, you will be able to:

14.1 Define and spell the word parts used to create terms for the special senses of sight and hearing.

14.2 Identify the major structures of sight and hearing.

14.3 Break down and define common medical terms used for symptoms, diseases, disorders, procedures, treatments, and devices associated with the special senses of sight and hearing.

14.4 Build medical terms from the word parts associated with the special senses of sight and hearing.

14.5 Pronounce and spell common medical terms associated with the special senses of sight and hearing.

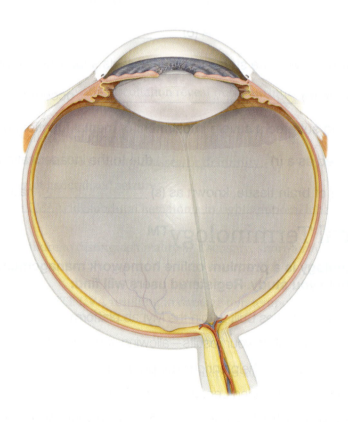

Anatomy and Physiology Terms

The following table provides the combining forms that commonly apply to the anatomy and physiology of the eyes and ears. Note that the combining forms are colored red to help you identify them when you see them again later in the chapter.

Combining Form	Definition	Combining Form	Definition
blephar/o	eyelid	ocul/o	eye
conjunctiv/o	to bind together, conjunctiva	ophthalm/o	eye
cor/o	pupil	opt/o	eye
dacry/o	tear	ot/o	ear
ir/o	iris	retin/o	retina
kerat/o	hard, cornea	rhin/o	nose
myring/o	membrane, eardrum	scler/o	hard, sclera

sight

sensory receptors

ears

14.1 The special senses are a part of the nervous system that include sensory receptors, which are specialized neurons that respond to a change in the environment, called a *stimulus*. There are four special senses, each of which contains sensory receptors and supportive tissues. They are smell, or olfaction; taste, or gustation; _____, or vision; and hearing, or audition. In this chapter, you learn the medical terms of the two most important special senses, sight and hearing.

14.2 The special sense of sight, or vision, is performed by the eyes, organs located in the orbits of the skull. Each eye contains _____ _____ sensitive to light, called *photoreceptors*, and supportive structures. The special sense of hearing, or audition, is centered within the _____, which contain sensory receptors that respond to mechanical vibrations. Also within the ears are receptors providing you with the sense of equilibrium.

14.3 To review the anatomy of the eye and ear, study the labeled diagrams in ■ Figure 14.1 and ■ Figure 14.2.

KEY TERMS A–Z

asthenopia
AHS then OH pee ah

blepharoptosis
BLEF ah ropp TOH sis

blepharitis
BLEF ah RYE tiss

leukocoria
loo koh KOR ee ah

ophthalmalgia
off thal MAL jee ah

ophthalmorrhagia
off thal moh RAHJ ee ah

14.7 The combining form *asthen/o* means "weakness," and the suffix *-opia* means "condition of vision." Therefore, a symptom of eye weakness, commonly referred to as "eyestrain," is known as _____. It is a short-term, or acute, symptom usually resulting from reading a computer screen or book without frequent breaks. The constructed form is asthen/opia.

14.8 The combining form for eyelid is *blephar/o*. In some people of senior age, the eyelid droops over the eye abnormally. Because the suffix *-ptosis* means "drooping," when it is added to the combining form for "eyelid" it forms the sign _____. The word parts forming **blepharoptosis** can be shown as blephar/o/ptosis.

14.9 A common sign of an inflammation of an eyelid is called _____. If the inflammation or trauma damages the eyelid, it may be repaired in a procedure known as **blepharoplasty** (BLEF ah roh plass tee).

14.10 The pupil is the black opening through the iris that allows light to enter the posterior cavity of the eyeball. The abnormal appearance of a white film in the pupil is a sign of disease. It is called _____, which literally means "white in the pupil." The four word parts forming this term can be shown as leuk/o/cor/ia.

14.11 One combining form for eye is *ophthalm/o*. It is used to form many medical terms of the eye, which you are about to discover. In one of these, the suffix *-algia* is included and means "condition of pain." The symptom of eye pain is therefore called _____. It is a constructed term: ophthalm/algia.

14.12 A second medical term that includes the combining form *ophthalm/o* means "abnormal discharge of the eye." To build this term, the suffix for abnormal discharge, *-rrhagia*, is added. This term, meaning bleeding of the eye, is _____. The constructed form is ophthalm/o/rrhagia.

PRACTICE: Signs and Symptoms of the Eyes and Sight

The Right Match

Match the term on the left with the correct definition on the right.

_____ 1. asthenopia   a. white in the pupil

_____ 2. blepharoptosis   b. abnormal discharge of the eye

_____ 3. leukocoria   c. inflammation of an eyelid

_____ 4. ophthalmalgia   d. drooping of an eyelid

_____ 5. ophthalmorrhagia   e. pain associated with an eye

_____ 6. blepharitis   f. eyestrain

Linkup

Link the word parts in the list to create the terms that match the definitions. You may use word parts more than once. Remember to add combining vowels when needed and that some terms do not use any combining vowel. The first one is completed as an example.

Combining Form	Suffix
asthen/o	-algia
blephar/o	-ia
cor/o	-itis
leuk/o	-opia
ophthalm/o	-ptosis
	-rrhagia

Definition

1. white in the pupil
2. eyestrain
3. pain associated with an eye
4. abnormal discharge of an eye
5. drooping of an eyelid
6. inflammation of an eyelid

Term

leukocoria

_____

_____

_____

_____

_____

diplopia

dih PLOH pee ah

14.18 Because a prefix that means "double" is *dipl-*, the condition of double vision is called _____. It may result from weakened extrinsic eye muscles, defects in the lens, or a condition of the brain.

14.19 In the disease of the eye known as **glaucoma**, a loss of vision occurs when the fluid pressure within the anterior chamber of the eyeball (called intraocular pressure) rises above normal and spreads to the posterior chamber, thereby pushing against the delicate retina and optic nerve. The rise of fluid pressure in _____ is often caused by a blockage in a small opening that normally drains the fluid (■ Figure 14.5).

glaucoma

glaw KOH mah

■ **Figure 14.5**
Glaucoma. (a) A buildup of pressure within the eye cavities, often caused by a blockage of vessels that drain fluid, may damage the optic nerve at the back of the eyeball to result in a gradual loss of sight and blindness. (b) Glaucoma often causes reduced sight, such as the loss of the perimeter of a visual field as shown here. *Photo Source: B. Boissonnet/ BSIP SA/Alamy Stock Photo.*

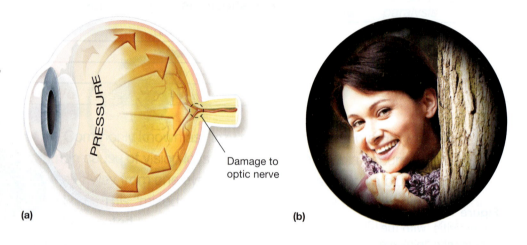

(a) (b)

Damage to optic nerve

hordeolum

hor DEE oh lum

14.20 A meibomian gland is a small gland in the eyelid that secretes lubricating fluid onto the conjunctiva. An infection of this gland produces a local swelling of the eyelid, known as a **hordeolum**. Also called a **sty**, the term _____ is derived from the Latin word *hordeum*, which means "barley" (■ Figure 14.6). A chronic form of this infection is often called a **chalazion** (kah LAY zee on), which is derived from *chalaza*, the Greek word that means "sty."

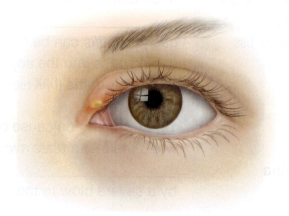

■ **Figure 14.6**
Hordeolum (or sty).

iritis
 eye RYE tiss
keratitis
 kair aht EYE tiss

14.21 During a bacterial infection of the eye, parts of the eye may become inflamed. When the iris is affected, the condition is known as _____, and when the cornea becomes inflamed, it is called _____. A common cause of both conditions is wearing contact lenses without careful cleaning. The word part construction of the term *iritis* is ir/itis and *keratitis* is kerat/itis. In addition to being caused by bacterial infections, both iritis and keratitis may also be caused by the herpes type I virus.

macular degeneration

14.22 The macula lutea is a small area of the retina that contains a high density of photoreceptors, known as cone cells. Because of the high concentration of cone cells, it is the area of sharpest vision. Progressive deterioration of the macula lutea leads to a loss of visual focus and is called **macular degeneration** (■ Figure 14.7). The abbreviated version of _____ _____ is **AMD** (age-related macular degeneration) because its most common cause is senior age.

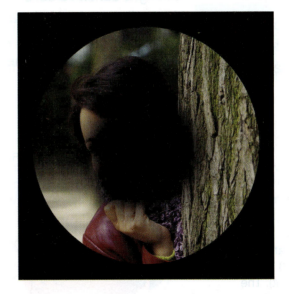

■ **Figure 14.7**
Vision with macular degeneration is experienced with an inability to focus in the center of the visual field, as shown here.
Source: B. Boissonnet/BSIP SA/Alamy Stock Photo.

Emmetropia and Refractive Errors

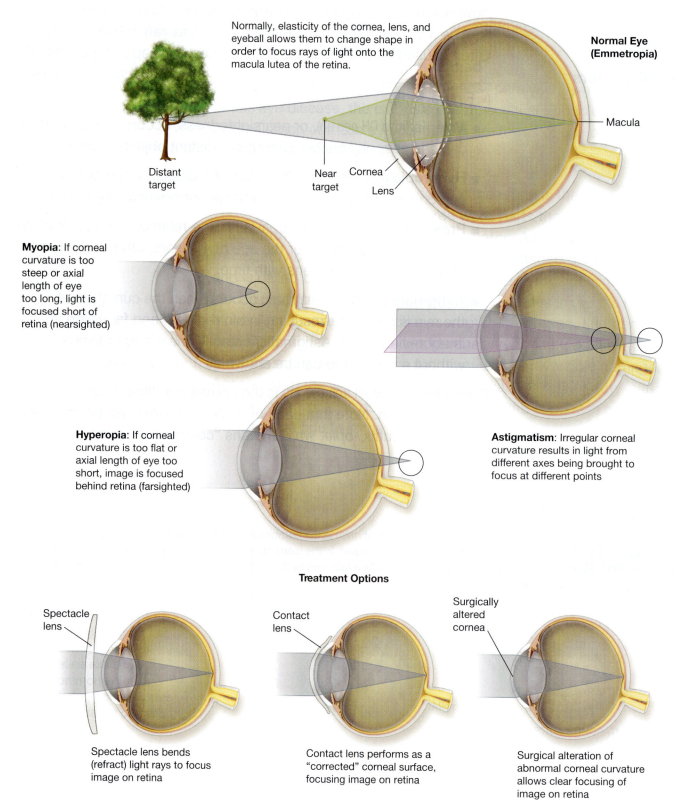

Normally, elasticity of the cornea, lens, and eyeball allows them to change shape in order to focus rays of light onto the macula lutea of the retina.

Normal Eye (Emmetropia)

Macula

Distant target

Near target Cornea Lens

Myopia: If corneal curvature is too steep or axial length of eye too long, light is focused short of retina (nearsighted)

Astigmatism: Irregular corneal curvature results in light from different axes being brought to focus at different points

Hyperopia: If corneal curvature is too flat or axial length of eye too short, image is focused behind retina (farsighted)

Treatment Options

Spectacle lens

Spectacle lens bends (refract) light rays to focus image on retina

Contact lens

Contact lens performs as a "corrected" corneal surface, focusing image on retina

Surgically altered cornea

Surgical alteration of abnormal corneal curvature allows clear focusing of image on retina

■ **Figure 14.9**
Vision. Normal vision (top), compared to common refractive errors and their treatment options.

PRACTICE: Diseases and Disorders of the Eyes and Sight

The Right Match

Match the vocabulary term on the left with the correct definition on the right.

_____ 1. glaucoma

_____ 2. cataract

_____ 3. macular degeneration

_____ 4. hordeolum

_____ 5. detached retina

_____ 6. ophthalmomalacia

a. occurs when the retina tears away from the choroid layer

b. progressive deterioration of the macula lutea

c. softening of the eye

d. loss of vision resulting from increased intraocular pressure

e. a condition in which the transparency of the lens is reduced

f. infection of the meibomian gland; also called a *sty*

Linkup

Link the word parts in the list to create the terms that match the definitions. You may use word parts more than once. Remember to add combining vowels when needed and that some terms do not use any combining vowel.

Prefix	Combining Form	Suffix
a-	conjunctiv/o	-ism
dipl-	ir/o	-itis
	ophthalm/o	-opia
	retin/o	-pathy
	stigmat/o	

Definition

1. bacterial infection of the conjunctiva

2. double vision

3. defective curvature of the eye that causes blurred vision

4. inflammation of the iris

5. disease of the retina

6. eye disease

Term

_____

_____

_____

_____

_____

_____

Treatments, Procedures, and Devices of the Eyes and Sight

Here are the word parts that commonly apply to eye treatments, procedures, and devices and are covered in the following section. Note that the word parts are color-coded to help you identify them: prefixes are yellow, combining forms are red, and suffixes are blue.

Prefix	Definition	Combining Form	Definition	Suffix	Definition
intra-	within	cyst/o	bladder, sac	-ar	pertaining to
		dacry/o	tear	-logist	one who studies
		kerat/o	hard, cornea	-metrist	one who measures
		ocul/o	eye	-stomy	surgical creation of an opening
		opt/o	eye	-tomy	incision, to cut
		radi/o	radius		
		rhin/o	nose		

KEY TERMS A–Z

cataract extraction

14.26 During **cataract extraction**, a lens damaged by a cataract is surgically removed and replaced with an artificial lens called an **intraocular lens (IOL)**. The most common technique in use for _____ _____ is **phacoemulsification** (FAY koh ee muhl sih fih KAY shun), or **phaco** (FAY koh). Illustrated in ■ Figure 14.10, phaco is the use of sound waves to break up the lens so that it can be removed by suction.

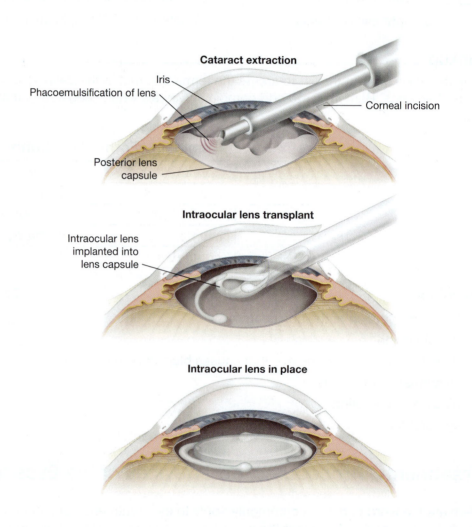

Cataract extraction

Iris
Phacoemulsification of lens
Corneal incision
Posterior lens capsule

Intraocular lens transplant

Intraocular lens implanted into lens capsule

Intraocular lens in place

■ **Figure 14.10**
Cataract extraction and the artificial intraocular lens. The procedure involves a surgical removal of a cataract lens and its replacement with an artificial lens. The artificial lens is made of silicone and acrylic. Artificial lenses are called *intraocular lenses (IOLs)*.

corneal grafting

14.27 The cornea is normally transparent, but may lose its transparency from exposure to ultraviolet light or become damaged from an injury. The most common treatment of corneal damage is **corneal grafting**. During _____ _____, the injured cornea is removed and replaced by implantation of a donor or synthetic cornea.

cryopexy
KRYE oh pek see

14.28 There are two primary treatments for the medical emergency of a detached retina (Frame 14.17), which are often needed to prevent blindness. In **cryopexy**, tiny holes are created through the retina by laser treatment, which "welds" the retina back into place. Freeze treatment may also be used, which is the origin of the term _____ and means "surgical fixation by freezing." The other technique to treat a detached retina is **scleral buckling**, in which a tiny synthetic band is attached to the white outside layer of the eyeball (called the *sclera*) to push the wall of the eye against the detached retina.

dacryocystorhinostomy
DAK ree oh SIS toh rye NOS toh mee

14.29 To treat dacryocystitis, described in Frame 14.16, antibiotic eyedrops are often used to defeat the bacterial infection. In some cases, a **dacryocystorhinostomy** may be needed. During a _____, a channel is surgically created between the nasal cavity and lacrimal sac to promote drainage. This term includes three combining forms: dacry/o/cyst/o/rhin/o/stomy.

LASIK
LAY sik

14.30 The acronym for **laser-assisted in situ keratomileusis** is _____. It is the use of a laser to reshape the corneal tissue beneath the surface of the cornea to correct refractive errors, such as myopia, hyperopia, and astigmatism (■ Figure 14.11).

Laser Eye Surgery Procedure

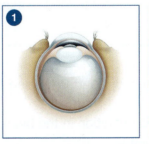
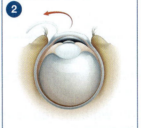
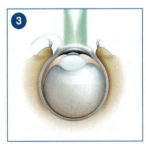
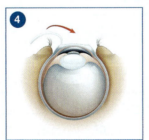
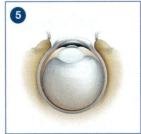

■ **Figure 14.11**
LASIK. The five steps in LASIK include (1) prepare patient; (2) expose the underside of the cornea by making an incision and folding it outward; (3) remove excess material with a programmable laser; (4) replace cornea; (5) close the incision.
Source: BlueRingMedia/Shutterstock.

optometrist ahp TOM eh trist	**14.31** Correcting refractive errors (Frame 14.25) is usually attempted with **corrective lenses** or **contact lenses** following a vision examination by an **optometrist**. An _____ is a health professional (not a physician) trained to examine eyes to correct vision problems and eye disorders.
ophthalmologist off thal MAH loh jist **radial keratotomy** RAY dee ahl * kair ah TOT oh mee	**14.32** As an alternative to using contact lenses for myopia, an **ophthalmologist** may perform a **radial keratotomy**, during which spokelike incisions are made into the cornea, which effectively flattens the cornea to correct for myopia. An _____ is a physician who specializes in the study and treatment of diseases associated with the eyes. A _____ _____ is a form of refractive surgery because it corrects the refractive error of myopia.

PRACTICE: Treatments, Procedures, and Devices of the Eyes and Sight

The Right Match

Match the vocabulary term on the left with the correct definition on the right.

_____ 1. cataract extraction   a. removal and replacement of an injured cornea

_____ 2. LASIK   b. surgical correction for myopia in which incisions flatten the cornea

_____ 3. radial keratotomy   c. surgical removal and replacement of a lens damaged by a cataract

_____ 4. corneal grafting   d. use of a laser to reshape the corneal tissue to correct vision

_____ 5. optometrist   e. a physician specializing in the study and treatment of eye diseases

_____ 6. ophthalmologist   f. a health professional trained to examine eyes to correct vision problems

Break the Chain

Analyze these medical terms:

a) Separate each term into its word parts; each word part is labeled for you (**p** = prefix, **r** = root, **cf** = combining form, and **s** = suffix).

b) For the Bonus Question, write the requested definition in the blank that follows.

The first set has been completed for you as an example.

1. a) optometrist   _opt/o/metrist_
                         cf   s

    b) *Bonus Question*: What is the definition of the combining form? _**eye**_____

2. a) dacryocystorhinostomy   _____/__/_____/__/_____/__/_____
                                    cf   cf   cf   s

    b) *Bonus Question*: What is the definition of the suffix? _____

3. a) ophthalmologist   _____/__/_____
                             cf   s

    b) *Bonus Question*: What is the definition of the combining form? _____

Signs and Symptoms of the Ears and Hearing

Here are the word parts that commonly apply to the signs and symptoms of the ears and hearing and are covered in the following section. Note that the word parts are color-coded to help you identify them: prefixes are yellow, combining forms are red, and suffixes are blue.

Prefix	Definition
an-	without, absence of
hyper-	excessive, abnormally high, above
para-	alongside, abnormal

Combining Form	Definition
ot/o	ear

Suffix	Definition
-acusis	condition of hearing
-algia	condition of pain
-rrhagia	abnormal discharge
-rrhea	discharge

KEY WORDS A–Z

anacusis
AN ah KYOO siss

hyperacusis
HIGH per ah KYOO siss

otalgia
oh TAHL jee ah

otorrhagia
oh toh RAJ ee ah

otorrhea
oh toh REE ah

14.33 The suffix that means "condition of hearing" is -acusis. When the prefix an- is included, the constructed term _____ is created, which literally means "condition of absence of hearing" and refers to a total loss of hearing. It can be written as an/acusis.

14.34 When the same suffix, -acusis, is used with the prefix that means "excessive, abnormally high, above," the term _____ is created, which literally means "condition of excessive hearing." It refers to a symptom of abnormally sensitive hearing. Replacing this prefix with another, para-, changes the meaning once again. The term **paracusis** (PAIR ah kyoo siss) is a symptom of partial loss of hearing.

14.35 The combining form that means "ear" is ot/o. When the suffix for a condition of pain, -algia, is included, the term _____ is created, which means "pain in the ear," or earache.

14.36 Another symptom of the ear using the combining form ot/o is **otorrhagia**. Because the meaning of the suffix -rrhagia is "abnormal discharge," the constructed term _____ means "abnormal ear discharge." The clinical meaning of the term is "bleeding from the external ear canal." The word parts are shown when the constructed form is written ot/o/rrhagia.

14.37 When the suffix -rrhea, which means "discharge," is added to the combining form for ear, the term _____ is created. This is a symptom of abnormal drainage (of pus) from the ear. The constructed form of this term is ot/o/rrhea.

tinnitus
  tinn EYE tuss
vertigo
  VER tih go
	14.38 Two common symptoms of the ears and hearing are not constructed of word parts. They are **tinnitus**, which is a ringing or buzzing sensation in the ears, and **vertigo**, which is a sensation of spinning or whirling motion. _____ is from the Latin word *tinnio*, which means "jingling sound," and _____ is derived from the Latin word *vertere*, which means "to turn."

PRACTICE: Signs and Symptoms of the Ears and Hearing

The Right Match

Match the term on the left with the correct definition on the right.

_____ 1. anacusis   a. partial hearing loss

_____ 2. otalgia   b. total hearing loss

_____ 3. hyperacusis   c. abnormal discharge from the ear

_____ 4. paracusis   d. pain in the ear, or earache

_____ 5. otorrhagia   e. a ringing in the ears

_____ 6. tinnitus   f. overly sensitive hearing

Linkup

Link the word parts in the list to create the terms that match the definitions. You may use word parts more than once. Remember to add combining vowels when needed and that some terms do not use any combining vowel.

Prefix	Combining Form	Suffix
an-	ot/o	-acusis
hyper-		-algia
para-		-rrhagia
		-rrhea

Definition   **Term**

1. partial loss of hearing   _____

2. abnormal drainage of pus from the ear   _____

3. pain in the ear   _____

4. bleeding from an ear   _____

5. total hearing loss   _____

6. overly sensitive hearing   _____

Diseases and Disorders of the Ears and Hearing

Here are the word parts that commonly apply to diseases and disorders of the ears and hearing and are covered in the following section. Note that the word parts are color-coded to help you identify them: combining forms are red and suffixes are blue.

Combining Form	Definition
extern/o	exterior
mastoid/o	resembling a breast
med/o	middle
ot/o	ear
presby/o	old age
scler/o	hard, sclera

Suffix	Definition
-acusis	condition of hearing
-itis	inflammation
-osis	condition of
-pathy	disease

KEY WORDS A–Z

cholesteatoma
koh LES tee ah TOH mah

14.39 A relatively common source of partial hearing loss (paracusis; Frame 14.34) and ear drainage (otorrhea; Frame 14.37) is called **cholesteatoma**. It is the formation of a cyst-like ball of epithelial cells in the middle ear. Although not a form of cancer, a _____ can enlarge to cause a complete loss of hearing (anacusis; Frame 14.33) in the affected ear and neurological complications. The term literally means "tumor of cholesterol" because it was once believed to be a benign tumor composed primarily of cholesterol.

mastoiditis
mas toyd EYE tiss

14.40 The term that literally means "inflammation of the part resembling a breast" is _____. The word part construction of this term is mastoid/itis. The mastoid process is an area of the temporal bone of the skull housing the middle and internal ear. Bacterial infections of the middle ear can travel into the mastoid area to produce mastoiditis, causing serious complications that can lead to impaired hearing or deafness.

Ménière's disease
MEN yerz

14.41 A chronic disease of the inner ear is known as **Ménière's disease**. _____ _____ includes symptoms of vertigo, or a spinning motion, and tinnitus, or ringing in the ears (Frame 14.38).

otitis
  oh TYE tiss

otitis media

ot/o/pathy

14.42 The general term for inflammation of the ear is
_____. In one form of this disease, the external auditory canal is involved, causing local sensations of pain, and is called **otitis externa** (oh TYE tiss * eks TER nah). In another form, the middle ear is involved to cause local pain and a temporary loss of hearing. Known as _____ _____
(oh TYE tiss * MEE dee ah), it is relatively common among children, is caused by bacterial infection, and often requires antibiotic therapy (see ■ Figure 14.12). It is abbreviated **OM**. It has been estimated that 80% of all children will have contracted otitis media by their third birthday, and it is the most common cause of partial hearing loss. Both otitis externa and otitis media are **otopathies** (OH toh path eez), which literally means "diseases of the ear." The word part construction of the term *otitis* is ot/itis and that of the term *otopathy* is ____/___/_____.

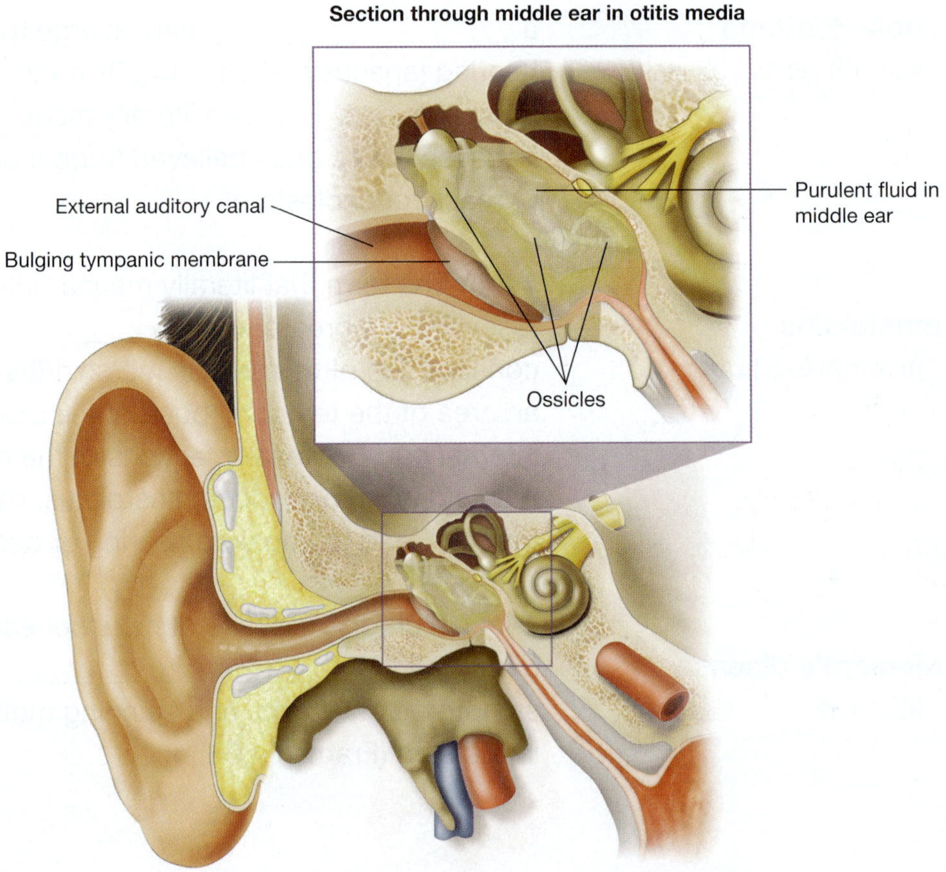

Section through middle ear in otitis media

External auditory canal

Bulging tympanic membrane

Purulent fluid in middle ear

Ossicles

■ **Figure 14.12**
Otitis media. This illustration shows an inflamed tympanic cavity, which is the most common source of ear pain in this infection. The eardrum may also become inflamed or bulge outward due to an accumulation of purulent fluid within the tympanic cavity.

otosclerosis

oh toh skler OH siss

14.43 An abnormal formation of bone within the ear, usually between the stapes and the oval window of the middle ear, is known as **otosclerosis**. The disease causes a progressive loss of hearing. Recall that the suffix *-osis* with the word root *scler* means "condition of hard." The term _____ includes four word parts, which can be shown by writing the word part construction as ot/o/scler/osis.

presbyacusis

pres bee ah KYOO siss

14.44 A gradual loss of hearing with advancing age is a very common condition. The term for this disease combines the word root that means "old age," *presby*, with the suffix that means "condition of hearing," which you learned is *-acusis*. The resulting term is _____.

PRACTICE: Diseases and Disorders of the Ears and Hearing

The Right Match

Match the vocabulary term on the left with the correct definition on the right.

_____ 1. Ménière's disease

_____ 2. presbyacusis

_____ 3. otitis media

_____ 4. otitis externa

_____ 5. mastoiditis

_____ 6. otopathy

a. any disease of the ear

b. inflammation of the middle ear

c. a chronic disease of the inner ear

d. inflammation of the mastoid area

e. inflammation of the external auditory canal

f. loss of hearing due to old age

Linkup

Link the word parts in the list to create the terms that match the definitions. You may use word parts more than once. Remember to add combining vowels when needed—and that some terms do not use any combining vowel.

Combining Form	Suffix
mastoid/o	-itis
ot/o	-osis
scler/o	-pathy

Definition

1. inflammation of the ear

2. an abnormal formation of bone within the ear

3. any disease of the ear

4. inflammation of the mastoid

Term

_____

_____

_____

_____

Treatments, Procedures, and Devices of the Ears and Hearing

Here are the word parts that commonly apply to ear treatments, procedures, and devices that are covered in the following section. Note that the word parts are color-coded to help you identify them: combining forms are red and suffixes are blue.

Combining Form	Definition
audi/o	hearing
labyrinth/o	maze, inner ear
mastoid/o	resembling a breast
myring/o	membrane, eardrum
ot/o	ear
tympan/o	eardrum

Suffix	Definition
-ectomy	surgical excision, removal
-logist	one who studies
-logy	study or science of
-metry	measurement, process of measuring
-plasty	surgical repair
-scope	instrument used for viewing
-scopy	process of viewing
-tomy	incision, to cut

KEY WORDS A–Z

audiologist
  aw dee AHL oh jist
audiometry
  aw dee AH meh tree

14.45 The combining form *audi/o* means "hearing." The study of hearing disorders is a field of practice called **audiology**. One who specializes in hearing disorders and treatment is called an _____. The procedure involving the measurement of hearing is usually performed by an **audiologist** and is called _____ (■ Figure 14.13). The constructed form of the term *audiology* is audi/o/logy, *audiologist* is audi/o/logist, and *audiometry* is audi/o/metry.

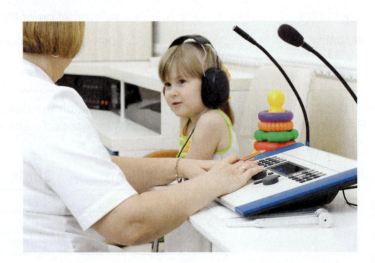

■ Figure 14.13
Audiometry. The child in this photograph is undergoing a hearing test with an audiologist.
Source: Capifrutta/Shutterstock.

cochlear implant

14.46 A **cochlear implant** is a small electronic device that helps to provide a sensation of sound to a person who is profoundly deaf or very hard of hearing. The _____ _____ contains an external part that is placed behind the outer ear and an internal part that is surgically implanted beneath the skin. The implant includes an array of electrodes placed within the cochlea that sends electrical signals to the auditory nerve when mechanical vibrations are amplified and received (■ Figure 14.14).

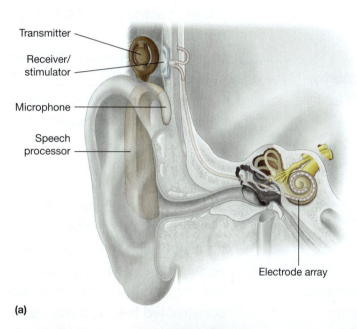

Transmitter

Receiver/ stimulator

Microphone

Speech processor

Electrode array

(a)

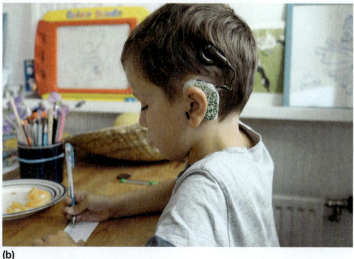

(b)

■ **Figure 14.14**
Cochlear implant. (a) Illustration of a cochlear implant. (b) Photograph of the external part of a cochlear implant.
Source: Kathy deWitt/Alamy Stock Photo.

labyrinthectomy
lab ee rin THEK toh mee

14.47 In some severe cases of permanent hearing loss, the inner ear, or labyrinth, is surgically removed and replaced with a synthetic hearing device. The surgical removal of the inner ear is called _____. Its constructed form is labyrinth/ectomy.

?　Did You KNOW

LABYRINTH

The combining form *labyrinth/o* is derived from the Greek word *labyrinth*, which means "a maze." It is believed to have originated from the ancient Lydian language that preceded the golden age of Greece. The term was used as the label for the *house of the double axe*, which was a maze designed to protect the inner sanctum of the throne room for Minos, the King of Crete. Over the years, the labyrinth became synonymous with the word *maze*. When early scientists first observed the twisting chambers of the inner ear, they were struck by its resemblance to a twisting maze, leading them to apply the term *labyrinth*.

---

mastoidectomy
mas toyd EK toh mee

mastoidotomy
mas toyd AHT oh mee

14.48 In some patients, it may become necessary to surgically remove part of the mastoid process of the temporal bone to treat severe mastoiditis (Frame 14.40). This procedure is called _____. The constructed form of this term is mastoid/ectomy. The procedure is preceded by making an incision into the mastoid process in a procedure called _____. The constructed form of this term is mastoid/o/tomy.

---

myringoplasty
mih RING oh plas tee
myringotomy
mih ring AH toh mee

14.49 The combining form *myring/o* means "membrane." Because the eardrum is a membrane, this combining form may be used in terms in which the eardrum is described. Therefore, a surgical repair of the eardrum is called _____. Similarly, an incision into the eardrum is called _____. Both are constructed terms, shown as myring/o/plasty and myring/o/tomy.

---

ot/o/logy

otoscope
OH toh skope

14.50 The medical field of ear disorders and their treatment is called **otology**. Write the constructed form of this term here: ___/__/____. The instrument that is used in a physical exam to view the ear canal and eardrum uses the same combining form and is called an _____. The exam procedure is called **otoscopy** (oh TOH skoh pee; ■ Figure 14.15).

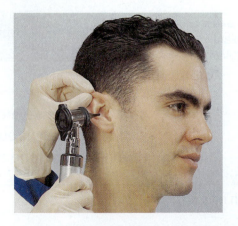

■ **Figure 14.15**
An ear exam, or otoscopy, using an otoscope.

tympanometry

tim pan AH meh tree

tympanoplasty

TIM pan oh plass tee

14.51 You may recall that the eardrum is also called the tympanic membrane. This alternate term uses the combining form *tympan/o*, which means "eardrum." A procedure that evaluates the elasticity of the eardrum by measuring its movement includes this combining form in the word _____. Another term that uses this combining form describes the surgical repair of the eardrum and is known as _____.

PRACTICE: Treatments, Procedures, and Devices of the Ears and Hearing

The Right Match

Match the vocabulary term on the left with the correct definition on the right.

_____ 1. mastoidectomy

_____ 2. otoscopy

_____ 3. tympanoplasty

_____ 4. labyrinthectomy

_____ 5. audiology

_____ 6. otology

a. physical examination of the ear canal and eardrum

b. the study of hearing disorders

c. surgical removal of part of the mastoid process

d. the medical field of ear disorders and treatment

e. surgical repair of the eardrum

f. surgical removal of the inner ear

Break the Chain

Analyze these medical terms:

a) Separate each term into its word parts; each word part is labeled for you (**p** = prefix, **r** = root, **cf** = combining form, and **s** = suffix).

b) For the Bonus Question, write the requested definition in the blank that follows.

1. a) otologist   _____/___/_____
                              cf   s

   b) *Bonus Question*: What is the definition of the combining form? _____

2. a) tympanometry   _____/___/_____
                              cf   s

   b) *Bonus Question*: What is the definition of the suffix? _____

3. a) myringoplasty   _____/___/_____
                              cf   s

   b) *Bonus Question*: What is the definition of the combining form? _____

Abbreviations of the Eyes and Ears

The abbreviations that are associated with the eyes and ears are summarized here. Study these abbreviations and review them in the exercise that follows.

Abbreviation	Definition	Abbreviation	Definition
AD	right ear; in Latin, *auris dexter*	IOL	intraocular lens
AMD	age-related macular degeneration	LASIK	laser-assisted in situ keratomileusis
AS	left ear; in Latin, *auris sinister*	OD	right eye; in Latin, *oculus dexter*
Ast	astigmatism	OM	otitis media
AU	both ears; in Latin, *aures unitas*	OS	left eye; in Latin, *oculus sinister*
EENT	eye, ear, nose, and throat	Oto	otology
Em	emmetropia	OU	each eye; in Latin, *oculus uterque*
ENT	ear, nose, and throat	Phaco	phacoemulsification
HEENT	head, eyes, ears, nose, and throat	TM	tympanic membrane

PRACTICE: Abbreviations

Fill in the blanks with the abbreviation or the complete medical term.

Abbreviation

1. _____
2. ENT
3. _____
4. AU
5. _____
6. Em
7. _____
8. AD
9. _____
10. TM
11. _____
12. HEENT
13. _____
14. LASIK
15. _____
16. OD_____

Medical Term

otitis media

_____

otology

_____

left ear

_____

age-related macular degeneration

_____

eye, ear, nose, and throat

_____

short for phacoemulsification

_____

astigmatism

_____

intraocular lens

_____

CHAPTER REVIEW

Word Building _____

Construct medical terms from the following meanings. The first question has been completed for you as an example.

1. inflammation of the cornea   kerat***itis***_____

2. a drooping eyelid   blepharo_____

3. a stone in the lacrimal apparatus   _____lithiasis

4. inflammation of the conjunctiva   conjunctiv_____

5. softening of the eye   _____malacia

6. paralysis of the eye   ophthalmo_____

7. a generalized disease of the retina   retino_____

8. a specialist who corrects vision disorders   _____metrist

9. inflammation of the lacrimal apparatus   _____itis

10. bleeding of the eye   ophthalmo_____

11. symptom of a white film in the pupil   _____coria

12. inflammation of the middle ear   _____itis media

13. condition of pain in the ear   ot_____

14. abnormal formation of bone in the ear   oto_____

15. pus discharge from the external ear canal   oto_____

Define the Combining Form _____

In the space provided, write the definition of the combining form, followed by one example of the combining form used to build a medical term in Chapter 14.

	Definition	**Use in a Term**
1. blephar/o	_____	_____
2. cor/o	_____	_____
3. ophthalm/o	_____	_____
4. conjunctiv/o	_____	_____
5. dacry/o	_____	_____
6. kerat/o	_____	_____
7. retin/o	_____	_____
8. ot/o	_____	_____
9. audi/o	_____	_____
10. labyrinth/o	_____	_____

Complete the Labels

Complete the blank labels in ■ Figures 14.16 and 14.17 by writing the labels in the spaces provided.

1. _____

2. _____

3. _____

4. _____

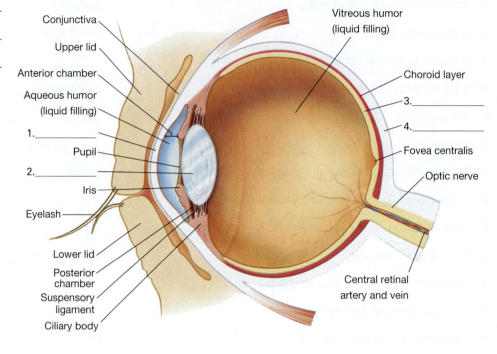

■ **Figure 14.16**
Anatomy of the eye. Lateral view of a sectioned eyeball in its socket.

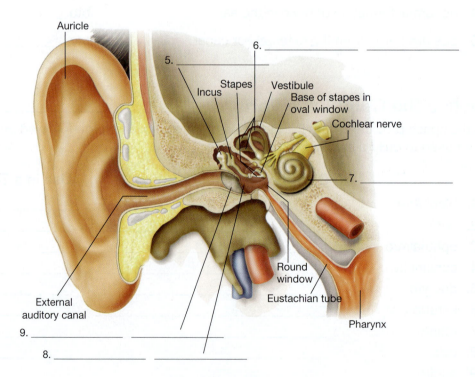

■ **Figure 14.17**
The ear. Lateral view of the ear region on one side of the head.

5. _____

6. _____

7. _____

8. _____

9. _____

MEDICAL REPORT EXERCISES

Salima Aziz

Read the following medical report, then answer the critical thinking questions that follow.

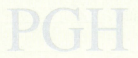

PEARSON GENERAL HOSPITAL

5500 University Avenue, Metropolis, New York
Phone: (211) 594-4000 • Fax (211) 594-4001

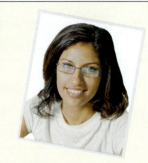

Medical Consultation: Ophthalmology   **Date**: 08/22/2017

Patient: Salima Aziz   **Patient ID**: 123456

Dob: 2/19/1999   **Age**: 18   **Sex**: Female   **Allergies**: NKDA

Provider: Jana Abashiri, MD

Subjective:

"My right eye has been hurting for the past week, especially when I rub it because it itches a lot. There is crustiness in the mornings when I wake up."

18 y/o female with ophthalmalgia, pruritis, swelling, and erythema in right eye for the past week. She also complains that, more recently, her left eye is beginning to redden and swell.

Objective:

Vital Signs: **T**: 98.6°F; **P**: 77; **R**: 21; **BP**: 120/75

Ht: 5'7"

Wt: 122 lb

General Appearance: Skin appears healthy, with no apparent masses or discolorations.

Heart: Rate at 77 bpm. Heart sounds with auscultation appear normal.

Lungs: Clear without signs of disease.

AbD: Bowel sounds normal all four quadrants.

MS: Joints and muscles symmetric. No swelling, masses, or deformity. ROM normal.

HEENT: Erythema of sclera, inflammation of conjunctiva in OD, spreading to OS and eyelids.

Assessment:

OU conjunctivitis with keratitis and blepharitis

Plan:

Antibiotic eyedrops with oral systemic antibiotic therapy. Follow-up visit in 2 weeks.

Photo Source: Michaeljung/Shutterstock.

Comprehension Questions

1. What patient complaints and evidence support the diagnosis of conjunctivitis? _____

   _____

   _____

2. Why would a treatment including antibiotics be prescribed for this ophthalmopathy? _____

   _____

   _____

3. What is the meaning of *OU ophthalmalgia*? _____

   _____

   _____

Case Study Questions

The following case study provides further discussion regarding the patient in the medical report. Fill in the blanks with the correct terms. Choose your answers from the following list of terms. (Note that some terms may be used more than once.)

conjunctivitis	keratitis	ophthalmologist
blepharitis	ophthalmalgia	OS

Salima Aziz, an 18-year-old female with no prior history of ophthalmic disease, complained to her parents

of eye pain or (a) _____ originating from the right eye and spreading to the left eye, or

(b) _____ (abbreviation), within a few days. She also noticed swelling of the eyelids, or

(c) _____, with a crusty exudate, and her parents became worried when they saw redness

of the eye, suggesting the condition of (d) _____. Her parents brought her to a physician

specializing in eye care, called an (e) _____, immediately. During the eye exam, the physician

diagnosed inflammation of the right eyelid, inflammation of the conjunctiva, or (f) _____, and

inflammation of the cornea, or (g) _____, and identified the probable cause to be bacterial. As

a result, antibiotic eyedrops and systemic antibiotics were prescribed with follow-up visits scheduled.

Reggie Fletcher

For a greater challenge, read the following medical report provided and answer the critical thinking questions that follow.

PEARSON GENERAL HOSPITAL

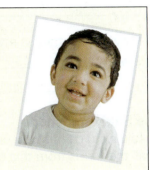

5500 University Avenue, Metropolis, New York
Phone: (211) 594-4000 • Fax (211) 594-4001

Medical Consultation: Pediatrics

Patient: Reggie Fletcher

Dob: 3/14/2015   **Age**: 2   **Sex**: Male

Provider: Judith N. VonTripp, MD

Date: 11/22/2017

Patient ID: 123456

Allergies: NKDA

Subjective:

Relayed by mother at visit: "Reggie has been whining and pulling at his right ear for the past week, with more crying and fussiness than usual. He's been having trouble sleeping too. I took his temperature this morning and it was 101°F, so I decided to bring him in to be seen."

2 y/o male brought in by his mother who complains that he is unusually distressed with pulling of the right ear. His records show he is current with vaccinations and has no abnormalities.

Objective:

Vital Signs: **T**: 101.6°F; **P**: 92; **R**: 28; **BP**: 118/70

Ht: 2'7"

Wt: 35 lb

General Appearance: Mild diaphoresis. Skin is otherwise healthy, with no apparent masses or discolorations.

Heart: Rate at 92 bpm. Heart sounds with auscultation appear normal.

Lungs: Clear without signs of disease.

AbD: Bowel sounds normal all four quadrants.

HEENT: Eyes clear, throat with mild erythema and swelling. Right TM with mild erythema and swelling, left ear normal.

Assessment:

AD myringitis with possible otitis media

Plan:

Antibiotic eardrops into right ear three times a day. Follow with return visit in 2 weeks. If not cleared, consult with EENT for possible myringotomy with tympanic cavity drainage.

Photo Source: Ami Parikh/Shutterstock.

Comprehension Questions

1. What evidence supports a diagnosis of AD myringitis with possible otitis media? _____
_____
_____

2. Why do you think a myringotomy may need to be performed if the child does not improve within 2 weeks? _____
_____

Case Study Questions

The following case study provides further discussion regarding the patient in the medical report. Recall the terms from this chapter to fill in the blanks with the correct terms.

Reggie Fletcher, a 2-year-old male, was brought to the medical clinic after his behavior during the preceding

several weeks indicated to his mother that he was experiencing ear pain, known as (h) _____,

of the right ear, abbreviated (i) _____. His behavior included pulling or tugging at his

right ear, an inability to sleep through the night, mild fever, and frequent fussiness. The general physician

examined his ears using an (j) _____ and observed inflammation of the tympanic membrane,

called (k) _____. Because this condition is often indicative of a potential infection within

the middle ear, called (l) _____ _____, the physician referred the patient to

(m) _____. Following an exam, the ear specialist, or (n) _____, determined a

course of treatment to include antibiotic eardrops with follow-up exams to ensure the infection is defeated.

Unfortunately, 2 weeks later the infection had spread into the tympanic cavity to produce the disease

(o) _____ _____. The tympanic membrane was then surgically incised in

a (p) _____ procedure and drainage tubes inserted into the tympanic cavity to drain the

purulent fluids. One month after the patient had recovered, a hearing test, or (q) _____, was

performed and found a 20% loss of hearing from the right ear.

MyLab Medical Terminology™

MyLab Medical Terminology is a premium online homework management system that includes a host of features to help you study. Registered users will find:

- A multitude of quizzes and activities built within the MyLab platform
- Powerful tools that track and analyze your results—allowing you to create a personalized learning experience
- Videos and audio pronunciations to help enrich your progress
- Streaming lesson presentations (Guided Lectures) and self-paced learning modules
- A space where you and your instructors can view and manage your assignments

Chapter 15

The Endocrine System

Learning Objectives

After completing this chapter, you will be able to:

15.1 Define and spell the word parts used to create terms for the endocrine system.

15.2 Identify the major organs of the endocrine system and describe their structure and function.

15.3 Break down and define common medical terms used for symptoms, diseases, disorders, procedures, treatments, and devices associated with the endocrine system.

15.4 Build medical terms from the word parts associated with the endocrine system.

15.5 Pronounce and spell common medical terms associated with the endocrine system.

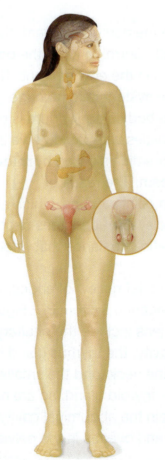

Anatomy and Physiology Terms

The following table provides the combining forms that commonly apply to the anatomy and physiology of the endocrine system. Note that the combining forms are colored red to help you identify them when you see them again later in the chapter.

Combining Form	Definition
aden/o	gland
adren/o	adrenal gland
crin/o	to secrete
gonad/o	sex gland
hormon/o	to set in motion

Combining Form	Definition
pancreat/o	sweetbread, pancreas
ren/o	kidney
thyr/o	shield, thyroid
thyroid/o	resembling a shield, thyroid

endocrine

  EN doh krin

gland

gonads

15.1 The **endocrine system** works hand in hand with the nervous system to regulate body functions. The primary organs of the _____ system include the pituitary gland, which is attached to the hypothalamus at the base of the brain, the thyroid _____ in the neck, the parathyroid glands embedded within the thyroid gland, the two adrenal glands located above each kidney, the pancreatic islets within the pancreas, and the _____, which include the ovaries of the female and testes of the male.

homeostasis

hormone

15.2 Like the nervous system, the endocrine system provides a method of control to keep the body functioning despite changing conditions in the environment. Thus, the primary role of the endocrine system is to manage _____, a state in which the body's equilibrium is maintained. Instead of regulating body activities with rapid nerve impulses, the endocrine organs secrete chemicals called **hormones** that are carried by the bloodstream. The result of _____ secretion is a change in cell functions, which alters body activities. When the endocrine system becomes deficient due to disease, the result is a homeostatic imbalance that often affects overall health.

15.3 As a brief review of endocrine anatomy, study the illustration of the endocrine system in ■ Figure 15.1. From this figure, note its major organs include the pituitary gland and pineal gland in the cranial cavity, the thymus gland in the thoracic cavity, the thyroid gland in the neck (and the smaller parathyroid glands embedded within the thyroid gland, so are not shown), the adrenal glands and pancreas in the abdominal cavity, and the testes in the scrotum of the male and ovaries in the pelvic cavity of the female.

?   Did You
Know

THYROID AND PARATHYROID

The shape of the thyroid gland must have reminded the Greeks of a shield because the term is derived from the Greek word for this defensive warrior gear, *thyreos*. Thus, the term *thyroid* literally means "resembling a shield." Although the four pea-sized parathyroid glands are not shaped like a Greek shield, their location within the much larger thyroid gland earns them their name because one meaning of the prefix *para-* is "alongside."

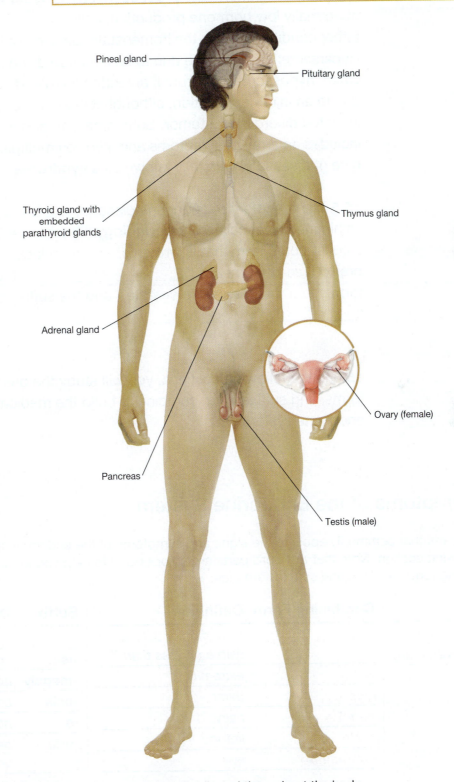

Pineal gland

Pituitary gland

Thyroid gland with embedded parathyroid glands

Thymus gland

Adrenal gland

Ovary (female)

Pancreas

Testis (male)

■ **Figure 15.1**
The endocrine glands of the endocrine system are distributed throughout the body.

Medical Terms for the Endocrine System

hyposecretion	**15.4** An array of disorders can occur when an endocrine gland fails to deliver the quantity of hormones needed to regulate body functions. In general, endocrine disease results from either abnormally high hormone production, called **hypersecretion**, or abnormally low hormone production, called _____. Either condition upsets the homeostatic balance of the body. Hypersecretion may arise due to an inherited disease or a tumor. Often, hyposecretion occurs if an endocrine gland suffers trauma due to an injury or infection, although it also may be caused by an inherited disorder or a tumor. Sometimes, an endocrine disorder includes an array of symptoms and involves multiple organs. This type of disease is generally known as a **syndrome**.
within **study** **science of**	**15.5** The treatment of endocrine diseases is a focused discipline within medicine, called **endocrinology** (EN doh krin ALL oh jee). This is a constructed term that is written endo/crin/o/logy and includes the prefix endo- that means "_____," the combining form crin/o that means "to secrete," and the suffix -logy that means "_____ or _____ _____."
	15.6 In the following sections, you will study the prefixes, combining forms, and suffixes that combine to build the medical terms of the endocrine system.

Signs and Symptoms of the Endocrine System

Here are the word parts that commonly apply to the signs and symptoms of the endocrine system and are covered in the following section. Note that the word parts are color-coded to help you identify them: prefixes are yellow, combining forms are red, and suffixes are blue.

Prefix	Definition
ex-	outside, away from
poly-	excessive, over, many

Combining Form	Definition
acid/o	a solution or substance with a pH less than 7
acr/o	extremity
dips/o	thirst
hirsut/o	hairy
ket/o	ketone
ophthalm/o	eye

Suffix	Definition
-ia	condition of
-ism	condition or disease
-megaly	abnormally large
-osis	condition of
-s	plural
-uria	pertaining to urine, urination

KEY TERMS A–Z

acidosis

ass ih DOH siss

15.7 Recall that the suffix *-osis* means "condition of." The sign of excess acid in the body is therefore known as _____, and the constructed form of the term is acid/osis. It occurs when carbon dioxide, the primary waste product from cellular metabolism, accumulates in tissues (including blood) to form carbonic acid. Acidosis is a symptom of diabetes mellitus (Frame 15.20) and may also be caused by respiratory or kidney disorders.

15.8 A sign of bone structure enlargement in an adult without a gain in height is known as **acromegaly**. The enlargement causes disfigurement, especially in the hands and face, and is a sign of hypersecretion of growth hormone (abbreviated **GH**) from the pituitary gland during adulthood (■ Figure 15.2). _____ literally means "abnormally large extremity." It is a constructed term that is written acr/o/megaly.

acromegaly

ak roh MEG ah lee

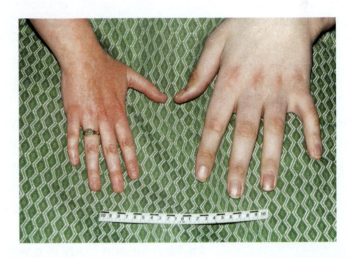

■ **Figure 15.2**
Acromegaly. Acromegaly is a metabolic disorder in which excessive amounts of growth hormone are secreted during adulthood, resulting in enlarged bones without increased height. The changes occur gradually and are often apparent mainly in the face and hands. In this photograph, a normal hand (left) is compared with the hand of a person of the same height, but with acromegaly (right).
Source: Biophoto Associate/Science Source.

15.9 The abnormal protrusion of the eyes is known as **exophthalmos**. It is a classic sign of excessive activity of the thyroid gland and literally means "outside eyes" (■ Figure 15.3). _____ is a constructed term: ex/ophthalm/o/s.

exophthalmos

eks off THAL mos

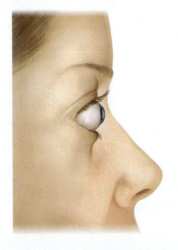

■ **Figure 15.3**
Exophthalmos. The protrusion of the eyes is a common symptom of hyperthyroidism.

goiter
GOY ter

15.10 A common sign of thyroid gland disease is a swelling on the anterior side of the neck in the location of the thyroid gland, known as a **goiter** (■ Figure 15.4). A _____ is an abnormal enlargement of the thyroid gland caused by a tumor, lack of iodine in the diet, or an infection. The term *goiter* is derived from the Latin word for throat, *guttur*.

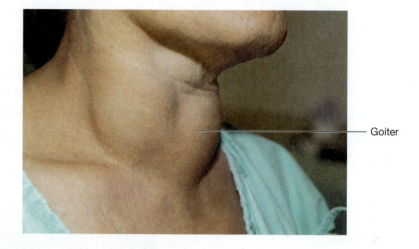
Goiter

■ **Figure 15.4**
Goiter. A goiter appears as a swelling in the anterior neck region, at the location of the thyroid gland.
Source: Karan Bunjean/ Shutterstock.

hirsutism
HER soot izm

15.11 A symptom of excessive body hair in a masculine pattern is known as **hirsutism**. The term is derived from the Latin word *hirsutus*, which means "hairy." When _____ occurs in women, it is caused by the hypersecretion of androgens by the adrenal cortex. Excessive production of androgens in women may also lead to muscle and bone growth. The resulting pattern of masculinization is known as **adrenal virilism** (add REE nal * VIHR ill izm).

ketosis
kee TOH siss

ketoacidosis
KEE toh ah sih DOH siss

15.12 A ketone body is a waste substance produced when cells are unable to metabolize carbohydrates. The condition called _____ is an excessive amount of ketone bodies in the blood and urine and is a sign of unmanaged diabetes mellitus (Frame 15.20) and starvation. Because **ketosis** produces an acidic condition of the body, it is also known as **ketoacidosis**. _____ contains four word parts and is shown as ket/o/acid/osis.

polydipsia
PALL ee DIP see ah

15.13 The prefix *poly-* means "excessive, over, many." It is sometimes used to indicate an abnormally excessive amount. The combining form *dips/o* means "thirst." Thus, the symptom called _____ literally means "condition of excessive thirst." An abnormal state of excessive thirst occurs during certain disorders of the pituitary gland or the pancreas, including diabetes mellitus (Frame 15.20).

15.14 As you learned in Chapter 11, the term **polyuria** includes the prefix *poly-* and means "excessive urination". It is a symptom of pituitary gland disease that arises when the hormone **ADH** is not produced normally. It is also a symptom of unmanaged diabetes mellitus (Frame 15.20). _____ is the production of abnormally large volumes of urine.

polyuria

PALL ee YOO ree ah

PRACTICE: Signs and Symptoms of the Endocrine System

The Right Match

Match the term on the left with the correct definition on the right.

_____ 1. acidosis

_____ 2. ketosis

_____ 3. goiter

_____ 4. adrenal virilism

_____ 5. hirsutism

a. enlargement at the throat

b. a pattern of masculinization and hair distribution in women

c. excessive body hair

d. abnormal accumulation of waste materials that are acidic

e. excessive amount of ketone bodies in the blood and urine

Break the Chain

Analyze these medical terms:

a) Separate each term into its word parts; each word part is labeled for you (**p** = prefix, **r** = root, **cf** = combining form, and **s** = suffix).

b) For the Bonus Question, write the requested definition in the blank that follows.

The first set has been completed as an example.

1. a) polydipsia   ___*poly/dips/ia*___
                              p   r   s

    b) *Bonus Question:* What is the definition of the suffix? ___*condition of*_____

2. a) exophthalmos   _____/_____/___/_____
                                 p   cf   s

    b) *Bonus Question:* What is the definition of the combining form? _____

3. a) polyuria   _____/_____
                             p   s

    b) *Bonus Question:* What is the definition of the suffix? _____

4. a) acromegaly   _____/___/_____
                               cf   s

    b) *Bonus Question:* What is the definition of the combining form? _____

5. a) ketoacidosis   _____/___/_____/_____
                                 cf   r   s

    b) *Bonus Question:* What is the definition of the combining form? _____

Diseases and Disorders of the Endocrine System

Here are the word parts that commonly apply to the diseases and disorders of the endocrine system and are covered in the following section. Note that the word parts are color-coded to help you identify them: prefixes are yellow, combining forms are red, and suffixes are blue.

Prefix	Definition
endo-	within
hyper-	excessive, abnormally high, above
hypo-	deficient, abnormally low, below
para-	alongside, abnormal

Combining Form	Definition
aden/o	gland
adren/o	adrenal gland
calc/i, calc/o	calcium
carcin/o	cancer
crin/o	to secrete
glyc/o	sweet, sugar
gonad/o	sex gland
myx/o	mucus
pancreat/o	sweetbread, pancreas
thyr/o	shield, thyroid
thyroid/o	resembling a shield, thyroid

Suffix	Definition
-al	pertaining to
-emia	condition of blood
-ism	condition or disease
-itis	inflammation
-megaly	abnormally large
-oma	tumor
-osis	condition of
-pathy	disease
-penia	abnormal reduction in number, deficiency

KEY TERMS A–Z

adenocarcinoma
ADD eh noh kar sih NOH mah

adenoma
ADD eh NOH mah

adrenalitis
add REE nah LYE tiss

adrenal insufficiency
add REE nal in suh FISH en see

adrenal hyperplasia
add REE nal high per PLAY zee a

15.15 A malignant tumor that arises from epithelial tissue to form a glandular or glandlike pattern of cells is called an _____. As a constructed term with four word parts, it is written aden/o/carcin/oma. An adenocarcinoma is a life-threatening form of cancer. It often develops from a benign tumor of glandular cells, known as an _____. An adenoma may cause excess secretion by the affected gland.

15.16 Adrenal gland failure leads to several disorders, some of which are due to genetic errors. For example, an inflammation of the adrenal gland is called _____. Clinically, it is known as **adrenal insufficiency**, in which one form is believed to be the result of a genetically based autoimmunity (the body's own white blood cells attack the organ). _____ _____ reduces the body's ability to manage stress and infection. Another dysfunction of the adrenal gland is **adrenal hyperplasia**, which means "excessive growth of the adrenal gland." It is caused by a genetic error resulting in a missing enzyme, and in women, it may cause virilism (Frame 15.11). _____ _____ may also be called **adrenomegaly**, which has three word parts: adren/o/megaly.

congenital hypothyroidism kon JEN ih tal *high poh THIGH royd izm	**15.17** A child suffering from the thyroid gland's inability to produce normal levels of growth hormone at birth may develop the condition called **congenital hypothyroidism**. Formerly known as *cretinism*, the condition _____ _____ results in reduced mental development and physical growth.
Cushing syndrome KUSH ing * SIN drohm	**15.18** A **syndrome** is a disease involving multiple organs that causes an array of symptoms. A syndrome caused by excessive secretion of the hormone cortisol by the adrenal cortex and affecting many organs is called **Cushing syndrome**. It is characterized by obesity, moon (round) face, hyperglycemia (Frame 15.24), and muscle weakness (■ Figure 15.5). A common cause of _____ _____ is an adenoma (Frame 15.15) of the adrenal cortex.

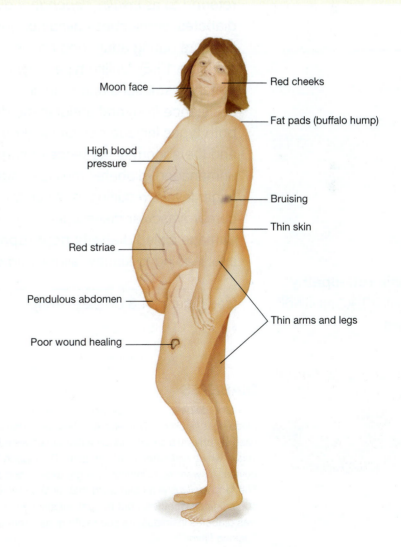

Moon face

High blood pressure

Red striae

Pendulous abdomen

Poor wound healing

Red cheeks

Fat pads (buffalo hump)

Bruising

Thin skin

Thin arms and legs

■ **Figure 15.5**
Cushing syndrome. Caused by excessive cortisol secretion by the adrenal cortex, this syndrome includes the symptoms of obesity, moon face, hyperglycemia, muscle weakness, and other symptoms shown here.

diabetes insipidus

DYE ah BEE teez * in SIP
ih duss

15.19 **Diabetes insipidus (DI)** is caused by hyposecretion of ADH by the pituitary gland. The disease _____ _____ is characterized by the symptoms of polydipsia (Frame 15.13) and polyuria (Frame 15.14).

15.20 Although the term *diabetes* is shared by two diseases, the chronic disorder of carbohydrate metabolism known as **diabetes mellitus (DM)** has very little in common with diabetes insipidus (Frame 15.19; see the Did You Know? box to read why). Diabetes mellitus is a result of resistance of body cells to insulin, or a deficiency or complete lack of insulin production by cells of the pancreas. Two major forms of _____

diabetes mellitus

DYE ah BEE teez * MELL
ih tuss

_____ strike human health. Type 1, which is less common, usually requires hormone replacement therapy with insulin and appears during childhood or adolescence. Because of the dependency of a type 1 diabetic to insulin therapy, it may also be referred to as *insulin-dependent diabetes*. The more common type 2 diabetes, sometimes called *non-insulin-dependent diabetes*, usually appears during adulthood and is often associated with obesity (■ Figure 15.6). Unlike type 1, type 2 can usually be managed with dietary restrictions and regular exercise, and usually with some assistance from oral antidiabetic drugs. Common symptoms of both types include polydipsia (Frame 15.13), polyuria (Frame 15.14), and the abnormal presence of sugar in the urine (glycosuria). If unmanaged, diabetes mellitus causes large fluctuations in blood sugar levels, resulting in circulatory deficiencies that result in cerebrovascular disease leading to heart failure or stroke, kidney damage called **diabetic nephropathy** (DYE ah BET ik * nef ROHP ah thee) leading to kidney failure, and damage to the eyes called

diabetic retinopathy

DYE ah BET ik * ret in NOP
ah thee

_____ _____ that leads to blindness (see Figure 14.8 on page 485).

? **Did You Know**

DIABETES

The term *diabetes* is a Greek word that means "to pass through" or "to pass over." Another meaning is "siphon." The term was first used during the Middle Ages when a siphon was used by physicians to withdraw a sample of urine from a patient to test for an excess of sugar, which was often done by taste. The siphon "passed urine through" to a collection device. A sweet taste indicated sugar excess and a crude diagnosis of diabetes mellitus. The term *mellitus* is a Latin word that means "sweetened with honey." If the "taste test" did not indicate sweetness, but the patient still complained of excessive urination, the diagnosis was diabetes insipidus. As you might guess, the term *insipidus* is a Latin word that means "lacking flavor."

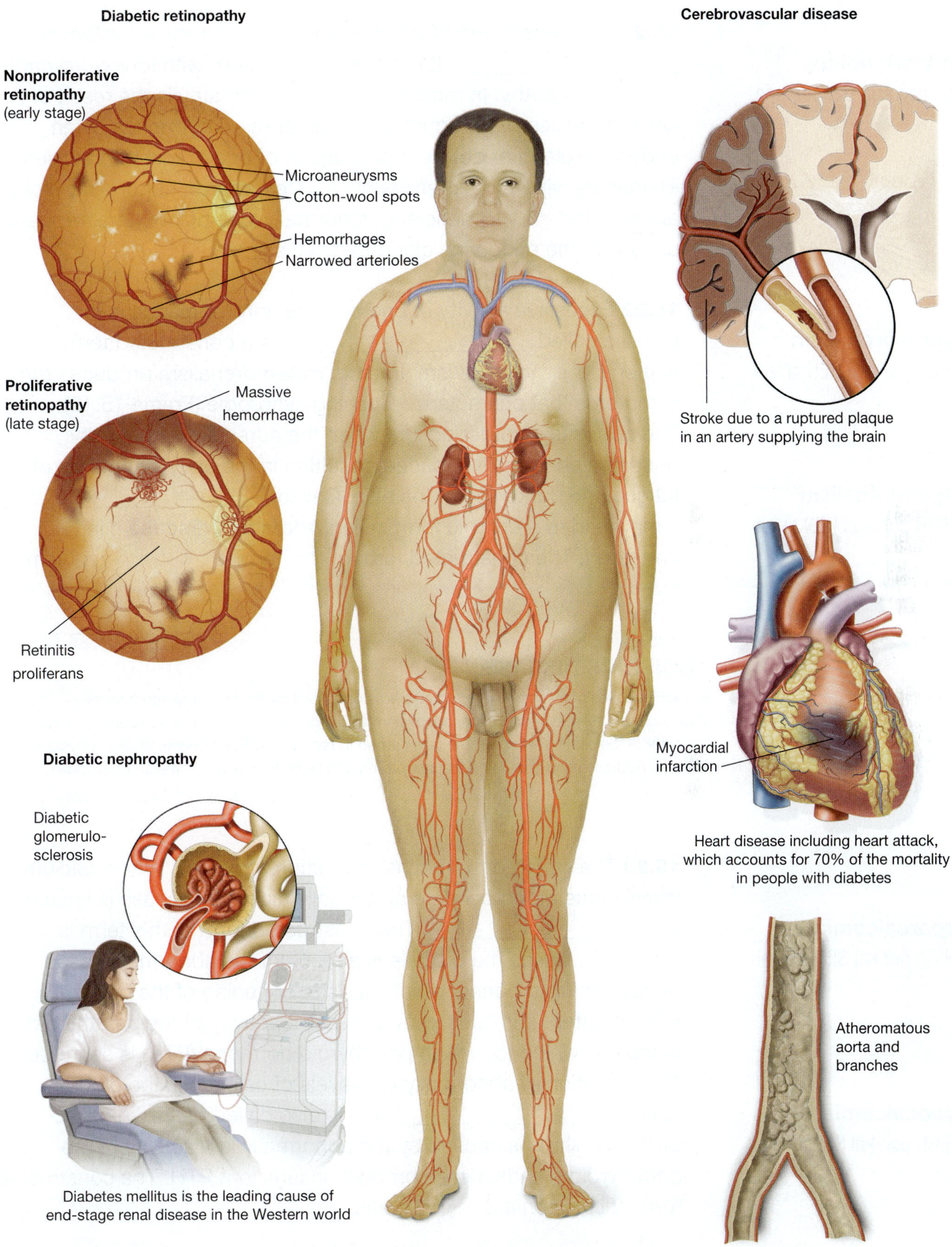

Diabetic retinopathy

Nonproliferative retinopathy
(early stage)

— Microaneurysms
— Cotton-wool spots

— Hemorrhages
— Narrowed arterioles

Proliferative retinopathy
(late stage)

Massive hemorrhage

Retinitis proliferans

Diabetic nephropathy

Diabetic glomerulo-sclerosis

Diabetes mellitus is the leading cause of end-stage renal disease in the Western world

Cerebrovascular disease

Stroke due to a ruptured plaque in an artery supplying the brain

Myocardial infarction

Heart disease including heart attack, which accounts for 70% of the mortality in people with diabetes

Atheromatous aorta and branches

■ **Figure 15.6**
Diabetes mellitus. The metabolic disease diabetes mellitus, with symptoms of polydipsia, polyuria, and widely ranging blood sugar levels, produces many chronic complications if not managed carefully. They include an increased risk of blindness (diabetic retinopathy), kidney disease (diabetic nephropathy), and heart attack or stroke (cerebrovascular disease).

endocrinopathy en doh krin OPP ah thee	**15.21** The general term for a disease of the endocrine system is _____. It is a constructed term with four word parts, endo/crin/o/pathy. In most cases, endocrinopathy is the result of either an excessive production of one or more hormones by an endocrine gland or deficient production of one or more hormones. To identify which, the prefixes *hyper-* ("excessive, abnormally high, above") and *hypo-* ("deficient, abnormally low, below") are frequently used with the endocrine gland that is diseased.
hyperadrenalism HIGH per add REN al izm **hypoadrenalism** HIGH poh add REN al izm	**15.22** Excessive activity of one or more adrenal glands is the disease called _____. It is a constructed term written hyper/adren/al/ism. In time, hyperadrenalism produces the symptoms that characterize Cushing syndrome (Frame 15.18). The opposite disorder occurs when the adrenal gland activity becomes abnormally reduced, resulting in the early symptoms of fatigue and darkening of the skin. Called _____, it may lead to a chronic form called **Addison's disease** if left untreated. The constructed form of this term is hypo/adren/al/ism.

? Did You Know

ADDISON'S DISEASE

In 1855, a series of signs and symptoms were connected for the first time into a disease. They included "feeble heart action, anemia, irritability of the stomach, and a peculiar change in the color of the skin." The syndrome was named to recognize its discoverer, English physician Thomas Addison, who correlated the symptoms and signs to a failure of the adrenal cortex.

hypercalcemia HIGH per kal SEE mee ah **hypocalcemia** HIGH poh kal SEE mee ah	**15.23** The suffix *-emia* means "condition of blood." When calcium levels in the blood become abnormally high, the disease is known as _____. The constructed form of this term is hyper/calc/emia. The disease is a result of the abnormal release of calcium from bones, which leads to softening of the bones if left untreated. It is caused by excessive activity of the parathyroid glands, in which too much parathyroid hormone (PTH) is secreted. The condition of abnormally low levels of calcium in the blood is called _____ and is also called **calcipenia** (KAL sih PEE nee ah). It is caused by the abnormally low activity of the parathyroid glands, which produce insufficient PTH. The constructed form of *calcipenia* is, calc/i/penia.

hypoglycemia

HIGH poh glye SEE mee ah

15.24 Another use of the suffix *-emia* is in the term **hyperglycemia**, which literally means "condition of blood excessive sugar." The constructed form of this term is hyper/glyc/emia. The chronic form of the disease often indicates the body may not be producing enough insulin or insulin receptor sites are resistant, resulting in the buildup of glucose in the blood as a characteristic of diabetes mellitus (Frame 15.20). In the opposite condition, _____, blood sugar levels fall to abnormally low levels. It is caused by excessive insulin administration or excessive production by the pancreas and is often accompanied by headache, malaise (weakness), tremors, hunger, and anxiety. If left untreated, it can lead to coma and death.

hypoparathyroidism

HIGH poh pair ah THIGH royd izm

hypo/para/thyroid/ism

15.25 The excessive production of PTH by the parathyroid glands is a disorder known as **hyperparathyroidism**. This lengthy term contains four word parts: hyper/para/thyroid/ism. Usually caused by a tumor, it results in excessive calcium levels in the blood, or hypercalcemia (Frame 15.23). In the opposite condition called _____, PTH levels are reduced and the condition of hypocalcemia (Frame 15.23) occurs. The constructed form of this term is ____/_____/_____/_____.

👁

WORDS TO Watch Out For

para-

Note that the prefix *para-* doesn't always appear at the beginning of a term. In the term *hypoparathyroid*, it appears in the middle of the term. But don't let that confuse you: it is still a prefix and it still means "alongside or abnormal."

hyperthyroidism

HIGH per THIGH royd izm

15.26 Excessive activity of the thyroid gland produces abnormally high levels of thyroid hormone in the disease _____, which accelerates metabolism. The constructed form of this term is hyper/thyroid/ism. Symptoms include exophthalmos (Frame 15.9), goiter (Frame 15.10), rapid heart rate, and weight loss. One form of chronic hyperthyroidism, called **Graves' disease**, is believed to be an autoimmune disease. Another form, known as **thyrotoxicosis** (THIGH roh toks ih KOH siss), is an acute event that is triggered by infection or trauma and can become life-threatening.

👁

WORDS TO Watch Out For

hyper- or *hypo-*?

The spelling of these two prefixes is very similar, but the difference in meaning is great. *Hyper-* means "excessive, abnormally high, above"; whereas *hypo-* means "deficient, abnormally low, below." An easy way to remember the difference is to think of the long *o* sound of the word "low," which matches the sound of the vowel in *hypo-*.

hypothyroidism
HIGH poh THIGH royd izm

15.27 When thyroid gland activity becomes deficient, thyroid hormone blood levels drop below normal in the disease called _____ (■ Figure 15.7). The constructed form is hypo/thyroid/ism. The most common cause of hypothyroidism is the autoimmune disorder in which the thyroid gland comes under attack by the body's own immune response, called **Hashimoto's disease**. The symptoms of hypothyroidism include a slow heart rate, dry skin, low energy, and weight gain. In the chronic form of hypothyroidism known as **myxedema** (miks eh DEE mah), the subcutaneous layer beneath the skin becomes thick and hard, and the body retains water, aging the skin prematurely while puffing the face and thickening the tongue and hands. _Myxedema_ literally means "swollen mucus."

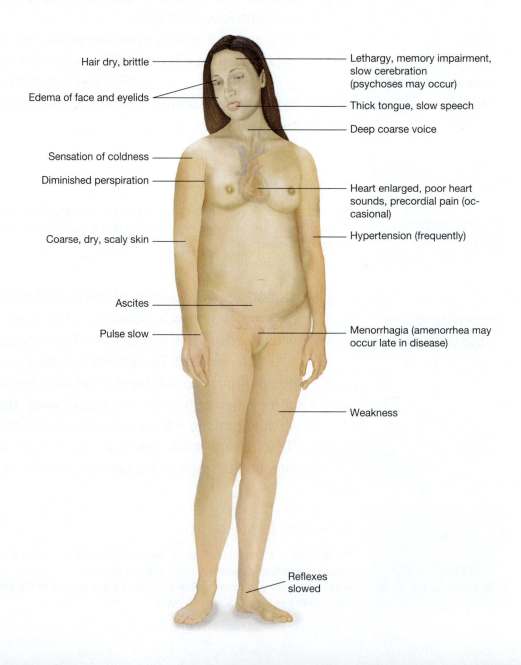

Hair dry, brittle

Edema of face and eyelids

Sensation of coldness

Diminished perspiration

Coarse, dry, scaly skin

Ascites

Pulse slow

Lethargy, memory impairment, slow cerebration (psychoses may occur)

Thick tongue, slow speech

Deep coarse voice

Heart enlarged, poor heart sounds, precordial pain (occasional)

Hypertension (frequently)

Menorrhagia (amenorrhea may occur late in disease)

Weakness

Reflexes slowed

■ **Figure 15.7**
Hypothyroidism. Hyposecretion of the thyroid gland produces the symptoms that are illustrated.

hypogonadism

HIGH poh GOH nad izm

hypo/gonad/ism

15.28 In the disease **hypogonadism**, abnormally low amounts of follicle-stimulating hormone (FSH) and luteinizing hormone (LH) are produced by the pituitary gland, which reduces the production of the sex hormones testosterone (produced by the male testes) and estrogen/progesterone (produced by the female ovaries). Also known as pituitary _____, it results in reduced sexual interest and reproductive capacity. If it occurs before puberty, the gonads (male testes and female ovaries) fail to develop, resulting in the failure of secondary sexual characteristics to form during adolescence such as body hair, muscle and bone growth (if male), or breasts (if female). *Hypogonadism* is a constructed term, which is written as _____/_____/_____.

pancreatitis

PAN kree ah TYE tiss

15.29 Inflammation of the pancreas is a disorder known as _____ (■ Figure 15.8). It often results in a deficient production of insulin, which leads to hyperglycemia (Frame 15.24). Pancreatitis may be an acute reaction to infection or trauma or a chronic condition resulting in progressive pancreatic failure, both of which can become life-threatening. The term includes only two word parts: pancreat/itis.

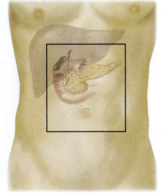

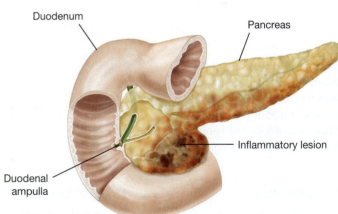

Duodenum

Pancreas

Duodenal ampulla

Inflammatory lesion

■ **Figure 15.8**
Pancreatitis. Inflammation of the pancreas may be the result of a bacterial infection, trauma, or chronic disease such as cancer.

pituitary gigantism
  pih TOO ih tair ee * JYE
  gant izm

15.30 Because the pituitary gland produces numerous hormones, a tumor or congenital defect of the pituitary can affect many body functions. In **pituitary dwarfism** (pih TOO ih tair ee * DWARF izm), the pituitary growth hormone is deficient at birth, resulting in short stature. An abnormally high production of pituitary growth hormone before adulthood results in _____ _____, and if it occurs after adulthood has begun, it results in acromegaly (Frame 15.8). A photograph comparing dwarfism and gigantism is provided in ■ Figure 15.9.

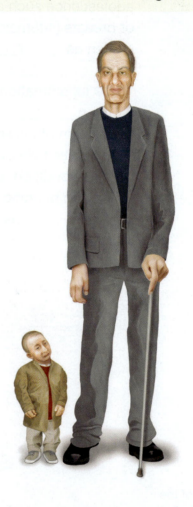

■ **Figure 15.9**
Growth hormone disorders. Illustration of a pituitary giant and a pituitary dwarf, both adults of about the same age. This illustration was rendered from an actual photograph.

thyroiditis
  THYE royd EYE tiss

15.31 Inflammation of the thyroid gland is called _____. The constructed form is thyroid/itis. Acute thyroiditis is usually caused by a local infection, whereas there are many forms of chronic thyroiditis that often lead to hyperthyroidism (Frame 15.26).

PRACTICE: Diseases and Disorders of the Endocrine System

Linkup

Link the word parts in the list to create the terms that match the definitions. You may use word parts more than once. Remember to add combining vowels when needed and that some terms do not use any combining vowel. The first one is completed as an example.

Prefix	Combining Form	Suffix
hyper-	aden/o	-al
hypo-	adren/o	-emia
para-	calc/o	-ism
	carcin/o	-itis
	glyc/o	-oma
	pancreat/o	-pathy
	thyroid/o	

Definition

1. inflammation of a gland
2. glandular disease
3. malignant tumor that arises from epithelial tissue to form a glandular or glandlike pattern of cells
4. excessive activity of one or both adrenal glands
5. a disease that results from abnormally high levels of calcium in the blood
6. abnormally low blood sugar levels
7. excessive production of parathyroid hormone by the parathyroid glands
8. a disease that results from abnormally low blood levels of thyroid hormone
9. inflammation of the pancreas
10. inflammation of the thyroid

Term

1. *adenitis*
2. _____
3. _____
4. _____
5. _____
6. _____
7. _____
8. _____
9. _____
10. _____

The Right Match

Match the term on the left with the correct definition on the right.

_____ 1. Addison's disease

_____ 2. diabetic nephropathy

_____ 3. diabetes insipidus

_____ 4. pituitary gigantism

_____ 5. Cushing syndrome

_____ 6. Graves' disease

_____ 7. diabetic retinopathy

_____ 8. diabetes mellitus

_____ 9. pituitary dwarfism

_____ 10. congenital hypothyroidism

a. caused by excessive secretion of the adrenal cortex

b. a form of chronic hyperthyroidism; may be an autoimmune disease

c. chronic disorder of carbohydrate metabolism

d. kidney damage caused by diabetes mellitus

e. potentially vision-threatening damage to the eye in diabetics

f. caused by hyposecretion of adrenal cortex

g. short stature resulting from a deficiency in pituitary growth hormone

h. caused by hyposecretion of ADH by the pituitary

i. reduced mental development and physical growth that results from a lack of thyroid hormone at birth

j. results from an abnormally high production of pituitary growth hormone before adolescence

Treatments, Procedures, and Devices of the Endocrine System

Here are the word parts that commonly apply to the treatments, procedures, and devices of the endocrine system and are covered in the following section. Note that the word parts are color-coded to help you identify them: prefixes are yellow, combining forms are red, and suffixes are blue.

Prefix	Definition		Combining Form	Definition		Suffix	Definition
endo-	within		adren/o	adrenal gland		-al	pertaining to
para-	alongside, abnormal		crin/o	to secrete		-ectomy	surgical excision, removal
			thyr/o	shield, thyroid		-logist	one who studies
			thyroid/o	resembling a shield, thyroid		-logy	study or science of
						-oma	tumor
						-tomy	incision, to cut

KEY TERMS A–Z

adrenalectomy
add REE nal EK toh mee

15.32 A procedure involving the surgical excision, or removal, of one or both of the adrenal glands is known as **adrenalectomy**. The constructed form of this term is adren/al/ectomy. An _____ may become necessary if hormone therapy fails to correct hyperadrenalism (Frame 15.22).

endocrinologist
en doh krin ALL oh jist

15.33 You learned at the beginning of this chapter that the term *endocrine* literally means "to secrete within," and the field of medicine focusing on the study and treatment of endocrine disorders is called **endocrinology**. A physician specializing in this field is known as an _____. It is a constructed term: endo/crin/o/logist.

fasting blood sugar

15.34 Measuring blood sugar levels provides information about how well the body manages carbohydrate metabolism. In a procedure called _____ _____ _____ **(FBS)**, blood sugar levels are measured after a 12-hour fast. In a **postprandial blood sugar (PPBS)** exam, blood sugar levels are measured about 2 hours after a meal (postprandial means "after a meal"). In both tests, extreme variations in blood sugar or abnormally high glucose levels (hyperglycemia) are an indication of diabetes mellitus (Frame 15.20). A common method of testing blood sugar levels is shown in ■ Figure 15.10.

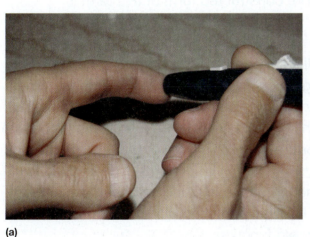
(a)

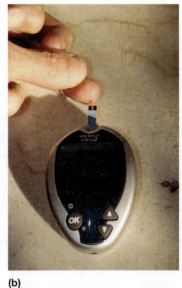
(b)

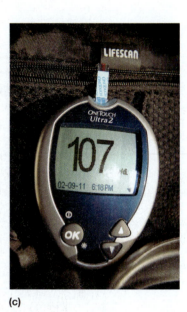
(c)

■ **Figure 15.10**
Blood glucose measurement. A fasting blood sugar test may be self-administered. (a) A lance pierces the skin of a finger. (b) A small blood sample is gently squeezed onto a reagent strip. (c) The glucose meter will display the glucose concentration in the blood sample. A reading of 80–100 mg/dL is a normal range. Note that the reading of 107 exceeds the normal values, suggesting the sample is from a diabetic patient.

glucose tolerance test

15.35 A test that may be used to confirm a diagnosis of diabetes mellitus examines a patient's tolerance of glucose. Known as a

_____ _____ _____ **(GTT)**, the patient is given glucose either orally or intravenously, then at timed intervals blood samples are taken and glucose levels measured and recorded. Large fluctuations of blood sugar confirm the diagnosis of diabetes mellitus.

hormone replacement therapy

15.36 A failure of an endocrine gland to produce sufficient levels of a hormone, or hyposecretion, can have a serious impact on health. A common therapy to counteract hyposecretion is called **hormone replacement therapy (HRT)**. Synthetic hormones or extracted hormones may be used in HRT. _____ _____ _____ may also be used following the surgical removal of an endocrine gland to restore homeostasis. It is an optional therapy for the treatment of symptoms associated with menopausal changes, although evidence suggests a slight risk of breast cancer with its use.

parathyroidectomy
PAIR ah THIGH royd EK toh mee

15.37 The surgical removal, or excision, of a parathyroid gland may be a treatment for parathyroid cancer, called **parathyroidoma**, or for hyperparathyroidism (Frame 15.25). The procedure is called _____. The constructed form of this term is para/thyroid/ectomy.

radioactive iodine

15.38 The producing cells of the thyroid gland use the element iodine as a necessary ingredient in forming thyroid hormones. One way in which thyroid function may be measured is to determine the amount of iodine taken into thyroid cells. In the diagnostic procedure known as **radioactive iodine uptake** (RAY dee oh AK tihv * EYE oh dyne * UP tayk), _____ _____ is used to track and measure its entry into thyroid gland cells with a scanning instrument. Abbreviated **RAIU**, a reduction of iodine uptake is an indication of deficient thyroid function.

radioiodine therapy
RAY dee oh EYE oh dyne *
THAIR ah pee

15.39 Because the thyroid gland is the only organ of the body that uptakes iodine, an effective treatment against a thyroid tumor, or thyroidoma (Frame 15.40), is the use of radioactive iodine. Called _____ _____, the radioactive iodine targets cells within the thyroid gland and destroys them.

thyroid scan
THIGH royd * skan

thyroidoma
THIGH royd OH mah

15.40 A procedure measuring thyroid function is called a **thyroid scan**, during which an image of the thyroid gland is obtained. The _____ _____ image is recorded with a scanning instrument following oral administration of a labeled substance, usually iodine (■ Figure 15.11). Thyroid scans are usually employed to detect a thyroid tumor, known as a _____.

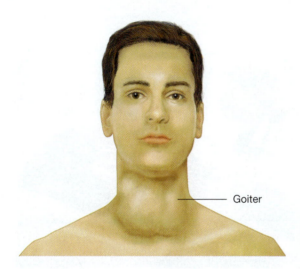
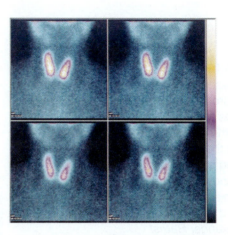

— Goiter

■ **Figure 15.11**
Thyroid scan. The right image is a colorized image from an abnormal thyroid scan, such as would occur in a patient with a goiter (illustrated on the left).
Source: Stefania Arca/Shutterstock.

thyroidectomy
THIGH royd EK toh mee
thyroidotomy
THIGH royd OTT oh mee

15.41 Recall the meaning of the suffix *-ectomy* is "surgical excision or removal." The surgical removal of the thyroid gland is therefore called _____. The constructed form is thyroid/ectomy. Because the suffix *-tomy* means "incision, to cut," a _____ is a procedure in which the thyroid gland is surgically entered. This constructed term is thyroid/o/tomy.

thyroid ultrasonography
THIGH royd* ul trah soh NAW grah fee

15.42 In addition to RAIU (Frame 15.38) and thyroid scan (Frame 15.40), the thyroid gland may also be evaluated for disease using ultrasound. The procedure is called _____ _____ and is shown in ■ Figure 15.12. The procedure can identify abnormalities of thyroid gland tissue, such as the presence of tumors or inflammation, and is often performed as a first step in running diagnostics of the thyroid gland. The words that build the term can be shown as thyroid ultra/son/o/graphy.

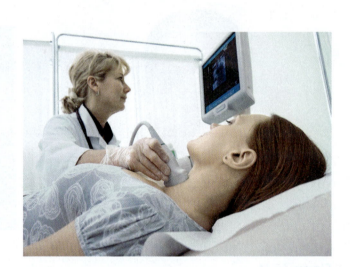

■ **Figure 15.12**
Thyroid ultrasonography. This diagnostic procedure sends sound waves generated by a transducer through a probe pressing on the anterior neck. The reflected sound waves are picked up and converted by a computer to a monitor to reveal thyroid gland abnormalities.
Source: Alexander Raths/ Shutterstock.

thyroparathyroidectomy
THIGH roh pair ah THIGH royd EK toh mee
thyr/o/para/thyroid/ectomy

15.43 In some cases, the parathyroid glands must be surgically removed with the thyroid gland. This procedure is called _____. Write the constructed form of this term: _____/___/_____/_____/_____.

thyroxine test
THIGH rox een

15.44 Thyroxine is one of several hormones produced by the thyroid gland. It regulates glucose metabolism and cell division in most cells of the body. A diagnostic test measuring thyroxine levels in the blood is simply called a _____ _____. It is often used as a diagnostic test for hyperthyroidism (Frame 15.26) or hypothyroidism (Frame 15.27).

PRACTICE: Treatments, Procedures, and Devices of the Endocrine System

The Right Match

Match the term on the left with the correct definition on the right.

_____ 1. fasting blood sugar

_____ 2. glucose tolerance test

_____ 3. hormone replacement therapy

_____ 4. radioactive iodine uptake

_____ 5. thyroid scan

_____ 6. thyroxine test

_____ 7. radioiodine therapy

a. synthetic or extracted hormones used to counteract hyposecretion

b. a procedure used to determine amount of iodine taken into thyroid cells

c. a test that examines a patient's tolerance of glucose

d. a procedure in which blood sugar levels are measured after a 12-hour fast

e. a diagnostic test that measures thyroxine levels in the blood

f. treatment for a thyroid tumor that targets cells within the thyroid gland and destroys them

g. a procedure that obtains an image of the thyroid to measure thyroid function

Break the Chain

Analyze these medical terms:

a) Separate each term into its word parts; each word part is labeled for you (**p** = prefix, **r** = root, **cf** = combining form, and **s** = suffix)

b) For the Bonus Question, write the requested definition in the blank that follows.

1. a) adrenalectomy _____/_____/_____
   r   s   s

   b) *Bonus Question:* What is the definition of the *first* suffix? _____

2. a) endocrinology _____/_____/___/_____
   p   cf   s

   b) *Bonus Question:* What is the definition of the combining form? _____

3. a) thyroidoma _____/_____
   r   s

   b) *Bonus Question:* What is the definition of the suffix? _____

4. a) thyroidotomy _____/___/_____
   cf   s

   b) *Bonus Question:* What is the definition of the suffix? _____

5. a) thyroparathyroidectomy _____/___/_____/_____/_____
   cf   p   r   s

   b) *Bonus Question:* What is the definition of the suffix? _____

Abbreviations of the Endocrine System

The abbreviations that are associated with the endocrine system are summarized here. Study these abbreviations and review them in the exercise that follows.

Abbreviation	Definition
ACTH	adrenocorticotropic hormone
ADH	antidiuretic hormone
DI	diabetes insipidus
DM	diabetes mellitus
FBS	fasting blood sugar
FSH	follicle-stimulating hormone
GH	growth hormone
GTT	glucose tolerance test
HRT	hormone replacement therapy
LH	luteinizing hormone
PPBS	postprandial blood sugar
PTH	parathyroid hormone
RAIU	radioactive iodine uptake
TSH	thyroid-stimulating hormone

PRACTICE: Abbreviations

Fill in the blanks with the abbreviation or the complete medical term.

Abbreviation

1. GTT

2. _____

3. PPBS

4. _____

5. FBS

6. _____

7. DM

8. _____

9. ADH

10. _____

Medical Term

_____

radioactive iodine uptake

_____

diabetes insipidus

_____

hormone replacement therapy

_____

parathyroid hormone

_____

follicle-stimulating hormone

CHAPTER REVIEW

Word Building _____

Construct medical terms from the following meanings. The first question has been completed as an example.

1. tumor of a gland — aden**oma**_____

2. excessive production of thyroid hormones — _____thyroidism

3. peripheral nerve damage during diabetes mellitus — diabetic neuro_____

4. inflammation of the adrenal gland — adrenal_____

5. disease of the endocrine system — _____pathy

6. excessive calcium levels in the blood — hyper_____

7. a tumor of the parathyroid gland — parathyroid_____

8. caused by too much GH prior to adulthood — pituitary gigant_____

9. abnormally reduced adrenal activity — _____adrenalism

10. excessive body hair — _____ism

11. deficient production of PTH — hypo_____

12. abnormally low blood sugar levels — hypo_____

13. acute form of hyperthyroidism triggered by infection or trauma — thyro_____

14. major cause of hypothyroidism — _____disease

15. caused by deficient FSH and LH that results in reduced reproductive capacity — _____gonadism

Define the Combining Form _____

In the space provided, write the definition of the combining form, followed by one example of the combining form used to build a medical term in Chapter 15.

	Definition	Use in a Term
1. aden/o	_____	_____
2. adren/o	_____	_____
3. crin/o	_____	_____
4. thyroid/o	_____	_____
5. glyc/o	_____	_____
6. pancreat/o	_____	_____
7. calc/o	_____	_____
8. acid/o	_____	_____

Complete the Labels _____

Complete the blank labels in Figure 15.13 by writing the labels in the spaces provided.

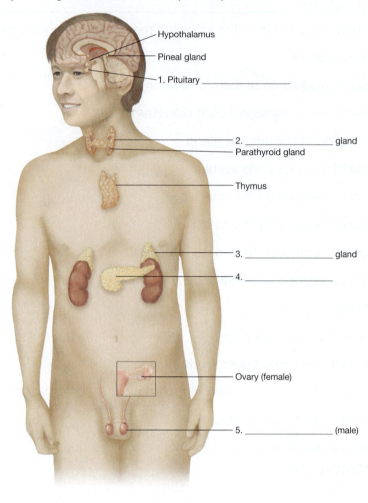

- Hypothalamus
- Pineal gland
1. Pituitary _____
2. _____ gland
- Parathyroid gland
- Thymus
3. _____ gland
4. _____
- Ovary (female)
5. _____ (male)

■ **Figure 15.13**
Organs of the endocrine system.

1. _____

2. _____

3. _____

4. _____

5. _____

MyLab Medical Terminology™

MyLab Medical Terminology is a premium online homework management system that includes a host of features to help you study. Registered users will find:

- A multitude of quizzes and activities built within the MyLab platform
- Powerful tools that track and analyze your results—allowing you to create a personalized learning experience
- Videos and audio pronunciations to help enrich your progress
- Streaming lesson presentations (Guided Lectures) and self-paced learning modules
- A space where you and your instructors can view and manage your assignments

MEDICAL REPORT EXERCISES

Anita Del Rio

Read the following medical report, then answer the questions that follow.

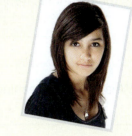

PEARSON GENERAL HOSPITAL

PGH

5500 University Avenue, Metropolis, New York
Phone: (211) 594-4000 • Fax (211) 594-4001

Medical Consultation: Pediatrics   **Date:** 09/07/2017

Patient: Anita Del Rio   **Patient ID:** 123456

Dob: 1/15/2004   **Age:** 13   **Sex:** Female   **Allergies:** NKDA

Provider: Jonathon McClary, MD

Subjective:

"I'm really tired most of the day, mostly between meals, and getting behind in school. I get real thirsty a lot, and it seems like I need to use the bathroom 20 times a day! Lately, I've also been getting headaches a lot and have trouble falling asleep at night."

13 y/o female complains of malaise, polydipsia, polyuria, cephalalgia, and insomnia. Although full of pep in the clinic during her visit, her mother supports her complaints and is very concerned with her lack of energy. No medical history available.

Objective:

Vital Signs: T: 98.6°F; **P:** 80; **R:** 22; **BP:** 120/75

Ht: 5'1"

Wt: 90 lb

General Appearance: Skin appears healthy, with no apparent masses or discolorations.

Heart: Rate at 80 bpm. Heart sounds with auscultation appear normal.

Lungs: Clear without signs of disease.

AbD: Bowel sounds normal all four quadrants.

HEENT: No abnormalities present.

Lab: Ketone bodies elevated, mild acidosis pH 7.3; FBS 220 confirmed with GTT

Assessment:

Diabetes mellitus type 1

Plan:

Treat as type 1 DM with regular insulin injection regimen and enroll with parent in diabetes management class.

Photo Source: Scott Griessel/Fotolia.

Comprehension Questions

1. What patient complaints are consistent with the signs? _____

   _____

   _____

2. Is the diagnosis temporary and capable of a cure with the prescribed treatment? _____

   _____

   _____

3. What are the meanings of the abbreviations FBS and GTT? _____

   _____

   _____

Case Study Questions

The following Case Study provides further discussion regarding the patient in the medical report. Fill in the blanks with the correct terms. Choose your answers from the following list of terms. (Note that some terms may be used more than once.)

acidosis	glucose	ketosis
endocrinology	hyperglycemia	polydipsia
fasting blood sugar	insulin	type 1 diabetes

A 13-year-old patient, Anita Del Rio, was referred by her personal physician for an endocrinological evaluation

in the (a) _____ department, following a 4-week history of symptoms of energy loss

between meals, excessive thirst, or (b) _____, headache, polyuria (excessive urination), and

sleeplessness. A routine blood test had also been recorded by the physician and had shown ketone bodies

in the blood, or (c) _____, combined with a lowered blood pH, or (d) _____.

Endocrinological evaluation included an FBS, or (e) _____ _____

_____ test, followed by a (f) _____ tolerance test, and a urinalysis. The tests

indicated the patient suffered from excessive sugar levels in the blood, or (g) _____, that

was due to a failure of islet beta cells to produce proper levels of the hormone (h) _____.

A diagnosis of (i) _____ _____ _____ was recorded. The

patient was treated with regular insulin, trained in self-glucose testing and insulin administration, and referred

to a local educational program in diabetes management to include her parents' participation.

Denaya Bellafonte

For a greater challenge, read the following medical report and answer the critical thinking questions that follow.

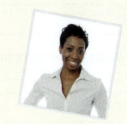

PGH PEARSON GENERAL HOSPITAL

5500 University Avenue, Metropolis, New York
Phone: (211) 594-4000 • Fax (211) 594-4001

Medical Consultation: Endocrinology **Date:** 04/22/2017

Patient: Denaya Bellafonte **Patient ID:** 123456

Dob: 10/23/1987 **Age:** 29 **Sex:** Female **Allergies:** NKDA

Provider: Joseph Ryan, MD

Subjective:

"I'm having headaches nearly every day and feel tired all the time. I'm gaining weight even though I'm not eating much. I'm also experiencing pain in my lower back and a strange growth of body hair on my face."

29 y/o female with no prior medical concerns. Her mother was diagnosed with thyrotoxicosis, treated with thyroidectomy at age 45 years. The patient complaints include lethargy, cephalalgia, unwanted weight gain, lower back pain, and hirsutism. All changes began at about the same time, approximately 3 months ago.

Objective:

Vital Signs: T: 98.8°F; **P:** 79; **R:** 22; **BP:** 122/80

Ht: 5'8"

Wt: 182 lb

General Appearance: Skin appears healthy, with no apparent masses or discolorations.

Heart: Rate at 79 bpm. Heart sounds with auscultation appear normal.

Lungs: Clear without signs of disease.

AbD: Bowel sounds normal all four quadrants.

HEENT: No abnormalities present.

Lab: Blood glucose elevated, at 165 mg/dL.

MRI: Tumor present at superior aspect of left adrenal gland, 1.2 cm × 2.0 cm, with damage to gland.

bx: Tumor is benign.

Assessment:

Adrenal hyperplasia, caused by left adrenal adenoma

Plan:

Schedule left adrenalectomy within 2 weeks.

Photo Source: Stockyimages/Shutterstock.

Comprehension Questions

1. Why would a tumor of the adrenal gland lead to hirsutism in the patient? _____
   _____
   _____

2. What is the correlation between the patient's hyperglycemia and weight gain? _____
   _____
   _____

3. What is adrenal hyperplasia? _____
   _____
   _____

Case Study Questions

The following case study provides further discussion regarding the patient in the medical report. Recall the terms from this chapter to fill in the blanks with the correct terms.

A 29-year-old patient, Denaya Bellafonte, was admitted for hospitalization following reports of symptoms that included frequent headaches, loss of energy, unexplained weight gain, and tenderness in the left lumbar region. More recently, increased body hair, or (j) _____, was an additional cause for concern. An early diagnosis was made of (k) _____, or an inflammation of the adrenals. Also, the attending physician believed that the lumbar pain could be explained by an abnormal enlargement of the adrenal glands, a condition known as (l) _____. In addition, the weight gain in the patient had produced a round "moon face" appearance that characterizes (m) _____ syndrome. This diagnosis also explained the elevated blood sugar levels, or (n) _____, combined with energy loss and muscle weakness. However, the actual cause remained a mystery until the patient's tender lumbar region was examined with MRI. This diagnostic tool revealed a tumor of the left adrenal gland. Apparently, the tumor had caused the adrenal cortex to hypersecrete male sex hormones known as (o) _____, which had caused the body hair, a sign of endocrine disease known as (p) _____. The tumor had also caused the hypersecretion of other adrenal cortex hormones, which led to the metabolic disturbance. A laparoscopic biopsy was performed, and the accompanying histology test confirmed the tumor was benign, and thereby called an (q) _____. Surgery was performed to remove the left adrenal gland, called a left (r) _____. Following the surgery the patient made a complete recovery with all symptoms abating within several weeks.

Appendices

Appendix A

Word Parts Glossary

The word parts that have been presented in this textbook are summarized with their definitions for quick reference. The chapter numbers correspond to the first chapter in which the word part is described. Prefixes are listed first, followed by combining forms and suffixes.

Prefix	Definition	Chapter	Prefix	Definition	Chapter
a-	without, absence of	1	intra-	within	3
ab-	away from	3	iso-	equal	7
ad-	toward	3	macro-	large	3
ambi-	both	3	mal-	bad	3
an-	without, absence of	3	mega-	large, great	3
ana-	up, toward	3	megalo-	large, great	3
ante-	before	3	meta-	after, change	3
anti-	against, opposite of	1	micro-	small	1
bi-	two	3	mono-	one	3
brady-	slow	1	multi-	many, more than once, numerous	3
circum-	around	3	neo-	new	1
con-	with, together, jointly	1	nulli-	none	3
contra-	counter, against	3	pan-	all	3
di-	double	3	par-	alongside, abnormal	5
dia-	through	3	para-	alongside, abnormal	3
dipl-	double	3	peri-	around	3
dis-	apart, away	3	poly-	excessive, over, many	2
dys-	bad, abnormal, painful, difficult	2	post-	to follow after	3
ec-	outside, out	3	pre-	to come before	1
ecto-	outside, out	3	primi-	first	3
en-	within, upon, on, over	11	pro-	before	4
endo-	within	1	pseudo-	false	3
ep-	upon, over, above, on top	3	quadri-	four	2
epi-	upon, over, above, on top	1	re-	back	10
eso-	inward	3	semi-	half, partial	3
eu-	normal, good	3	sub-	under, beneath, below	3
ex-	outside, away from	3	super-	above	3
exo-	outside, away from	3	supra-	above	3
extra-	outside	3	sym-	together, joined	3
hemi-	half	3	syn-	together, joined	2
heter-	different	3	tachy-	rapid, fast	3
hetero-	different	3	tetra-	four	3
hyper-	excessive, abnormally high, above	3	trans-	through, across, beyond	3
hypo-	deficient, abnormally low, below	2	tri-	three	3
infer-	below	3	ultra-	beyond normal	3
inter-	between	3	uni-	one	3

Combining Form	Definition	Chapter
abdomin/o	abdomen	4
abort/o	miscarry	12
abras/o	to rub away	5
acid/o	a solution or substance with a pH less than 7	10
acr/o	extremity	15
actin/o	radiation	5
aden/o	gland	5
adren/o	adrenal gland	15
albin/o	white	5
albumin/o	albumin (a protein)	11
alveol/o	air sac, alveolus	9
amni/o	amnion	12
an/o	anus	10
andr/o	male	12
angi/o	blood vessel	8
ankyl/o	crooked	6
anter/o	front	4
aort/o	aorta	8
append/o	appendix	1
appendic/o	appendix	1
arter/o	artery	8
arteri/o	artery	8
arthr/o	joint	6
articul/o	joint	6
asthen/o	weakness	14
atel/o	incomplete	9
ather/o	fatty plaque	8
atri/o	atrium	8
audi/o	hearing	14
aut/o	self	5
azot/o	urea, nitrogen	11
bacteri/o	bacteria	7
balan/o	glans penis	12
bi/o	life	1
bil/i	bile	10
blast/o	germ, bud, developing cell	7
blephar/o	eyelid	14
botul/o	sausage	7
brachi/o	arm	4
bronch/i	airway, bronchus	9
bronch/o	airway, bronchus	9
burs/o	purse or sac, bursa	6
calc/i	calcium	15
calc/o	calcium	15
carcin/o	cancer	5
cardi/o	heart	1
carp/o	wrist	6
caud/o	tail	4
cec/o	blind intestine, cecum	10
cellul/o	little cell	5
cephal/o	head	4
cerebell/o	little brain, cerebellum	13

Combining Form	Definition	Chapter
cerebr/o	brain, cerebrum	1
cervic/o	neck, cervix	4
cheil/o	lip	10
chol/e	bile, gall	10
cholecyst/o	gallbladder	10
choledoch/o	common bile duct	10
chondr/i	gristle, cartilage	4
chondr/o	gristle, cartilage	6
chori/o	membrane, chorion	12
chron/o	time	4
chym/o	juice	5
cirrh/o	orange	10
coccidioid/o	*Coccidioides immitis* (a fungus)	9
col/o	colon	10
colon/o	colon	10
colp/o	vagina	12
coni/o	dust	9
condyl/o	knuckle of a joint	6
conjunctiv/o	to bind together, conjunctiva	14
cor/o	pupil	14
coron/o	crown or circle, heart	8
cost/o	rib	6
cran/o	skull, cranium	4
crani/o	skull, cranium	4
crin/o	to secrete	15
crypt/o	hidden	5
cutane/o	skin	5
cyan/o	blue	5
cyes/o	pregnancy	12
cyesi/o	pregnancy	12
cyst/o	bladder, sac	9
cyt/o	cell	2
dacry/o	tear	14
dent/o	teeth	10
derm/o	skin	1
dermat/o	skin	1
dilat/o	to widen	9
dips/o	thirst	15
dist/o	distant	4
diverticul/o	diverticulum	10
dors/o	back	4
duoden/o	twelve, duodenum	10
dur/o	hard	12
ech/o	sound	8
electr/o	electricity	1
embol/o	plug	8
embry/o	embryo	12
encephal/o	brain	1
enter/o	small intestine	1
epididym/o	epididymis	12
episi/o	vulva	12
erythr/o	red	7

Combining Form	Definition	Chapter
esophag/e	gullet, esophagus	10
esophag/o	gullet, esophagus	10
esthesi/o	sensation	13
extern/o	exterior	14
fasci/o	fascia	6
fec/o	feces	10
femor/o	thigh, femur	4
fet/o	fetus	12
fibr/o	fiber	6
fibul/o	fibula	6
flux/o	flow	10
follicul/o	little follicle	5
fung/o	fungus	7
gangli/o	swelling, knot	13
ganglion/o	swelling, knot	13
gastr/o	stomach	1
gingiv/o	gums	10
gli/o	glue	13
globin/o	protein	7
glomerul/o	little ball, glomerulus	11
gloss/o	tongue	10
glott/o	opening into the windpipe	9
gluc/o	sweet, sugar	11
glute/o	buttock	4
glyc/o	sweet, sugar	11
glycos/o	sweet, sugar	11
gnos/o	knowledge	13
gonad/o	sex gland	15
gravid/o	pregnancy	12
gravidar/o	pregnancy	12
gyn/o	woman	12
gynec/o	woman	12
halit/o	breath	10
hem/o	blood	1
hemat/o	blood	7
hepat/o	liver	1
hidr/o	sweat	5
hirsut/o	hairy	15
hom/o	same	4
home/o	sameness, unchanging	4
hormon/o	to set in motion	15
hydr/o	water	7
hyster/o	uterus	1
iatr/o	physician	7
idi/o	individual	7
ile/o	to roll, ileum	10
ili/o	flank, hip, groin, ilium of the pelvis	4
immun/o	exempt, immunity	7
infer/o	below	4
inguin/o	groin	4
ir/o	iris	14
isch/o	hold back	8

Combining Form	Definition	Chapter
ischi/o	haunch, hip joint, ischium	6
jejun/o	empty, jejunum	10
kerat/o	hard, cornea	5
ket/o	ketone	11
keton/o	ketone	11
kinesi/o	motion	6
kyph/o	hump	6
labyrinth/o	maze, inner ear	14
lact/o	milk	12
lamin/o	thin, lamina	6
lapar/o	abdomen	10
laryng/o	voice box, larynx	1
later/o	side	4
lei/o	smooth	12
leuk/o	white	1
lingu/o	tongue	10
lip/o	fat	2
lith/o	stone	1
lob/o	a rounded part, lobe	9
lord/o	bent forward	6
lumb/o	loin, lower back	4
lymph/o	clear water or fluid	7
mamm/o	breast	1
man/o	thin, scanty	8
mast/o	breast	1
mastoid/o	resembling a breast	14
maxim/o	biggest, highest	1
meat/o	opening, passage	11
med/o	middle	14
medi/o	middle	4
melan/o	black	5
men/o	month, menstruation	12
mening/i	membrane	13
mening/o	membrane	13
menisc/o	meniscus	6
menstru/o	month, menstruation	12
ment/o	mind	1
metr/i	uterus	12
metr/o	uterus	12
muc/o	mucus	9
muscul/o	muscle	1
my/o	muscle	6
myc/o	fungus	5
myel/o	bone marrow; spinal cord, medulla, myelin	6
myos/o	muscle	6
myring/o	membrane, eardrum	14
myx/o	mucus	15
narc/o	numbness	13
nas/o	nose	9
nat/o	birth	1
necr/o	death	7
nephr/o	kidney	11

Combining Form	Definition	Chapter
neur/o	nerve	1
noct/o	night	11
nosocom/o	hospital	7
nucle/o	kernel, nucleus	7
obstetr/o	midwife	12
ocul/o	eye	14
olig/o	few in number	11
onych/o	nail	5
oophor/o	ovary	12
ophthalm/o	eye	14
opt/o	eye	14
or/o	mouth	10
orchi/o	testis	12
orchid/o	testis	12
orex/o	appetite	10
organ/o	tool	4
orth/o	straight	6
ost/o	bone	6
oste/o	bone	6
ot/o	ear	9
ovar/o	ovary	12
ox/i	oxygen	9
pancreat/o	sweetbread, pancreas	10
pariet/o	wall	6
parot/o	parotid gland	10
patell/o	patella	6
path/o	disease	1
pect/o	chest	8
pector/o	chest	8
ped/o	child	6
pedicul/o	body louse	5
pelv/o	bowl, basin	4
pen/o	penis	12
peps/o	digestion	10
pept/o	digestion	10
peritone/o	to stretch over, peritoneum	10
petr/o	stone	6
phag/o	eat, swallow	10
phalang/o	phalanges	6
pharyng/o	throat, pharynx	9
phasi/o	to speak	13
phleb/o	vein	8
phragm/o	partition	9
phragmat/o	partition	9
phren/o	mind	13
phys/o	growth	6
physi/o	nature	4
plasm/o	form	12
pleur/o	pleura, rib	4
pneum/o	air, lung	9
pneumon/o	air, lung	9
poikil/o	irregular	7

Combining Form	Definition	Chapter
poli/o	gray	13
polyp/o	small growth	10
por/o	hole	6
poster/o	back	4
presby/o	old age	14
proct/o	rectum or anus	1
prostat/o	prostate gland	12
protein/o	protein	11
proxim/o	near	4
pseud/o	false	12
psych/o	mind	1
pub/o	pubis	6
pulmon/o	lung	1
py/o	pus	9
pyel/o	renal pelvis	11
pylor/o	pylorus	10
radi/o	radius	6
radic/o	nerve root	13
radicul/o	nerve root	13
rect/o	rectum	10
ren/o	kidney	11
retin/o	retina	14
rhin/o	nose	1
rhiz/o	nerve root	13
rhythm/o	rhythm	8
rhytid/o	wrinkle	5
rrhythm/o	rhythm	8
sacr/o	sacred, sacrum	6
salping/o	trumpet, fallopian tube	12
sarc/o	flesh, meat	6
schiz/o	to divide, split	13
scler/o	hard, sclera	5
scoli/o	curved	6
scop/o	viewing instrument	1
seb/o	sebum, oil	5
semin/o	seed, sperm	12
sept/o	putrefying; wall, partition	7
sial/o	saliva	10
sigm/o	the letter *s*, sigmoid colon	10
sinus/o	cavity	9
skelet/o	skeleton	1
somat/o	body	13
son/o	sound	8
spadias/o	rip, tear	11
sperm/o	seed, sperm	12
spermat/o	seed, sperm	12
sphygm/o	pulse	8
sphyx/o	pulse	9
spir/o	breathe	9
splen/o	spleen	7
spondyl/o	vertebra	6
staphylococc/o	*Staphylococcus* (a bacterium)	7

Combining Form	Definition	Chapter
steat/o	fat	10
sten/o	narrow	8
stern/o	chest, sternum	6
stigmat/o	point	14
stomat/o	mouth	10
streptococc/o	Streptococcus (a bacterium)	7
super/o	above	4
syn/o	connect	6
synov/o	synovial	6
synovi/o	synovial	6
tampon/o	plug	8
tars/o	tarsal bone	6
tax/o	reaction to a stimulus	6
ten/o	stretch, tendon	6
tendon/o	stretch, tendon	6
tens/o	pressure	8
test/o	testis, testicle	12
testicul/o	little testis, testicle	12
thorac/o	chest, thorax	4
thromb/o	clot	7
thym/o	wartlike, thymus gland	7
thyr/o	shield, thyroid	15
thyroid/o	resembling a shield, thyroid	15
toc/o	birth	12
tom/o	to cut	4
tonsill/o	almond, tonsil	1
tox/o	poison	7

Combining Form	Definition	Chapter
trache/o	windpipe, trachea	9
trich/o	hair	5
troph/o	development	6
tubercul/o	little swelling	9
tympan/o	eardrum	14
umbilic/o	navel, umbilicus	4
ur/o	urine	11
ureter/o	ureter	11
urethr/o	urethra	11
urin/o	urine	11
vag/o	vagus nerve	10
vagin/o	sheath, vagina	12
valvul/o	little valve	8
varic/o	dilated vein	8
vas/o	vessel	1
vascul/o	little vessel	8
ven/o	vein	8
ventr/o	belly	4
ventricul/o	little belly, ventricle	8
vertebr/o	vertebra	6
vesic/o	bladder	11
vesicul/o	small bag	12
volv/o	to roll	10
vulv/o	vulva	12
xer/o	dry	5
zo/o	animal, living	12

Suffix	Definition	Chapter
-a	singular	2
-ac	pertaining to	2
-acusis	condition of hearing	14
-ad	toward	2
-ade	process	8
-ae	plural	2
-al	pertaining to	1
-algesia	pain	13
-algia	condition of pain	2
-ar	pertaining to	2
-ary	pertaining to	1
-asthenia	weakness	2
-atresia	closure or absence of a normal body opening	2
-capnia	condition of carbon dioxide	9
-cele	hernia, swelling, protrusion	2
-centesis	surgical puncture	2
-clasia	break apart	2
-clasis	break apart	2

Suffix	Definition	Chapter
-clast	break apart	2
-crit	to separate	7
-cyesis	pregnancy	12
-desis	surgical fixation, fusion	2
-drome	run, running	2
-dynia	condition of pain	2
-ectasis	expansion, dilation	9
-ectomy	surgical excision, removal	1
-emesis	vomiting	2
-emetic	pertaining to vomiting	10
-emia	condition of blood	1
-genesis	origin, cause	6
-genic	pertaining to producing, forming	7
-gnosis	knowledge	4
-gram	a record or image	1
-graph	instrument for recording	2
-graphy	recording process	2
-hemia	condition of blood	2

Abbreviation	Definition
Bx	biopsy
bx	biopsy
C	Celsius
C1–C7	seven cervical vertebrae
C&S	stool culture and sensitivity
c/o	complains of
Ca	calcium
CA	cancer
CA-125	cancer antigen-125 tumor marker
CABG	coronary artery bypass graft
CAD	coronary artery disease
cal	calorie
cap	capsule
CAPD	continuous ambulatory peritoneal dialysis
CAT	computed (axial) tomography
cath	catheter, catheterization
CBC	complete blood count
CBR	complete bedrest
CBS	chronic brain syndrome
cc	cubic centimeter
CC	colony count
CCU	coronary care unit
CDH	congenital dislocation of the hip
CEA	carcinoma embryonic antigen
CF	cystic fibrosis
CHB	complete heart block
CHD	coronary heart disease
chemo	chemotherapy
CHF	congestive heart failure
CHO	carbohydrate
chol	cholesterol
CI	coronary insufficiency
CIN	cervical intraepithelial neoplasia
circ	circumcision
CIS	carcinoma in situ
cl	clinic
Cl	chloride
cl liq	clear liquid
CLD	chronic liver disease
CLL	chronic lymphocytic leukemia
cm	centimeter
CML	chronic myelogenous leukemia
CNS	central nervous system
CO	carbon monoxide
CO_2	carbon dioxide
COLD	chronic obstructive lung disease
cond	condition
COPD	chronic obstructive pulmonary disease

Abbreviation	Definition
CP	chest pain
CP	cerebral palsy
CPAP	continuous positive airway pressure
CPK	creatine phosphokinase
CPN	chronic pyelonephritis
CPR	cardiopulmonary resuscitation
CRD	chronic respiratory disease
creat	creatinine
CRF	chronic renal failure
CRNA	certified registered nurse-anesthetist
C-section	cesarean section
CSF	cerebrospinal fluid
CT	calcitonin
CT (CAT) scan	computed (axial) tomography scan
CTS	carpal tunnel syndrome
Cu	copper
CVA	cerebrovascular accident (stroke)
CVP	central venous pressure
CXR	chest x-ray
D&C	dilation and curettage
D/S	dextrose in saline
D/W	dextrose in water
DAT	diet as tolerated
DC	discontinued
del	delivery
DI	diabetes insipidus
DIC	diffuse intravascular coagulation
diff	differential (blood count)
DJD	degenerative joint disease
DLE	discoid lupus erythematosus
DM	diabetes mellitus
DMD	Duchenne muscular dystrophy
DNA	deoxyribonucleic acid
DO	physician specializing in osteopathy
DOA	dead on arrival
DOB	date of birth
Dr	dram
DRE	digital rectal exam
DRG	diagnosis-related group
DT	delirium tremens
DTR	deep tendon reflexes
DVT	deep vein thrombosis
Dx	diagnosis
E	enema
EBL	estimated blood loss
ECG	electrocardiogram
ECHO	echocardiogram
EchoEG	echoencephalography
ECT	electroconvulsive therapy

Abbreviation	Definition
ED	erectile dysfunction
EDD	expected date of delivery
EEG	electroencephalography
EENT	eye, ear, nose, and throat
EGD	esophagogastroduodenoscopy
EKG	electrocardiogram
Em	emmetropia
EMG	electromyography
ENT	ear, nose, and throat
EP studies	ectopic pregnancy studies
EP studies	evoked potential studies
ERCP	endoscopic retrograde cholangiopancreatography
ERT	estrogen replacement therapy
ESKD	end-stage kidney disease
ESR	erythrocyte sedimentation rate
ESWL	extracorporeal shock wave lithotripsy
etio	etiology
EtOH	ethanol
EUS	endoscopic ultrasound
ex	external
F	Fahrenheit
FACP	Fellow of the American College of Physicians
FACS	Fellow of the American College of Surgeons
FAS	fetal alcohol syndrome
FASD	fetal alcohol spectrum disorder
FBD	fibrocystic breast disease
FBS	fasting blood sugar
Fe	iron
FHT	fetal heart tones
flu	influenza
FOBT	fetal occult blood test
FSH	follicle-stimulating hormone
FTT	failure to thrive
FUO	fever of undetermined origin
Fx	fracture
g	gram
GB series	gallbladder series
GC	gonorrhea
GER	gerontology
GERD	gastroesophageal reflux disease
GH	growth hormone
GI	gastrointestinal
GSW	gunshot wound
GTT	glucose tolerance test
GU	genitourinary
GYN	gynecology
h	hour

Abbreviation	Definition
H	hypodermic
H&H	hemoglobin and hematocrit
H&P	history and physical examination
H_2O	water
H_2O_2	hydrogen peroxide
HB	heart block
HBV	hepatitis B virus
HCl	hydrochloric acid
HCO^{3-}	bicarbonate
HCT, Hct	hematocrit
HCVD	hypertensive cardiovascular disease
HD	hemodialysis
HEENT	head, eyes, ears, nose, and throat
Hg	mercury
HGB, Hgb	hemoglobin
HHD	hypertensive heart disease
HIV	human immunodeficiency virus
HNP	herniated nucleus pulposus; a herniated intervertebral disk
HOB	head of bed
HPI	history of present illness
HPV	human papillomavirus
HRT	hormone replacement therapy
hs	hour of sleep
HSG	hysterosalpingogram
HSV	herpes simplex virus
HSV-2	herpes simplex virus type 2
ht	height
HTN	hypertension
Hx	history
hypo	hypodermic
I&D	incision and drainage
I&O	intake and output
IBD	inflammatory bowel disease
IBS	irritable bowel syndrome
ICD	implantable cardioverter defibrillator
ICU	intensive care unit
IDC	infiltrating ductal carcinoma
IDDM	insulin-dependent diabetes mellitus
IHD	ischemic heart disease
IM	intramuscular
inf	inferior
INR	international normalized ratio
IOL	intraocular lens
IPPR	intermittent positive pressure breathing
irrig	irrigation
isol	isolation
IUD	intrauterine device
IV	intravenous

Abbreviation	Definition
IVC	intravenous cholangiogram
IVP	intravenous pyelogram
K	potassium
KCl	potassium chloride
kg	kilogram
KUB	kidney, ureter, and bladder x-ray
KVO	keep vein open
L	liter
L&D	labor and delivery
L1–L5	five lumbar vertebrae
LA	left atrium
lac	laceration
LAP	laparotomy
LAS	lymphadenopathy syndrome
LASIK	laser-assisted in situ keratomileusis
lat	lateral
LE	lupus erythematosus
LEEP	loop electrosurgical excision procedure
LGI	lower GI series
LH	luteinizing hormone
LI	lactose intolerance
LLL	left lower lobe (of lung)
LLQ	left lower quadrant
LMP	last menstrual period
LOC	loss of consciousness
LP	lumbar puncture
LPN	licensed practical nurse
LR	lactated Ringer's
LTB	laryngotracheobronchitis
LUL	left upper lobe
LUQ	left upper quadrant
LV	left ventricle
LVN	licensed vocational nurse
mcg	microgram
MCH	mean corpuscular hemoglobin
MCV	mean corpuscular volume
MD	medical doctor
MD	muscular dystrophy
mEq	milliequivalent
Mets	metastasis
MG	myasthenia gravis
mg	milligram
MI	myocardial infarction
MI	milliliter
mm	millimeter
MM	multiple myeloma
MOM	milk of magnesia
MR	may repeat
MRA	magnetic resonance angiography

Abbreviation	Definition
MRCP	magnetic resonance cholangiopancreatography
MRI	magnetic resonance imaging
MRSA	methicillin-resistant *Staphylococcus aureus*
MS	multiple sclerosis
MSH	melanocyte-stimulating hormone
MVP	mitral valve prolapse
N&V	nausea and vomiting
Na	sodium
NA	nursing assistant
NaCl	sodium chloride (salt)
NB	newborn
neuro	neurology
NG	nasogastric
NHL	non-Hodgkin lymphoma
NICU	neonatal intensive care unit
NICU	neurology intensive care unit
NIDDM	non-insulin-dependent diabetes mellitus
NIVA	noninvasive vascular assessment
NKDA	no known drug allergies
noc	night
noct	night
NPO	nothing by mouth
NRDS	neonatal respiratory distress syndrome
NS	normal saline
NSAIDs	nonsteroidal anti-inflammatory drugs
NSR	normal sinus rhythm
NVS	neurovital signs
O	objective
O_2	oxygen
OA	osteoarthritis
OB	obstetrics
OB/GYN	obstetrics/gynecology
OD	right eye (in Latin, *oculus dexter*)
OM	otitis media
OP	outpatient
Ophth	ophthalmic
OR	operating room
ortho	orthopedics
OS	left eye (in Latin, *oculus sinister*)
OSA	obstructive sleep apnea
OT	occupational therapy
OT	oxytocin
Oto	otology
OU	each eye (in Latin, *oculus uterque*)
oz	ounce
P	phosphorus

Abbreviation	Definition
PA	physician's assistant
PA	posteroanterior
PAC	premature atrial contractions
Pap smear (test)	Papanicolaou smear (or test)
PAT	paroxysmal atrial tachycardia
pc	after meals
PCOS	polycystic ovary syndrome
PCU	progressive care unit
PCV	packed cell volume
PD	Parkinson's disease
PDA	patent ductus arteriosus
PDR	*Physician's Desk Reference*
PE	pulmonary embolism
PE	physical examination
PED	pediatrics
PEG	percutaneous endoscopic gastrostomy
per	by
PERRLA	pupils equal, round, reactive to light and accommodation
PET	positron emission tomography
PFT	pulmonary function test
PICC	peripherally inserted central catheter
PICU	pediatric intensive care unit
PID	pelvic inflammatory disease
PIH	pregnancy-induced hypertension
PKU	phenylketonuria
PLT	platelet count
PMS	premenstrual syndrome
PNS	peripheral nervous system
po	postoperation
po	orally
post-op	postoperatively
PP	postpartum
PPBS	postprandial blood sugar
PPD	purified protein derivative
pr	per rectum
PRBC	packed red blood cells
pre-op	preoperation
PRK	photorefractive keratotomy
PRL	prolactin
prn	as needed
PSA	prostate-specific antigen
pt	patient
PT	prothrombin time
PT	physical therapy
PTCA	percutaneous transluminal coronary angioplasty
PTH	parathyroid hormone

Abbreviation	Definition
PTSD	posttraumatic stress disorder
PTT	partial thromboplastin time
PUL	percutaneous ultrasound lithotripsy
PVC	premature ventricular contractions
PVD	peripheral vascular disease
Px	prognosis
q	every
qd	every day
qid	four times a day
qn	every night
qod	every other day
qt	quart
R	rectal
R	right
RA	right atrium
RA	rheumatoid arthritis
RAIU	radioactive iodine uptake
RBC	red blood cell or red blood count
RDS	respiratory distress syndrome
reg	regular
REM	rapid eye movement
resp	respiration
RHD	rheumatic heart disease
RICE	rest, ice, compression, elevation
RK	radial keratotomy
RLL	right lower lobe
RLQ	right lower quadrant
RN	registered nurse
ROM	range of motion
RP	retrograde pyelogram
RR	recovery room
rt	right
rt	routine
RT	respiratory therapy
RUL	right upper lobe
RUQ	right upper quadrant
RV	right ventricle
Rx	prescription
SA	sinoatrial
SAB	spontaneous abortion
SARS	severe acute respiratory syndrome
SBE	subacute bacterial endocarditis
SBE	self breast examination
SCA	sudden cardiac arrest
SCI	spinal cord injury
SG	specific gravity
SHG	sonohistogram
SICU	surgical intensive care unit
SIDS	sudden infant death syndrome

Abbreviation	Definition
SL	semilunar (pertaining to the heart valve)
SLE	systemic lupus erythematosus
SMR	submucous resection
SO	salpingo-oophorectomy
SOAP	subjective, objective, assessment, and plan
SOB	shortness of breath
SPECT	single-photon emission computed tomography
SqCCa	squamous cell carcinoma
ss	one-half
SSE	soapsuds enema
St	stage (of cancer development)
staph	*Staphylococcus*
stat	immediately
STI	sexually transmitted infection
strep	*Streptococcus*
subq	subcutaneous
sup	superior
supp	suppository
surg	surgery
SVD	spontaneous vaginal delivery
T&A	tonsillectomy and adenoidectomy
T1–T12	12 thoracic vertebrae
T3	triiodothyronine
T4	thyroxine
TAB	therapeutic abortion
tab	tablet
TAH	total abdominal hysterectomy
TAH/BSO	total abdominal hysterectomy/bilateral salpingo-oophorectomy
TAT	tetanus antitoxin
TB	tuberculosis
TBI	traumatic brain injury
TBSA	total body surface area
TCDB	turn, cough, deep breathe
TCT	thrombin clotting time
TEE	transesophageal echocardiogram
temp	temperature
THA	total hip arthroplasty
THR	total hip replacement
TIA	transient ischemic attack
tid	three times a day
TKA	total knee arthroplasty
TKR	total knee replacement
TM	tympanic membrane
TMJ	temporomandibular joint disease

Abbreviation	Definition
TNM	tumor, node, metastasis
TPN	total parenteral nutrition
tr	tincture
trach	tracheostomy
TSH	thyroid-stimulating hormone
TSS	toxic shock syndrome
TUIP	transurethral incision of the prostate
TULIP	transurethral laser incision of the prostate
TUMT	transurethral microwave thermotherapy
TURP	transurethral resection of the prostate
TV	tidal volume
TVH	total vaginal hysterectomy
TVS	transvaginal sonography
TWE	tapwater enema
Tx	treatment
U	unit
UA	urinalysis
UGI	upper GI series
UNG	ointment
UPPP	uvulopalatopharyngoplasty
URI	upper respiratory infection
US	ultrasound
UTI	urinary tract infection
UV	ultraviolet
UVR	ultraviolet radiation
VA	visual acuity
vag	vaginal
VBAC	vaginal birth after cesarean section
VC	vital capacity
VCUG	voiding cystourethrogram
Vertebrae	
C1 through C7	seven cervical vertebrae
T1 through T12	12 thoracic vertebrae
L1 through L5	five lumbar vertebrae
VLAP	visual ablation of the prostate
V/Q scan	ventilation-perfusion scanning
VS	vital signs
VSD	ventricular septal defect
W/C	wheelchair
WA	while awake
WBC	white blood cell or white blood count
WNL	within normal limits
Wt	weight
XRT	radiation therapy

Appendix C

Word Parts for Describing Color, Number, and Plurals

Combining Forms for Terms Describing Color

Combining Form	Meaning
albin/o	white
chlor/o	green
chrom/o	color
cirrh/o	orange
cyan/o	blue
erythr/o	red
jaund/o	yellow
leuk/o	white
melan/o	black
xanth/o	yellow

Prefixes for Terms Describing Numbers

Prefix	Meaning
mono-	one
uni-	one
bi-	two
di-	two
tri-	three
quadri-	four
tetra-	four

Singular versus Plural Endings

Singular Endings	Plural Endings	Example: Singular	Example: Plural
-a	-ae	fistula	fistulae
-ax	-aces	hemothorax	hemothoraces
-ex	-ices	cortex	cortices
-is	-es	diagnosis	diagnoses
-ix	-ices	cicatrix	cicatrices
-ma	-mata	fibroma	fibromata
-on	-a	ganglion	ganglia
-um	-a	bacterium	bacteria
-us	-i	fungus	fungi
-y	-ies	episiotomy	episiotomies

Glossary-Index

Note: Terms that appear in boldface are Key Terms from the chapters. Definitions are provided here for these terms. Page numbers with *f* indicate figures; those with *t* indicate tables.

respiratory tract disease; also called an *otolaryngologist*, 237

Ecchymosis, condition caused by leaking blood vessels in the dermis, producing purplish patches of purpura, 93

ECG. *See* **Electrocardiogram**

Echocardiogram, recorded data resulting from echocardiography, an ultrasound procedure that directs sound waves through the heart to evaluate heart function, 219

Echocardiography, an ultrasound procedure that directs sound waves through the heart to evaluate heart function; recorded data is typically called an *echocardiogram*, 219

EchoEG. *See* **Echoencephalography**

Echoencephalography, a procedure that uses ultrasound technology to record brain structures, 451

Eclampsia, a condition of high blood pressure associated with a pregnancy that may worsen to cause convulsions and possibly coma and death, 410

Ectopic pregnancy, a pregnancy occurring outside the uterus, 46, 410, 410*f*

Eczema, a skin disease marked by severe chronic pruritus and deep scaliness; also called atopic dermatitis, 92

ED. *See* **Erectile dysfunction**

Edema, swelling due to leakage of fluid from the bloodstream into the interstitial space between body cells, 84, 163, 163*f*, 252

EEG. *See* **Electroencephalography**

Effectual drug therapy, a general type of treatment to manage neurological disorders, 452

EKG. *See* **Electrocardiogram**

Electrical bone stimulation, a procedure that applies electricity to stimulate the healing process of a fracture, 139

Electrocardiogram (ECG or EKG), recorded data resulting from electrocardiography, a procedure in which electrodes are pasted to the skin of the chest to detect and measure the electrical events of the heart conduction system, 220, 220*f*

Electrocardiography, a procedure in which electrodes are pasted to the skin of the chest to detect and measure the electrical events of the heart conduction system and used to evaluate heart function; the record or image of the data is called an *electrocardiogram* (*ECG* or *EKG*), 220, 220*f*

Electroencephalography (EEG), a diagnostic procedure that records electrical impulses of the brain to measure brain activity, 452, 452*f*

Electromyography, a procedure that provides electrical stimulation of a muscle and records and analyzes the contractions, 139

Em. *See* **Emmetropia**

Embolectomy, the surgical removal of a floating blood clot, or embolus, 221

Embolism, a blockage or occlusion caused by a blood clot or foreign particle (including air or fat), an embolus, that moves through the circulation, 26, 206, 252

Embolus, an abnormal particle or blood clot that moves along with the bloodstream, 206, 252

Emmetropia (Em), the normal condition of the eye, 480, 481*f*

Emollient, a chemical agent that softens or smoothes the skin, 101

Emphysema, chronic lung disease characterized by dyspnea, chronic cough, barrel chest, and chronic hypoxemia and hypercapnia, 248, 248*f*

Empyema, another term for pyothorax, or the presence of pus in the pleural cavity, 253

Encephalitis, inflammation of the brain, 441

Encephalomalacia, an abnormal softening of brain tissue, 441

End-stage kidney disease (ESKD), life-threatening condition in which both kidneys fail to form urine; also called *renal failure*, 336

Endarterectomy, the surgical removal of the inner lining of an artery to remove a fatty plaque, 221

Endocarditis, inflammation of the endocardium, 20, 206

Endocervicitis, a form of cervicitis that occurs when the inner lining of the cervix becomes inflamed, 389

Endocrine system, 63, 503–525
  abbreviations of, 525
  anatomy and physiology terms, 503–504
  diseases and disorders of, 509–17
  medical report exercises, 505–8
  medical terms for, 506
  signs and symptoms of, 506–518
  treatments, procedure, devices of, 520–524

Endocrinologist, a physician specializing in endocrinology, 520

Endocrinology, the field of medicine that focuses on the study and treatment of endocrine disorders, 506, 520

Endocrinopathy, a general term for disease of the endocrine system, 514

Endometrial ablation, a procedure in which lasers, electricity, or heat is used to destroy the endometrium, 308

Endometrial cancer, a malignant tumor arising from the endometrial tissue lining the uterus, 300
  stages of, 300*f*

Ventral, 64*t*

Ventral cavity, the body cavity on the anterior side of the body that includes the thoracic cavity and abdominopelvic cavity, 67, 68*f*

Ventricular fibrillation, the condition of uncoordinated, rapid contractions of the muscle forming the ventricles that results in circulatory collapse due to the failure of the ventricles to expel blood, 218

Ventricular septal defect (VSD), a congenital disease in which an opening in the septum separating the right and left ventricles of the heart is present at birth, 211

Ventriculitis, inflammation of the ventricles of the brain, 448

Verruca, a wart that is a sign of infection by a papillomavirus, 88

Vertebrae, the bones that form the spinal column, 14

Vertebral cavity, the dorsal body cavity that houses the spinal cord; also called *spinal cavity*, 67, 67*f*

Vertebroplasty, a surgical procedure that repairs damaged or diseased vertebrae, 142

Vertigo, a sensation of dizziness, 488

Vesicle, small skin elevation filled with fluid; a blister, 84*f*, 88*f*, 88

Vesicotomy, another name for cystotomy, which is an incision through the urinary bladder wall, 347

Vesicourethral, 354

Vesicourethral suspension, a surgery that stabilizes the position of the urinary bladder, 354

Vesicovaginal fistula, a fistula occurring between the urinary bladder and the vagina, 391

Vesiculectomy, a surgical procedure to remove the seminal vesicles, 382

Viral hepatitis, a viral-induced inflammation of the liver, 298

Virology, the study of viruses, a subspecialty of immunology, or infectious disease, 157

Viscera, internal contents of body cavities, which include organs and supporting structures, 67

Vision disorders. *See* **Refractive error**

Voiding cystourethrogram (VCUG), a cystourethrogram procedure that includes x-rays taken before, during, and after urination to observe bladder function, 345

Volvulus, severe twisting of the intestine that leads to obstruction, 303, 303*f*

VPS. *See* **Ventilation-perfusion scanning**

V/Q scan, another term for ventilation-perfusion scanning (VPS), a diagnostic tool that uses nuclear medicine or radioactive material to evaluate pulmonary function; also called *lung scan*, 269

VSD. *See* **Ventricular septal defect**

Vulvectomy, the surgical removal of the vulva, 404

Vulvitis, inflammation of the external genitals, or vulva, 395

Vulvovaginitis, inflammation of the external genitals and vagina, 395

W

Warfarin, the most common anticoagulant agent (Coumadin), 173

Wheal, a temporary, itchy elevation of the skin, 84*f*, 88

White blood count (WBC), 180

Whooping cough, common term for pertussis, an acute infectious disease that causes inflammation of the larynx, trachea, and bronchi with spasmodic coughing that produces a distinct noise, 249

Wilms' tumor, another name for nephroblastoma, which is a tumor originating from kidney tissue that includes developing embryonic cells, 338

Word parts, 6–12
    forming words from, 13–15
    prefix, 6
    suffix, 6, 8, 10
    word root, 6, 8

Word root, 6, 8, 13

Words, forming from word parts, 11–14

World Health Organization, 170

X

Xeroderma, condition characterized by abnormally dry skin, 98

Y

Yersinia pestis, 172